Decisi
Neurocritical Care

Christa Swisher

699-0902

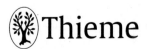 Thieme

Decision Making in Neurocritical Care

Jennifer A. Frontera, MD
Assistant Professor
Departments of Neurology and Neurosurgery
Medical Director
Neuroscience Intensive Care Unit
Mount Sinai School of Medicine
New York, New York

Thieme
New York • Stuttgart

**Dedicated to my parents, Alfred and Veronica Frontera,
who have guided me both intellectually and spiritually.**

Thieme Medical Publishers, Inc.
333 Seventh Ave.
New York, NY 10001

Executive Editor: Kay D. Conerly
Editorial Assistant: Dominik Pucek
Vice President, Production and Electronic Publishing: Anne T. Vinnicombe
Production Editor: Frank Weihenig
Vice President, International Marketing and Sales: Cornelia Sculze
Chief Financial Officer: Peter van Woerden
President: Brian D. Scanlan
Compositor: Prepare Inc.
Printer: The Maple-Vail Book Manufacturing Group

Library of Congress Cataloging-in-Publication Data

Decision making in neurocritical care / [edited by] Jennifer Frontera.
   p. ; cm.
   Includes bibliographical references and index.
   ISBN 978-1-60406-047-8
   1. Neurological intensive care—Decision making. [DNLM: 1. Nervous System Diseases—
   diagnosis. 2. Nervous System Diseases—therapy. 3. Critical Care—methods. 4. Trauma,
   Nervous System—diagnosis. 5. Trauma. I. Frontera, Jennifer. Nervous System—
   therapy. WL 141 D294 2009]
   RC350.N49D43 2010
   616.8'0428—dc22
                                        2008042540

Important note: Medical knowledge is ever-changing. As new research and clinical
experience broaden our knowledge, changes in treatment and drug therapy may be
required. The authors and editors of the material herein have consulted sources believed
to be reliable in their efforts to provide information that is complete and in accord with
the standards accepted at the time of publication. However, in view of the possibility of
human error by the authors, editors, or publisher of the work herein or changes in
medical knowledge, neither the authors, editors, nor publisher, nor any other party who
has been involved in the preparation of this work, warrants that the information
contained herein is in every respect accurate or complete, and they are not responsible
for any errors or omissions or for the results obtained from use of such information.
Readers are encouraged to confirm the information contained herein with other sources.
For example, readers are advised to check the product information sheet included in the
package of each drug they plan to administer to be certain that the information contained
in this publication is accurate and that changes have not been made in the recommended
dose or in the contraindications for administration. This recommendation is of particular
importance in connection with new or infrequently used drugs.

Some of the product names, patents, and registered designs referred to in this book are in
fact registered trademarks or proprietary names even though specific reference to this
fact is not always made in the text. Therefore, the appearance of a name without
designation as proprietary is not to be construed as a representation by the publisher
that it is in the public domain.

Printed in the United States

10 9 8 7 6 5 4 3 2

ISBN   978-1-60406-047-8

Contents

Foreword

Neurocritical care is one of the newest and most exciting specialties in medicine today. As recently as the late 1980s, neurocritical care in the modern sense did not exist. Neurosurgical intensive care units (ICUs) had been established in larger teaching hospitals, but the patient's ticket into the unit was via the operating room. Neurosurgeons understood that close clinical monitoring during the postoperative period was essential for attaining good outcomes; it would be tragic if all of their hard work and surgical skill would go for naught because a postoperative complication was not picked up and managed in a timely fashion. In those days, neurosurgeons directed the care of their patients, the units were open, and consultants were abundant. Apart from specially trained neuro-nurses, intracranial pressure monitors, and the novel use of a pulmonary artery catheter to apply hypertensive hypervolemic therapy for vasospasm, there was little to differentiate the neurologic ICU from any medical or surgical ICU.

Things could not be more different today. Neurocritical care is now recognized as a bona fide subspecialty of medicine. The Neurocritical Care Society was incorporated in 2002, the journal *Neurocritical Care* began publication in 2004, and the first U.S. Neurocritical Care Board Examination was given in 2007. The past 20 years have witnessed an explosion of therapies for conditions that were long considered untreatable, including reperfusion therapies for acute ischemic stroke, hypothermia for cardiac arrest, and hemostatic and local thrombolytic therapy for intracerebral hemorrhage. Proof of effectiveness varies for these treatments, but clearly the rules have changed, and new battle lines have been drawn. Even more exciting are the transformational insights into the comatose human brain that have come from the application of newer sophisticated neuromonitoring modalities. It is now feasible to continuously monitor brain tissue oxygenation and blood flow, neurochemistry, and electrical function in real time. The challenge that confronts us today is how to make optimal use of this information in ways that can improve clinical outcomes.

Perhaps nothing reflects the spirit of neurocritical care more, however, than the forward-looking attitudes that neurointensivists have regarding prognosis. Our patients are the sickest of the sick. A devastating injury to the brain—unlike any other organ—threatens a person's "being" like nothing else can. The diseases that we now consider to be our greatest challenges are exactly those that were typically considered untreatable just 10 or 20 years ago. We have discarded the therapeutic nihilism of older days and replaced it with hope and a newfound respect for the resilience of the human brain. We still have a long, long way to go, but as we continue to challenge, probe, explore, and test new approaches to treating severe brain injury, we have every reason to be optimistic.

Dr. Frontera's *Decision Making in Neurocritical Care* is a succinct and highly utilitarian introduction to the basics of managing patients in the neurologic ICU. The emphasis is on rapid, focused clinical evaluation and evidence-based management strategies. Medication dosages and management protocols are spelled out in a clear and direct fashion. When there is a lot of variability and controversy regarding how a disease state or condition should best be treated, this is highlighted and the therapeutic options are spelled out. Whether you are a nurse, medical student, resident, fellow, or attending physician, it is the perfect quick reference for managing critically ill neurologic patients.

Stephan A. Mayer, MD, FCCM
Associate Professor
Director of the Division
of Neurocritical Care
Columbia University
New York, New York

Preface

The aim of this book is to provide a basic overview of the new and rapidly developing subspecialty of neurocritical care in a format that is easily accessible. As neurocritical care develops and becomes more specialized with new diagnostic, monitoring and therapeutic modalities, neurologists, neurosurgeons, and critical care medicine physicians will find themselves managing patients with unique physiologic needs. In addition, with the trend toward an increased number of beds in intensive care units, more physicians will be treating more patients with a critical illness.

This book is structured to deal with adult neurocritical care diagnosis, evaluation, and therapeutic decision-making as it would arise for the typical provider. The focus on flowchart algorithms and decision trees allows for a streamlined overview of each topic. The book contains all of the important evidence-based elements essential to management in a format that is portable and allows for easy reference. Each chapter begins with a case example and provides bulleted essentials of diagnosis, including epidemiologic data and a differential diagnosis, examination features and suggestions for laboratory, imaging, and special diagnostic studies. Evaluation and treatment options are discussed and each chapter ends with "Pearls and Pitfalls" in evaluation and management.

Decision Making in Neurocritical Care will also prove to be a useful study guide, as it covers specific topics that appear on the United Council of Neurological Subspecialties Neurocritical Care Board Examination.

Contributors

Moses Bachan, MD
Critical Care Fellow
Critical Care Medicine
Mount Sinai School of Medicine
New York, New York

Joshua B. Bederson, MD
Professor and Chairman
Department of Neurosurgery
Mount Sinai School of Medicine
New York, New York

Sherry Hsiang-Yi Chou
Instructor
Division of Cerebrovascular Diseases
    and Neuro-Critical Care
Department of Neurology
Brigham and Women's Hospital
Harvard Medical School
Boston, Massachusetts

Tanvir Choudhri, MD
Assistant Professor
Department of Neurosurgery
Mount Sinai School of Medicine
New York, New York

Jan Claassen
Assistant Professor
Division of Neurocritical Care
Department of Neurology
Columbia University
New York, New York

Valerie Dechant, MD
Resident
Department of Neurology
Thomas Jefferson University
Philadelphia, Pennsylvania

Eduardo Adonias de Sousa, MD
Assistant Professor
Department of Neurology
Thomas Jefferson University
Philadelphia, Pennsylvania

Andres Fernandez, MD
Resident
Department of Neurology
Jackson Memorial Hospital
University of Miami
Miami, Florida

Isabel Fragata, MD
Neurointerventional Fellow
Department of
    Neurosurgery/Radiology
Mount Sinai School of Medicine
New York, New York

Jennifer A. Frontera, MD
Assistant Professor
Departments of Neurology and
    Neurosurgery
Medical Director
Neuroscience Intensive Care Unit
Mount Sinai School of Medicine
New York, New York

Meagen Gaddis
Department of Anesthesia
Mount Sinai School of Medicine
New York, New York

Lawrence J. Hirsch, MD
Associate Clinical Professor of
    Neurology
Comprehensive Epilepsy Center
Columbia University
New York, New York

Arthur Jenkins III, MD
Assistant Professor
Department of Neurosurgery
Mount Sinai School of Medicine
New York, New York

Zinobia Khan, MD
Critical Care Fellow
Critical Care Medicine
Mount Sinai School of Medicine
New York, New York

Roopa Kohli-Seth, MD
Assistant Professor
Division of Surgical Critical Care
Department of Surgery
Mount Sinai School of Medicine
New York, New York

David C. Kramer, MD
Assistant Professor
Department of Anesthesiology
Mount Sinai School of Medicine
New York, New York

Stephen Krieger, MD
Assistant Professor
Department of Neurology
Mount Sinai School of Medicine
New York, New York

Kiwon Lee, MD
Assistant Professor
Departments of Clinical Neurology
    and Neurological Surgery
Columbia University
New York, New York

Stephan A. Mayer, MD FCCM
Associate Professor
Director of the Division of
    Neurocritical Care
Columbia University
New York, New York

Scott Meyer, MD
Resident
Department of Neurosurgery
Mount Sinai School of Medicine
New York, New York

Chad Miller, MD
Assistant Professor
Division of Neurosurgery
UCLA Medical Center
Los Angeles, California

Mariana Nunez, MD
Critical Care Fellow
Critical Care Medicine
Mount Sinai School of Medicine
New York, New York

Irene Osborn, MD
Assistant Professor
Department of Anesthesiology
Mount Sinai School of Medicine
New York, New York

Aman Patel, MD
Associate Professor
Department of Neurosurgery
Mount Sinai School of Medicine
New York, New York

Fred Rincon, MD
Fellow
Department of Critical Care and
    Neurology
Columbia University
New York, New York

Owen Samuels, MD
Assistant Professor
Departments of Neurosurgery and
    Neurology
Emory University
Atlanta, Georgia

David Seder, MD
Assistant Professor
Pulmonary Medicine Division
Maine Medical Center
Portland, Maine

Harshpal Singh, MD
Resident
Department of Neurosurgery
Mount Sinai School of Medicine
New York, New York

Mark Sivak, MD
Assistant Professor
Department of Neurology
Mount Sinai School of Medicine
New York, New York

Stanley Tuhrim, MD
Professor
Department of Neurology
Mount Sinai School of Medicine
New York, New York

Chitra Venkatasubramanian, MD
Assistant Professor
Department of Neurology
Stanford University
Palo Alto, California

Katja E. Wartenberg, MD
Assistant Professor
Department of Neurology
University of Dresden
Dresden, Germany

Adam Webb, MD
Fellow
Department of Neurology
Emory University
Atlanta, Georgia

Christine A. Wijman, MD
Associate Professor
Department of Neurology
Stanford University
Palo Alto, California

1 Subarachnoid Hemorrhage

Harshpal Singh, Joshua B. Bederson, and Jennifer A. Frontera

Subarachnoid hemorrhage (SAH) is defined as the presence of blood within the subarachnoid space between the arachnoid membrane and the pia mater. SAH may be categorized as traumatic or nontraumatic. Nontraumatic or spontaneous SAH accounts for 1 to 7% of all strokes; ~80 to 90% of the time they can be attributed to the rupture of a cerebral aneurysm. Approximately 5% of the population harbors an intracranial aneurysm, and 20 to 30% of this population will have multiple aneurysms.[1] However, the vast majority of aneurysms never rupture. The annual incidence of spontaneous SAH is 2 to 25 per 100,000 people, and ~30,000 spontaneous SAHs occur in the United States per year.[2] The peak age range for aneurysmal SAH is 50 to 60 years, and it is more common in women and blacks. Although it is unclear why, aneurysmal SAH occurs more commonly in the winter and spring (**Table 1.1**).

Previous SAH is one of the strongest predictors of SAH. Patients with previously ruptured aneurysms should undergo repair of additional unruptured aneurysms. The International Study of Unruptured Intracranial Aneurysms (ISUIA)[3] addressed treatment of unruptured aneurysms detected in patients with and without previous SAH. In patients without a history of SAH, patients >50 years of age with large posterior circulation aneurysms are at the greatest risk for both rupture and repair complications (**Table 1.2**).

The decision whether to treat an unruptured aneurysm should involve a discussion of the risks of rupture and the risks and benefits associated with treatment. Considerations include aneurysm size and location, as well as the patient's age and comorbidities. Often, patients without a history of SAH and with aneurysms <7 mm are observed and followed with serial imaging.

Table 1.1 Risk Factors for Aneurysm Formation

Modifiable Risk Factors	Nonmodifiable Risk Factors
Cigarette smoking (dose-dependent effect on aneurysm formation; the most important modifiable risk factor)	Previous SAH (new aneurysm formation rate 1–2% per year)
Hypertension	Polycystic kidney disease
Moderate to heavy EtOH use	Connective tissue disease (Ehlers–Danlos syndrome, Marfan syndrome)
Cocaine use	Aortic coarctation
Endocarditis (mycotic aneurysm)	Pseudoxanthoma elasticum Moyamoya disease Arteriovenous malformation Fibromuscular dysplasia Dissection with pseudoaneurysm Vasculitis Neurofibromatosis 1 Glucocorticoid remediable hyperaldosteronism Family history (Japanese and Finnish cohorts. Familial intracranial aneurysm syndrome: Two 1st- to 3rd-degree relatives with intracranial aneurysms; 8% risk of having an unruptured aneurysm. These patients tend to have SAH at a younger age and have multiple aneurysms.)

Abbreviations: EtOH, ethyl alcohol; SAH, subarachnoid hemorrhage.

Table 1.2 Five-Year Rupture Risk for Patients with No History of Subarachnoid Hemorrhage Stratified by Aneurysm Location and Size

Aneurysm Location	Aneurysm Size			
	<7 mm %	7–12 mm %	13–24 mm %	≥25 mm %
Cavernous carotid artery	0	0	3.0	6.4
ACOMM/MCA/ICA	0	2.6	14.5	40
PCOMM/posterior circulation	2.5	4.5	18.4	50

Abbreviations: ACOMM, anterior communicating artery; ICA, internal cerebral artery; MCA, middle cerebral artery; PCOMM, posterior communicating artery.
Data from: Kassell NF, Torner JC, Jane JA, Haley EC Jr, Adams HP. The International Cooperative Study on the Timing of Aneurysm Surgery. Part 2: Surgical results. J Neurosurg 1990;73:37–47.

Case Example

A 56-year-old woman had a sudden onset of "the worst headache of my life and neck stiffness." She had no known past medical history.

Questions

- What is the patient's level of consciousness?
- Are there any focal deficits?
- When was the time of onset or when was the patient last seen at her baseline?
- Were there any sentinel headaches?
- Did the patient have a seizure at ictus?
- Is the patient taking any antiplatelet or anticoagulant medications?

Urgent Orders

- Check ABCs (airway, breathing, circulation—always address airway issues, particularly in the context of decompensated mental status)
- Order noncontrast head computed tomography (CT) scan
- Maintain blood pressure control (use nimodipine, and nicardipine or labetalol infusion if needed)
- Confirm infusion of anticonvulsant medication
- Consider antifibrinolytic therapy to prevent rebleeding if the time from SAH onset is <72 hours
- Reverse a coagulopathy, if present. (See chapter 4)

■ History and Examination

History

The most common presenting complaint is that of a severe headache. Often patients present with a warning or "sentinel" headache that precedes the "thunderclap" headache. Some patients complain of pain radiating down the legs; this is due to pooling of blood in the lumbar cistern and the irritation of nerve roots. Neck stiffness, photophobia, and meningeal symptoms occur. Diplopia (due to cranial nerve palsy) is also common. Loss of consciousness at ictus can occur due to a sudden rise in intracranial pressure (ICP) with a consequent drop in cerebral perfusion pressure (CPP). This should be distinguished from seizure.

Twelve percent of those with SAH die before reaching medical attention. The misdiagnosis of SAH is thought to be as high as 12% (particularly in patients with mild symptoms).[4] Because treatment is urgent and the consequences of misdiagnosis are severe, a high index of suspicion for SAH should be maintained.

Physical Examination

Kernig's or Brudzinski's sign may signify meningismus from SAH. Assess for external signs of trauma to evaluate for traumatic versus spontaneous SAH.

Neurologic Examination

- A full neurologic examination, including assessment of mental status, cranial nerves, motor skills, and reflexes, as well as a sensory and cerebellar examination, should be performed on all patients.
- Cranial nerve III compression classically occurs from an aneurysm of the posterior communicating artery, but it can also occur with posterior cerebral artery or superior cerebellar artery aneurysms. Uncal herniation causing pupillary dilatation, third nerve palsy, and deteriorating mental status is an ominous sign. Lateral rectus (6th nerve) palsy may signify an increased ICP, but it is generally nonlocalizing.
- Retinal examination: subhyaloid hemorrhages occur in 13% of SAH patients (Terson syndrome).[5]
- The Hunt and Hess[6] and the World Federation of Neurological Surgeons (WFNS) clinical grading scales for SAH are commonly employed. (**Table 1.3, Table 1.4**).

■ Differential Diagnosis

1. *Ruptured saccular cerebral aneurysm.* Ninety percent of aneurysms develop in the anterior circulation, most commonly the anterior communicating artery (ACOMM, 30%), the posterior communicating artery (PCOMM, 25%), the middle cerebral artery (MCA) bifurcation (20%), the internal carotid artery (ICA) bifurcation (8%), and 7% from other locations. Ten percent of aneurysms arise from the posterior circulation.

Table 1.3 Hunt and Hess Grading Scale for Subarachnoid Hemorrhage

Grade	Clinical Examination	Associated Mortality %	Mean Glasgow Outcome Score[†]
1	Asymptomatic, mild headache, slight nuchal rigidity	1	4
2	Cranial nerve palsy, moderate to severe headache, severe nuchal rigidity	5	4
3	Mild focal deficit, lethargy, confusion	19	3
4	Stupor, moderate to severe hemiparesis, early decerebrate rigidity	40	2
5	Deep coma, decerebrate rigidity, moribund appearance	77	2

Data from: Hunt WE, Hess RM. Surgical risk as related to time of intervention in the repair of intracranial aneurysms. J Neurosurg 1968;28:14–20. Oshiro EM, Walter KA, Piantadosi S, Witham TF, Tamargo RJ. A new subarachnoid hemorrhage grading system based on the glasgow coma scale: A comparison with the hunt and hess and world federation of neurological surgeons scales in a clinical series. Neurosurgery. 1997;41:140–147; discussion 147–148.

[†] See table 1.7

Table 1.4 World Federation of Neurological Surgeons Subarachnoid Grade

Grade	GCS Score	Major Focal Deficit (Aphasia, Hemiparesis)	Associated Mortality %	Mean Glasgow Outcome Score[†]
1	15	−	5	4
2	13–14	−	9	4
3	13–14	+	20	3
4	7–12	±	33	2
5	3–6	±	77	2

Abbreviation: GCS, Glasgow Coma Scale.

Data from: Report of World Federation of Neurological Surgeons Committee on a Universal Subarachnoid Hemorrhage Grading Scale. J Neurosurg 1988;68:985–986. Oshiro EM, Walter KA, Piantadosi S, Witham TF, Tamargo RJ. A new subarachnoid hemorrhage grading system based on the glasgow coma scale: A comparison with the hunt and hess and world federation of neurological surgeons scales in a clinical series. Neurosurgery. 1997;41:140–147; discussion 147–148.

[†] See table 1.7

2. *Traumatic SAH.* Typically convexity SAH, often accompanied by a clear history of trauma and other signs of injury such as orbital frontal contusions, skull fracture, or external scalp trauma.

3. *Vascular malformation*

   - *Arteriovenous malformation (AVM).* AVMs are congenital malformations comprised of direct fistulas from arteries to veins without any intervening capillary bed. The interposed brain tissue is nonfunctional. Patients may present with SAH, intracerebral hemorrhage, intraventricular hemorrhage, seizures, headache, or neurologic deficits. The bleeding rate of an AVM is 2 to 4% per year, and the recurrent bleeding rate is 6 to 18% per year (highest during the first year after an initial bleed).[7,8,9] The lifetime risk of hemorrhage is 105 minus the patient's age (in years).[10] Risk factors for rupture include previous rupture, high pressure over the malformation, small nidus, deep brain location, intranidal or feeding artery aneurysms, deep venous drainage, and venous occlusions. Patients with no risk factors have a bleeding rate as low as 0.9% annually.[11] Repair options include embolization with subsequent resection or gamma knife obliteration (for lesions <3 cm). The Spetzler–Martin AVM grading scale assesses surgical risk.[12] Grading is based on size, location, and venous drainage pattern: <3 cm = 1 point, 3 to 6 cm = 2 points, >6 cm = 3 points; eloquent location = 1 point, noneloquent location = 0 point; deep venous drainage = 1 point, superficial venous drainage = 0 point. Increasing points correlate with a higher surgical risk for resection.

   - *Cavernous malformations* are vascular lesions with closely spaced sinusoidal vessels lacking a smooth muscle layer and without interspaced neural tissue. They appear as "popcorn-like" lesions on gradient echo magnetic resonance imaging (MRI) with differing ages of blood products. The annual bleeding rate is 0.25 to 1.1% in the anterior circulation with a rebleed rate of 4.5% per year.[13] The annual bleeding rate for posterior fossa cavernous malformations is 2 to 3% with a 17 to 21% rebleed rate.[14] The high rate of rebleeding for posterior fossa lesions may be related to a higher likelihood of symptoms from small bleeds in very eloquent tissue. Cavernous malformations are angiographically occult, but they may be associated with developmental venous anomalies.

4. *Intracranial dissection with pseudoaneurysm rupture*

5. *Vasculopathy-related SAH.* Vasculopathy may present with multiple strokes, cognitive changes, psychiatric symptoms, seizure, headache, and rarely SAH. Etiologies include primary central nervous system (CNS) angiitis, polyarteritis nodosa, Churg–Strauss syndrome, Wegener's granulomatosis, lupus, cryoglobulinemia, Kawasaki disease, bacterial meningitis, viral infections (hepatitis B and C, cytomegalovirus [CMV], Epstein–Barr virus [EBV], parvovirus B19, varicella, and human immunodeficiency virus [HIV]), syphilis, CNS tuberculosis, drug-induced vasculopathy (e.g. SSRI), and cocaine- and methamphetamine-induced vasculopathy.

6. *Oncotic aneurysm rupture*

7. *Endocarditis with mycotic aneurysm rupture* (typically distal fusiform artery aneurysms; may be accompanied by vasculitis).

8. *Meningitis/encephalitis.* Can be mistaken for SAH with symptoms of headache and meningeal findings. Look for fever, lumbar puncture results.

9. *Thunderclap headache and benign coital headache*

Life-Threatening Diagnoses Not to Miss

- *Aneurysmal SAH*
- *Dissection with pseudoaneurysm rupture*
- *Endocarditis with mycotic aneurysm rupture*
- *Meningitis/encephalitis*

■ Diagnostic Evaluation

- *Imaging studies.*
  - *Noncontrast CT scan.* SAH is radiographically visible in 90% of patients within 24 hours of ictus, but the sensitivity of CT drops to 60% 5 days after ictus.[15] The thickness of SAH clot and the presence of intraventricular hemorrhage (IVH) both predict the risk of vasospasm. The modified Fisher scale

Table 1.5 Modified Fisher and Fisher Grading Scale for Subarachnoid Hemorrhage

Grade	Modified Fisher	% with Vasospasm	Fisher	% with Vasospasm
0	No SAH or IVH	—	—	
1	Thin SAH, no IVH	24	No SAH or IVH	21
2	Thin SAH with IVH	33	Focal or diffuse, thin SAH	25
3	Thick SAH, no IVH	33	Diffuse thick or localized clot +/− ICH or IVH	37
4	Thick SAH with IVH	40	No or diffuse thin SAH + ICH or IVH	31

Note: ~1 mm vertical thickness as the cutoff between thin and thick.
Abbreviations: ICH, intracranial hemorrhage; IVH, intraventricular hemorrhage; SAH, subarachnoid hemorrhage.

Data from: Fisher CM, Kistler JP, Davis JM. Relation of cerebral vasospasm to subarachnoid hemorrhage visualized by computerized tomographic scanning. Neurosurgery 1980; 6:1–9. Claassen J, Bernadini GL, Kreiter K, Bates J, Du YE, Copeland D, Connolly ES, Mayer SA. Effect of cisternal and ventricular blood on risk of delayed cerebral ischemia after subarachnoid hemorrhage: The fisher scale revisited. Stroke 2001;32:2012–2020. Frontera JA, Claassen J, Schmidt JM, Wartenberg KE, Temes R, Connolly ES, Jr., MacDonald RL, Mayer SA. Prediction of symptomatic vasospasm after subarachnoid hemorrhage: the modified Fisher scale. Neurosurgery 2006;59:21–27; discussion 21–27.

incorporates the risk of vasospasm due to both SAH and IVH into its grading system (**Table 1.5, Fig. 1.1**).[16,17,18]

- ◦ *Cerebral angiogram.* Gold standard for ruling out a ruptured cerebral aneurysm, for defining the relevant neuroanatomy, and possibly providing immediate endovascular treatment. Fifteen to 20% of SAH patients have negative angiograms. Repeat angiography detects an abnormality in 1 to 2%.[19]
- ◦ *CT angiography (CTA).* >5 mm aneurysm = 95 to 100% sensitive, <5 mm aneurysm = 64 to 83% sensitive.[20,21]
- ◦ *Magnetic resonance angiography (MRA).* >5 mm aneurysm = 85 to 100% sensitive, <5 mm aneurysm = 56% sensitive.[22]
- • *Lumbar puncture.* A lumbar puncture must be performed if the history is suspicious for SAH and the head CT is negative. Always check an opening pressure. Look for clearing of blood between

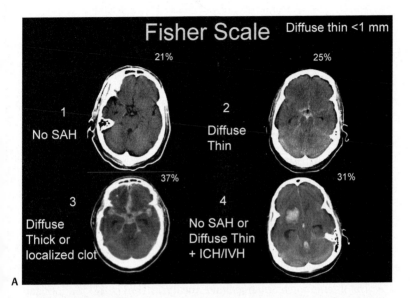

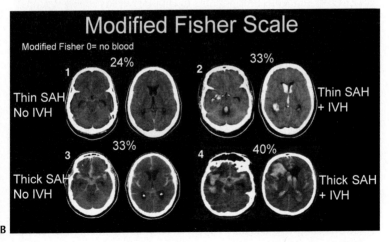

Fig. 1.1 **(A)** Fisher[18] and modified **(B)**[15,16] Fisher computed tomography (CT) rating scales. The percentage of patients who developed symptomatic vasospasm is listed next to each grade. ICH, intracerebral hemorrhage; IVH, intraventricular hemorrhage; SAH, subarachnoid hemorrhage.

tubes 1 and 4 and spin for xanthochromia (may not be present within 12 hours of ictus, but it remains for ~2 weeks).

- *Laboratory studies.* Perform toxicology screen in at-risk populations.
- See 2009 AHA/ASA guidelines on pages 337–340 for the management of Aneurysmal Subarachnoid Hemorrhage (Addendum).[23]

■ Treatment

Secure the Aneurysm

- *Open microsurgical or endovascular methods.* The optimal method for each patient should be individualized based on several factors, including: (1) aneurysm morphology, (2) patient characteristics, and (3) the experience of the treating facility. Early treatment is recommended to decrease the 67% mortality rate that is associated with rebleeding.[23]

- *The International Subarachnoid Aneurysm Trial (ISAT)* randomized 2143 spontaneous SAH patients to clipping versus coiling within 28 days of SAH onset. The majority of patients were World Federation of Neurological Surgeons (WFNS) grade 1–2; 97% had anterior circulation aneurysms, and most aneurysms were <10 mm. At 1 year, 24% of endovascular treated patients had disability or death (modified Rankin Scale 3–6) compared with 31% of surgically treated patients (p = .0019). At 7-year follow-up, the mortality was significantly higher in the surgical group (p = .03), and seizure rates were higher in the surgical group. The early rebleeding risk (up to 30 days after the initial procedure) was higher with endovascular repair, but at 7 years the rebleeding rates between the two groups was similar.[24,25]

Manage Complications of SAH

- *Rebleeding.* There is a 3–4% risk of rebleeding during the first 24 hours, 2% risk the second day, and 0.3% risk each subsequent day, or a 15 to 20% rebleeding risk within the first 2 weeks and up to 50% risk during the first 6 months if the aneurysm is not repaired.[26] Rebleeding is the most treatable cause of poor outcome after SAH. Risk factors for rebleeding include aneurysm size, the severity of the initial bleed, elevated blood pressure (which may be causative or secondary to the rebleeding), seizure, loss of consciousness at ictus, sentinel bleed, and the presence of intracranial hemorrhage (ICH) or IVH. Although placement of an external ventricular drain (EVD) may change the pressure dynamics of an aneurysm leading to rebleeding, this is a rare complication, and an EVD should nonetheless be placed if it is indicated.

- *Prevention of rebleeding.* The only definitive method to prevent rebleeding is to secure the aneurysm by excluding it from the intracranial circulation by neurosurgical clipping or endovascular obliteration. Antifibrinolytics (epsilon-aminocaproic acid: 4 mg intravenous (IV) load, then 1 g/hour continuous infusion or tranexamic acid: 1 g IV loading dose then 1 g every 6 hours until aneurysm occlusion) have been used to reduce the incidence of early rebleeding when early definitive treatment is not available. In some studies, these medications have reduced rebleeding from 10 to 2%.[27] Because antifibrinolytics can cause vasospasm, their use should be limited to within 72 hours of ictus (prior to typical vasospasm onset period) and should not be used in patients with coagulopathies, history of myocardial infarction (MI), ischemic stroke, pulmonary embolism (PE), or deep vein thrombosis (DVT). Blood pressure lowering to a systolic blood pressure (SBP) of 140 to 160 mm Hg is reasonable prior to securing the aneurysm and is usually done with a titratable drip such as nicardipine or labetalol. Seizure prophylaxis prior to aneurysm repair is reasonable since seizures have been associated with rebleeding in unsecured aneurysms.

- *Hydrocephalus* is associated with worse clinical grade and increased blood on CT. It occurs in 15% of patients radiographically, 40% of whom are symptomatic. Temporary cerebrospinal fluid (CSF) diversion is achieved by external ventricular drainage (EVD). Typical indications for EVD include ventriculomegaly on CT with symptoms of hydrocephalus, a noncommand following exam, and suspicion of elevated ICP. Most EVDs are set to drain at 15 to 20 cm H_2O initially with a goal ICP of <20 mm Hg. Forty to 80% of patients have some improvement in exam with EVD placement. Patients who undergo surgical clipping of their aneurysm may also be treated with a third ventriculostomy, which may ameliorate hydrocephalus. A ventriculoperitoneal shunt is needed in roughly 30%.[28,29]

- *Elevated ICP* can be treated initially with CSF diversion, mannitol 20% 1 g/kg IV bolus or 23% saline IV push (30 cc over 10 to 20 minutes via a central line; see Chapter 15).

- *Seizures* occur in 10% of patients at ictus, 4% during hospital stay, and another 7% have late seizures. Risk factors include ICH, MCA aneurysm, hypertension (HTN), and infarct. All patients who have seizures should receive anticonvulsants. Prior to securing an aneurysm, antiepileptic prophylaxis is reasonable because seizures can lead to aneurysm rebleeding. Many practitioners treat patients who have not seized for a period of 7 days to prevent early seizure. Some data have shown that patients exposed to phenytoin have worse cognitive outcomes at 3 months, although eventually these patients slowly recover to the level of those not exposed once anticonvulsants are discontinued.[30] Phenytoin has been the anticonvulsant traditionally used; however, newer generations of anticonvulsants are undergoing evaluation.

- *Hyponatremia* is commonly seen in SAH patients; it was originally thought to be secondary to the syndrome of inappropriate antidiuretic hormone (SIADH), but is most often due to cerebral salt wasting (CSW). CSW has been postulated to be related to neural humoral control of atrial natriuretic factor (ANF) and brain natriuretic peptide (BNP). SIADH results from excess release of antidiuretic hormone (ADH), which acts at the distal collecting duct of the nephron. Differentiation between SIADH and CSW can be determined by volume status because SIADH is associated with normovolemia/hypervolemia, whereas CSW results in volume depletion. Urine output that exceeds input in SAH patients should alert physicians to the possibility of CSW. Sodium should be monitored every 6 to 12 hours and urine output replaced such that "ins" and "outs" are matched.

  ○ Sodium supplementation can be administered by oral salt tablets (3 to 9 g/day), hypertonic saline (2 or 3% saline infusion), or fludrocortisone acetate (2 mg by mouth [PO] or IV twice daily [b.i.d.]). Rapid overcorrection may result in central pontine myelinolysis (CPM), although this is rare in patients with hyponatremia for less than 24 hours. Avoid overcorrection by not exceeding 8 meq/24 hours in patients who are chronically hyponatremic. Fluid restriction of SAH patients should be strictly avoided because this has been shown to exacerbate the development of infarcts related to vasospasm. Avoid $1/2$ normal saline (NS) or 5% dextrose in water (D5W) IV fluids. Conivaptan, an inhibitor of vasopressin V1a and V2 receptors, can be used to treat SIADH.

- *Vasospasm* typically occurs between days 3 to 14 after ictus, but timing can be variable. Symptomatic vasospasm occurs in 20 to 40% of patients and is defined as a clinical deterioration due to vasospasm when other causes (seizure, hydrocephalus, edema, etc.) have been excluded. Angiographic vasospasm occurs in 30 to 70% of patients, but its significance is unclear. Delayed cerebral ischemia is defined as symptomatic vasospasm or new infarct on CT or MRI due to vasospasm. Risk factors for vasospasm include poor clinical grade, thick blood on CT (SAH and IVH), fever, admission hypertension, sentinel bleed, ultra-early angiographic spasm, volume depletion, low cardiac output, and smoking.

- Diagnosing vasospasm:
  - Cerebral angiography is the gold standard.
  - Transcranial Doppler ultrasound (TCD) shows elevated velocities that may precede clinical symptoms by 24 to 48 hours. An inability to insonate intracranial vessels occurs in ~10% of patients. For angiographic spasm, the positive predictive value of MCA mean flow velocity (MFV) >200 cm/s is 87%, and the negative predictive value for MCA MFV <120 cm/s is 94%.[31] However, the predictive value in other territories, such as the ACA, is poor, and the association of TCD velocities and symptomatic vasospasm is limited.[32] The Lindegaard ratio corrects the MFV for hyperemia (due to increased cardiac output, pressor use, or anemia) and is defined as the MCA/ICA velocity (**Table 1.6**).

Table 1.6 Lindegaard Ratio

Lindegaard Ratio	Angiographic Vasospasm
<3	No spasm
3–4.5	Mild spasm
4.5–6	Moderate spasm
>6	Severe spasm

Data from: Lindegaard KF, Nornes H, Bakke SJ, Sorteberg W, Nakstad P. Cerebral vasospasm after subarachnoid haemorrhage investigated by means of transcranial Doppler ultrasound. Acta Neurochir Suppl (Wien) 1988;42:81–84.

TCD is typically performed on a daily basis and serves to indicate which patients may require closer observation for impending symptomatic vasospasm/ischemia. Treatment for vasospasm should not be initiated based on TCD values: patients should be maintained in a normovolemic state, and if symptoms of vasospasm/ischemia develop, further evaluation and treatment should be initiated. In patients with marginal exams in whom it is difficult to detect symptomatic spasm, additional testing such as digital subtraction angiography, CT or MR angiography may be useful when TCD velocities are elevated or increasing. Hypercalcemia can cause or exacerbate vasospasm and should be avoided or corrected. TCD does have a reasonable negative predictive value for angiographic and symptomatic spasm.

- Alternatively, CT angiography/CT perfusion, MR perfusion, MRA, xenon CT, and single-photon emission computed tomography (SPECT) scan can be used to detect vasospasm/ischemia. These modalities may be particularly useful for detecting small vessel distal spasm.

• Vasospasm prophylaxis:

- Nimodipine is the only medication proven in large trials to improve outcome after SAH. In a meta-analysis of 10 studies, nimodipine reduced death or severe disability, symptomatic vasospasm, and CT-documented infarction from vasospasm. However, nimodipine does not reduce rates of angiographic vasospasm.[33,34]

Nimodipine is given for 21 days and typically dosed as 60 mg every 4 hours for SBP >140 mm Hg, 30 mg every 4 hours for SBP 120 to 140 mm Hg, and held for an SBP <120 mm Hg.

- Fever is associated with the development of symptomatic spasm and should be controlled aggressively.

- Volume-depleted patients are at increased risk for symptomatic vasospasm, and normovolemia should be maintained.

- Prophylactic hypervolemic-hypertensive-hemodilution (HHH) therapy (in those *without* symptoms of vasospasm) has not been shown to reduce rates of symptomatic vasospasm or improve outcome and is not recommended.

• Treatment of symptomatic vasospasm:

- HHH therapy is typically employed by elevating blood pressure with either phenylephrine or norepinephrine to at least

20 mm Hg above baseline blood pressure to a maximum pressure of 220/120 mm Hg. Pressor use can be limited by the development of end organ damage (myocardial infarction, congestive heart failure [CHF], renal insufficiency, digital ischemia, etc.). Patients similarly receive volume in the form of normal saline or colloid. Hemodilution using phlebotomy is typically not used. There are no randomized trials proving the efficacy of HHH therapy, and certain studies have questioned the value of hypervolemia.[35]

○ Endovascular treatment of vasospasm can reverse symptoms of delayed cerebral ischemia (DCI) in 30 to 70% of patients. Options include intra-arterial vasodilators such as papaverine, verapamil, and nicardipine, or angioplasty. Vasodilators are short-lived, and angioplasty has a more durable effect but also carries the risk of vessel rupture. Endovascular treatment is most successful if performed early, preferably within 2 hours of symptom onset.[36]

Sample Admission Order Set for SAH

- Prescribe fosphenytoin 20 mg/kg IV load, then phenytoin 100 mg IV every 8 hours.
- Prescribe nimodipine 60 mg PO every 4 hours for SBP ≥140, 30 mg for SBP 120 to 140, hold for SBP ≤120 mm Hg.
- Keep SBP between ≤160 mm Hg with labetalol drip or Cardene (Roche Laboratories, Inc., Nutley, NJ) drip (avoid nitroprusside, as this can raise ICP) and ≥90 mm Hg with norepinephrine or phenylephrine 2 to 10 mg/kg/min as needed.
- Assess need for aminocaproic acid (Wyeth-Ayerst Pharmaceuticals, Radnor, PA) administration if prior to SAH day 3 and aneurysm treatment will be delayed >12 hours and no history of stroke, MI, peripheral vascular disease (PVD), or abnormal electrocardiogram (EKG).
  - ○ Give 4 g IV over first hour, then 1 g IV every hour; hold aminocaproic acid 1 to 3 hours prior to angiogram.
- Order noncontrast head CT; consider CT angio/CT perfusion.
- Assess for hydrocephalus; consider EVD.
- Schedule cerebral angiogram. In patients with renal insufficiency, preangiogram treatment with hydration (NS at 1 mL/kg/h) before and after the angiogram can be nephroprotective. Some advocate acetylcysteine (600 mg PO b.i.d. x 2 days).

■ Prognosis

Major predictors of outcome include Hunt–Hess grade, age, aneurysm size, and rebleeding. Overall, approximately 10% of patients die before reaching the hospital, and 65% have some cognitive impairment.[37] There are several causes of poor outcome following SAH. These include, in order of decreasing importance: (1) deleterious effects on the brain of the initial bleed; (2) aneurysm rerupture; (3) cerebral vasospasm; (4) hydrocephalus; and (5) hyponatremia, seizures, and other causes. Two commonly used measures of outcome are the Glasgow Outcome Score (**Table 1.7**) and the Modified Rankin Scale (mRS) (**Table 1.8**).

Table 1.7 Glasgow Outcome Score

Glasgow Outcome Score	Function
1	Dead
2	Persistent vegetative state
3	Severe disability, conscious but limited communication skills, dependent for daily activities of living
4	Independent but with disabilities; able to work
5	Resumption of normal life despite minor physical or mental deficits

Data from: Jennett B, Bond M. Assessment of outcome after severe brain damage. Lancet 1975;1:480–484.

Table 1.8 Modified Rankin Scale

Score	Description
0	No symptoms at all
1	No significant disability despite symptoms; able to carry out all usual duties and activities
2	Slight disability; unable to carry out all previous activities, but able to look after own affairs without assistance
3	Moderate disability; requiring some help, but able to walk without assistance

(Continued)

Table 1.8 Modified Rankin Scale *(continued)*

Score	Description
4	Moderately severe disability; unable to walk without assistance and unable to attend to own bodily needs without assistance
5	Severe disability; bedridden, incontinent and requiring constant nursing care and attention
6	Dead
Total (0–6):	

Data from: Rankin J. Cerebral vascular accidents in patients over the age of 60. Scott Med J 1957;2:200–15. Bonita R, Beaglehole R. Modification of Rankin Scale: Recovery of motor function after stroke. Stroke 1988 Dec;19(12):1497–1500. Van Swieten JC, Koudstaal PJ, Visser MC, Schouten HJ, van Gijn J. Interobserver agreement for the assessment of handicap in stroke patients. Stroke 1988;19(5):604–7.

Pearls and Pitfalls

- All practitioners should maintain a high index of suspicion for subarachnoid hemorrhage, even when the initial CT is negative. A lumbar puncture should be performed to assess for CSF xanthochromia in CT-negative patients.

- Early treatment of a ruptured aneurysm is strongly recommended to prevent the mortality and morbidity associated with rerupture.

- Symptomatic vasospasm is a significant contributor to morbidity and must be treated early and aggressively.

References

1. Stehbens WE. Aneurysms and anatomical variation of cerebral arteries. Arch Pathol 1963;75:45–64
2. Report of World Federation of Neurological Surgeons Committee on a Universal Subarachnoid Hemorrhage Grading Scale. J Neurosurg 1988;68:985–986
3. Wiebers DO, Whisnant JP, Huston J III, et al. Unruptured intracranial aneurysms: natural history, clinical outcome, and risks of surgical and endovascular treatment. Lancet 2003;362(9378):103–110
4. Kowalski RG, Claassen J, Kreiter KT, et al. Initial misdiagnosis and outcome after subarachnoid hemorrhage. JAMA 2004;291:866–869
5. McCarron MO, Alberts MJ, McCarron P. A systematic review of Terson's syndrome: frequency and prognosis after subarachnoid haemorrhage. J Neurol Neurosurg Psychiatry 2004;75:491–493
6. Hunt WE, Hess RM. Surgical risk as related to time of intervention in the repair of intracranial aneurysms. J Neurosurg 1968;28:14–20

7. Mast H, Young WL, Koennecke HC, et al. Risk of spontaneous haemorrhage after diagnosis of cerebral arteriovenous malformation. Lancet 1997;350:1065–1068

8. Stapf C, Mast H, Sciacca RR, et al. Predictors of hemorrhage in patients with untreated brain arteriovenous malformation. Neurology 2006;66:1350–1355

9. Yamada S, Takagi Y, Nozaki K, Kikuta K, Hashimoto N. Risk factors for subsequent hemorrhage in patients with cerebral arteriovenous malformations. J Neurosurg 2007;107:965–972

10. Brown RD Jr. Simple risk predictions for arteriovenous malformation hemorrhage. Neurosurgery 2000;46:1024

11. Stapf C, Mast H, Sciacca RR, et al. Predictors of hemorrhage in patients with untreated brain arteriovenous malformation. Neurology 2006;66(9):1350–1355

12. Spetzler RF, Martin NA. A proposed grading system for arteriovenous malformations. J Neurosurg 1986;65:476–483

13. Robinson JR, Awad IA, Little JR. Natural history of the cavernous angioma. J Neurosurg 1991;75:709–714

14. Fritschi JA, Reulen HJ, Spetzler RF, Zabramski JM. Cavernous malformations of the brain stem: a review of 139 cases. Acta Neurochir (Wien) 1994;130(1–4):35–46

15. Sidman R, Connolly E, Lemke T. Subarachnoid hemorrhage diagnosis: lumbar puncture is still needed when the computed tomography scan is normal. Acad Emerg Med 1996;3:827–831

16. Claassen J, Bernadini GL, Kreiter K, Bates J, Du YE, Copeland D, Connolly ES, Mayer SA. Effect of cisternal and ventricular blood on risk of delayed cerebral ischemia after subarachnoid hemorrhage: The Fisher Scale revisited. Stroke 32:2012–2020, 2001.

17. Frontera JA, Claassen J, Schmidt JM, et al. Prediction of symptomatic vasospasm after subarachnoid hemorrhage: the modified Fisher scale. Neurosurgery 2006;59(1):21–27

18. Fisher CM, Kistler JP, Davis JM. Relation of cerebral vasospasm to subarachnoid hemorrhage visualized by computerized tomographic scanning. Neurosurgery 1980 Jan; 6:1–9

19. Rinkel GJ, Wijdicks EF, Hasan D, et al. Outcome in patients with subarachnoid haemorrhage and negative angiography according to pattern of haemorrhage on computed tomography. Lancet 1991;338:964–968

20. Chappell ET, Moure FC, Good MC: Comparison of computed tomographic angiography with digital subtraction angiography in the diagnosis of cerebral aneurysms: a meta-analysis. Neurosurgery 2003;52:624–631; discussion 630–621

21. van Gelder JM. Computed tomographic angiography for detecting cerebral aneurysms: implications of aneurysm size distribution for the sensitivity, specificity, and likelihood ratios. Neurosurgery 2003;53:597–605; discussion 605–596

22. Huston J III, Nichols DA, Luetmer PH, et al. Blinded prospective evaluation of sensitivity of MR angiography to known intracranial aneurysms: importance of aneurysm size. AJNR Am J Neuroradiol 1994;15:1607–1614

23. Bederson JB, Connolly ES, Jr., Batjer HH, Dacey RG, Dion JE, Diringer MN, Duldner JE, Jr., Harbaugh RE, Patel AB, Rosenwasser RH. Guidelines for the management of aneurysmal subarachnoid hemorrhage. A statement for healthcare professionals from a special writing group of the stroke council, American Heart Association. Stroke 2009

24. Molyneux A, Kerr R, Stratton I, et al. International Subarachnoid Aneurysm Trial (ISAT) of neurosurgical clipping versus endovascular coiling in 2143 patients with ruptured intracranial aneurysms: a randomised trial. Lancet 2002;360(9342):1267–1274

25. Molyneux AJ, Kerr RS, Yu LM, et al. International subarachnoid aneurysm trial (ISAT) of neurosurgical clipping versus endovascular coiling in 2143 patients with ruptured intracranial aneurysms: a randomised comparison of effects on survival, dependency, seizures, rebleeding, subgroups, and aneurysm occlusion. Lancet 2005;366(9488):809–817

26. Naidech AM, Janjua N, Kreiter KT, et al. Predictors and impact of aneurysm rebleeding after subarachnoid hemorrhage. Arch Neurol 2005;62:410–416

27. Hillman J, Fridriksson S, Nilsson O, et al. Immediate administration of tranexamic acid and reduced incidence of early rebleeding after aneurysmal subarachnoid hemorrhage: a prospective randomized study. J Neurosurg 2002;97(4):771–778

28. Jartti P, Karttunen A, Isokangas JM, Jartti A, Koskelainen T, Tervonen O. Chronic hydrocephalus after neurosurgical and endovascular treatment of ruptured intracranial aneurysms. Acta Radiol 2008;49:680–686

29. Varelas P, Helms A, Sinson G, Spanaki M, Hacein-Bey L. Clipping or coiling of ruptured cerebral aneurysms and shunt-dependent hydrocephalus. Neurocrit Care 2006;4:223–228

30. Naidech AM, Kreiter KT, Janjua N, et al. Phenytoin exposure is associated with functional and cognitive disability after subarachnoid hemorrhage. Stroke 2005;36(3):583–587

31. Vora YY, Suarez-Almazor M, Steinke DE, et al. Role of transcranial Doppler monitoring in the diagnosis of cerebral vasospasm after subarachnoid hemorrhage. Neurosurgery 1999;44(6):1237–1247

32. Suarez JI, Qureshi AI, Yahia AB, et al. Symptomatic vasospasm diagnosis after subarachnoid hemorrhage: evaluation of transcranial Doppler ultrasound and cerebral angiography as related to compromised vascular distribution. Crit Care Med 2002;30(6):1348–1355

33. Allen GS, Ahn HS, Preziosi TJ, et al. Cerebral arterial spasm—a controlled trial of nimodipine in patients with subarachnoid hemorrhage. N Engl J Med 1983;308(11):619–624

34. Feigin VL, Rinkel GJ, Algra A, et al. Calcium antagonists in patients with aneurysmal subarachnoid hemorrhage: a systematic review. Neurology 1998;50(4):876–883

35. Muench E, Horn P, Bauhuf C, et al. Effects of hypervolemia and hypertension on regional cerebral blood flow, intracranial pressure, and brain tissue oxygenation after subarachnoid hemorrhage. Crit Care Med 2007;35(8):1844–1851

36. Rosenwasser RH, Armonda RA, Thomas JE, et al. Therapeutic modalities for the management of cerebral vasospasm: timing of endovascular options. Neurosurgery 1999;44(5):975–979

37. Tidswell P, Dias PS, Sagar HJ, Mayes AR, Battersby RD. Cognitive outcome after aneurysm rupture: relationship to aneurysm site and perioperative complications. Neurology 1995;45:875–882

2 Traumatic Brain Injury

Chad Miller

Trauma accounts for over 150,000 deaths in the United States each year. A frequent cause of mortality for this group is head injury, for which over 230,000 patients require hospital care.[1] The most common source of traumatic brain injury (TBI) changes with age and includes motor vehicle accidents, physical assault, and falls. The impact of TBI is substantial, considering the disability resulting from injury and the propensity for young individuals to be affected. These facts underscore the importance of prompt and comprehensive treatment for those suffering head injury. Although prevention remains the most effective treatment, recent studies have highlighted the contribution of secondary injury to overall disability in TBI. Standardization of care following evidence-based guidelines has been shown to improve patient outcomes. Level 1 trauma centers are best equipped to deliver this comprehensive care.

Case Example

A 34-year-old passenger in a motor vehicle is brought to the emergency department after a moderate-speed collision with an automobile at a busy intersection. The patient is found unconscious at the scene. Emergency services personnel arrived within 5 minutes of the accident and found the patient nonverbal, without eye opening, and withdrawing to noxious stimuli.

Questions

- Is the patient currently intubated, and if so, were cervical spine precautions taken?
- Is cervical spine stabilization in place?
- Are there other injuries?
- What are the vital signs?

Urgent Orders

- Perform primary survey (airway, breathing, circulation [ABCs])
- Order a focused abdominal sonogram for trauma (FAST exam evaluates pericardium, right and left upper abdomen, and pelvic region for blood)
- Obtain a complete blood count (CBC), chemistry panel, coagulation studies, type and cross, toxicology screen, arterial blood gas, and pregnancy test (if indicated)
- Maintain PaO_2 >60 mm Hg and systolic blood pressure (SBP) ≥90 mm Hg or mean arterial pressure (MAP) ≥65 mm Hg
- Perform a noncontrast head computed tomography (CT), spine CT, CT of chest, abdomen, and pelvis when patient is stabilized.

■ History and Examination

History

- Determine events surrounding the accident—use of a seatbelt or helmet, position of the patient in the vehicle, type of vehicle (motorcycle or automobile), direction from which the vehicle was hit, speed of collision, windshield or steering wheel damage (may indicate concomitant injury such as aortic rupture or other systemic injury).
- Assess for use of ethyl alcohol (EtOH) or illicit drugs, as these may confound the examination.
- Passive rewarming of hypothermic trauma patients is crucial prior to assessing the neurologic examination.
- Inquire about seizure activity following the accident.

Physical Examination

- Look and palpate for scalp lacerations, depressed skull fractures, and cerebrospinal fluid (CSF) drainage from nares and ears, while keeping in mind that significant head injury can occur without external stigmata. Most skull fractures are nondisplaced. Raccoon's eyes and Battle's sign are classically associated with basilar skull fracture.

Neurologic Examination

- A full neurologic examination, including assessment of mental status, cranial nerves, motor skills, and reflexes, as well as a sensory and cerebellar exam, should be performed on all patients.

- The Glasgow Coma Scale (GCS) provides a succinct assessment of the neurologic examination and is widely used to give an overview of the patient's neurologic status. Coma is defined as a GCS ≤8, and the minimal score is 3. The GCS is scored using the best response in any limb (**Table 2.1**).

- Long track signs and weakness ipsilateral to the lesion and ipsilateral third nerve palsy (i.e., right hemiparesis and right blown pupil in a patient with a right subdural hematoma) is an ominous sign that may represent Kernohan's notch phenomenon (compression of the contralateral cerebral peduncle against the incisura of the tentorium due to transtentorial herniation and stretching of the ipsilateral third nerve).

Table 2.1 The Glasgow Coma Scale

Assessment		Score
Verbal		
	Alert, oriented, and conversant	5
	Confused, disoriented, but conversant	4
	Intelligible words, not conversant	3
	Unintelligible sounds	2
	No verbalization	1
Eye opening		
	Spontaneous	4
	To verbal stimuli	3
	To painful stimuli	2
	None	1
Motor		
	Follows commands	6
	Localizes	5
	Withdraws from stimulus	4
	Flexor posturing	3
	Extensor posturing	2
	No response to noxious stimulus	1

■ Differential Diagnosis

1. *Traumatic brain injury.* May include subdural, epidural, subarachnoid hemorrhage, traumatic parenchymal lesion, diffuse axonal injury, posterior fossa mass lesion, depressed skull fracture. TBI is classified as mild (GCS ≥13), moderate (GCS 9–12) or severe (GCS ≤8).

2. *Spinal cord injury.* May include sensory level, spinal shock (bradycardia, hypotension), initial absence of reflexes

3. *In falls or when a patient is "found down" with intracranial hemorrhage (ICH), the inciting event could be an aneurysm or AVM rupture, or ischemic stroke with hemorrhagic conversion with secondary trauma.* The physician must keep an open mind while caring for patients with unwitnessed events, as the treatment priorities may be quite different from those undertaken for TBI.

Life-Threatening Diagnoses Not to Miss

- *Lesions requiring surgical treatment.* These include subdural hemorrhage, epidural hemorrhage, depressed skull fracture, posterior fossa lesions, certain parenchymal contusions, elevated intracranial pressure refractory to medical management, and certain spinal cord injuries.

- *Elevated intracranial pressure (ICP)* (if in doubt, insert an ICP monitor).

■ Diagnostic Evaluation

- *Imaging studies*
  - Head CT:
    - For mild TBI (patients with GCS 15 with loss of consciousness and no neurologic deficit, age >3 years), according to New Orleans Criteria,[2] a noncontrast head CT to evaluate for the presence of any abnormality is recommended in patients with headache, vomiting, seizure, intoxication, short-term memory deficit, age >60 years, or injury above the clavicle. According to the Canadian CT Head Rule,[3] in patients with GCS 13–15 with loss of consciousness but no neurologic

deficit, no seizure, no history of anticoagulation, and age >16 years: patients at high risk for neurosurgical intervention and abnormal head CT include those with GCS <15 at 2 hours postinjury, suspected skull fracture, any sign of basal skull fracture, vomiting (≥2 times), and aged ≥65 years. Medium-risk patients for neurosurgical intervention and abnormal head CT are those with retrograde amnesia >30 minutes, or a dangerous mechanism of injury (pedestrian vs motor vehicle, ejected from motor vehicle, fall from height >1 m or five stairs.)

- All moderate-severe TBI patients require a noncontrast head CT, and, when in doubt, it is appropriate to check a head CT. Head CT can be classified using the Marshall Classification system (**Table 2.2**).[4]

- In severe TBI, head CT abnormalities are found in 93% of patients. For severe TBI patients, the absence of abnormalities on head CT is associated with, but does not guarantee, a favorable prognosis. Conversely, obliteration of the basal cisterns confers an unfavorable outcome with a positive predictive value of 97%.[5]

Table 2.2 The Marshall Classification of Head Injury

Category	Definition
Diffuse injury I	No visible pathology on CT
Diffuse injury II	Cisterns present with MLS <5 mm; no high-density lesion >2.5 cm
Diffuse injury III	Cisterns compressed or absent; no high-density lesion >2.5 cm
Diffuse injury IV	MLS >5 mm; no high-density lesion >2.5 cm
Evacuated mass	Any lesion surgically evacuated
Nonevacuated mass	High-density lesion >2.5 cm; not surgically evacuated

Abbreviations: CT, computed tomography; MLS, midline shift.

Data from: Marshall LF, Marshall SB, Klauber MR, et al. The diagnosis of head injury requires a classification based on computed axial tomography. J Neurotrauma 1992;9(Suppl 1):S287–S292.

- Contusions and subdural hemorrhage (SDH) are the most common CT findings in severe TBI, each occurring in about one-fourth of patients, typically at locations where the brain collides with the adjacent skull (orbital frontal, temporal regions). Fluid-fluid levels may indicate coagulopathy.

- SDH results from tearing of bridging veins and has a propensity to expand over time. These concave lesions do not cross the falx but cross suture lines. Mixed density lesions may be seen, indicating aging blood products.

- Traumatic SAH is common and may lead to angiographic vasospasm if extensive (>1 mm in thickness) in 20 to 40% of cases.[6] For these reasons, daily assessment of vascular narrowing with transcranial Doppler (TCD) ultrasound is performed at many institutions.

- Epidural hematomas (EDH) occur infrequently (1 to 2%)[7] and result from temporal or parietal skull fractures, which damage underlying arteries. These lesions are concave and do not cross suture lines. Despite the classical teachings, these bleeds seldom result in a period of lucidity following loss of consciousness.

- Progressive hemorrhagic injury occurs in over 40% of patients with TBI (DTICH—delayed traumatic intracerebral hematoma).[8] Neurologic deterioration accompanies many of these changes; however, this progression can be latent, particularly in severe TBI patients with a compromised baseline exam. As a result, severe TBI patients should receive routine head CT scans at 4 to 6 hour intervals until stability of the lesion is confirmed.

- Traumatic arterial dissection can lead to perfusion failure or embolic stroke and can be evaluated by CT angiogram, magnetic resonance imaging (MRI), or magnetic resonance angiography (MRA) of the brain and neck or by digital subtraction angiography if there is sufficient suspicion.

◦ MRI:
  - Shearing axonal injury of the brain (diffuse axonal injury) results from torsional traumatic forces and often accounts for disability disproportionate to the CT radiological injury. Gradient echo (GRE) MRI and susceptibility weighted imaging changes, particularly in the corpus callosum and brainstem, represent hemorrhage and diffuse axonal injury (DAI).

- Fluid attenuated inversion recovery (FLAIR) sequences may demonstrate cerebral edema; diffusion-weighted image (DWI) and apparent diffusion coefficient imaging (ADC) abnormalities may show infarction.

○ ICP monitoring

- According to 2007 Brain Trauma Foundation guidelines,[9] ICP monitoring should occur in all patients with GCS <9 and an abnormal head CT (e.g. hematomas, contusions, swelling, herniation, or compressed basal cisterns). ICP monitoring is indicated in patients with GCS <9 and a normal CT if two or more of the following are met at admission: age >40, unilateral or bilateral posturing, SBP < 90 mm Hg.

- If the patient is comatose and has an abnormal CT, 50 to 60% will have abnormal ICP. If the patient is comatose with a normal CT, 10 to 15% will have abnormal ICP. If two of the following factors are present (age >40, unilateral or bilateral posturing, SBP <90 mm Hg), 33% will have an abnormal ICP.[10]

○ Additional testing

- Focused abdominal sonogram for trauma (FAST) exam evaluates pericardium, right and left upper abdomen, and pelvic region for blood.

- CT of chest, abdomen, and pelvis

- In patients with long bone fracture, evaluate creatine kinase (CK), and check compartment pressures for compartment syndrome if CK is elevated.

■ Treatment

Medical Treatment

- Maintenance of ABCs are of paramount importance and supersede all other neurologic concerns. Patients with poor airway protection, GCS <9, or hypoxemia refractory to supplemental oxygen should generally be intubated. Intubation should occur with removal of the C-spine collar and manual stabilization of the C-spine.

If intubation is not emergent, options include use of video laryngoscopes or fiberoptic intubation. Unless increased ICP and/or herniation are suspected, normal ventilation ($PaCO_2$ 35 to 40 mm Hg) should be targeted.

- Hypoxia and hypotension affect over one-third of all trauma patients and have a disastrous impact on outcome. A single episode of hypotension (SBP < 90 mm Hg) doubles mortality.[9] In a randomized trial of TBI patients, initial resuscitation with 7.5% hypertonic saline compared with lactated Ringer revealed no difference in neurologic outcome at 6 months.[11] However, hypotonic and dextrose-containing solutions should be avoided to minimize cerebral swelling and hyperglycemia. In a post hoc analysis of TBI patients enrolled in the Saline versus Albumin Fluid Evaluation (SAFE) study, fluid resuscitation with albumin was associated with higher mortality than saline resuscitation.[12] Hypoxemia (PaO_2 <60 mm Hg) is also associated with increased morbidity and mortality.

- Elevations in ICP occur in many patients with severe TBI. These elevations correlate with poor outcome and must be identified and appropriately treated. See Chapter 15.

- Dysautonomia or sympathetic storming is characterized by episodic hypertension, tachypnea, fever, diaphoresis, dystonia, and posturing. Dysautonomia can persist for months or years and may be due to loss of GABA (gamma-aminobutyric acid) inhibition of cortical projections. These episodes can be managed with β blockers (centrally acting propranolol), clonidine, opiates, benzodiazepines (midazolam, clonazepam, etc.), gabapentin, pregabalin, bromocriptine, dantrolene, levodopa, chlorpromazine, or baclofen.

- See the 2007 Brain Trauma Foundation Guidelines in **Table 2.3** [9,13,14] for specific treatment guidelines.

Table 2.3 2007 Brain Trauma Foundation Guidelines for the Assessment of Traumatic Brain Injury

	Level I	Level II	Level III
Blood pressure and oxygenation	None	Blood pressure should be monitored and BP <90 mm Hg avoided	Oxygenation should be monitored and PaO$_2$ <60 mm Hg or O$_2$ sat <90% avoided
Hyperosmolar therapy	None	Mannitol is effective to control ICP at doses of 0.25–1 g/Kg; SBP <90 mm Hg should be avoided	Restrict mannitol use prior to ICP monitoring to patients with signs of herniation or progressive neurologic deterioration not attributable to extracranial causes
Prophylactic induced hypothermia	None	None	Prophylactic induced hypothermia is not significantly associated with decreased mortality, but 48 h of hypothermia treatment suggests a decrease in mortality risk
Infection prophylaxis	None	Periprocedural antibiotics for intubation should be administered to reduce the incidence of pneumonia. However, this does not change length of stay or mortality. Early tracheostomy should be performed to reduce mechanical ventilation days.	Routine ventricular catheter (EVD) exchange or prophylactic antibiotic use for EVD placement is not recommended to reduce infection. Early extubation in qualified patients can be done without increased risk of pneumonia.
Deep vein thrombosis prophylaxis	None	None	Graduated compression stockings or intermittent pneumatic compression stockings are recommended. LMWH or unfractionated heparin should be used in combination with mechanical prophylaxis. However, there is an increased risk of expanded ICH. There is insufficient data to recommend preferred agent, timing or dose of prophylaxis.

(Continued)

Table 2.3 2007 Brain Trauma Foundation Guidelines for the Assessment of Traumatic Brain Injury *(continued)*

	Level I	Level II	Level III
ICP monitoring	None	GCS <9 with abnormal head CT	GCS<9 with normal head CT and two of the following: age >40, uni- or bilateral posturing, SBP <90 mm Hg
ICP thresholds	None	Treatment should be initiated for ICP >20 mm Hg	A combination of ICP values, clinical and head CT findings should be used to determine treatment.
Cerebral perfusion thresholds	None	Aggressive attempts to maintain CPP >70 mm Hg with fluids and pressors should be avoided because of the risk of ARDS.	CPP <50 mm Hg should be avoided. Patients with intact autoregulation tolerate higher CPP values. Goal CPP 50–70 mm Hg. Monitoring of CBF, oxygenation, and metabolism facilitates CPP management.
Brain oxygen monitoring and thresholds	None	None	Jugular venous saturation <50% or brain oxygen tension <15 mm Hg are treatment thresholds.
Anesthetics, analgesics, and sedatives	None	Prophylactic barbiturates to induce burst suppression EEG is not recommended. High-dose barbiturates are recommended to control elevated ICP refractory to maximum standard medical and surgical treatment. Hemodynamic stability is essential before and during barbiturate therapy. Propofol is recommended to control ICP but not for improvement in 6-month mortality	None

(Continued on next page)

Table 2.3 2007 Brain Trauma Foundation Guidelines for the Assessment of Traumatic Brain Injury *(continued)*

	Level I	Level II	Level III
		or outcome. High-dose propofol can cause significant morbidity (propofol infusion syndrome).	
Nutrition	None	Patients should be fed to attain full caloric replacement by day 7 postinjury.	None
Antiseizure prophylaxis	None	Prophylactic use of phenytoin and valproic acid is not recommended for preventing late posttraumatic seizures. Anticonvulsants are indicated to decrease the incidence of early posttraumatic seizures (within 7 days of injury). Early seizures are not associated with worse outcomes.	
Hyperventilation	None	Prophylactic hyperventilation (PaCO$_2$ ≤25 mm Hg) is not recommended.	Hyperventilation is recommended as a temporizing measure for the reduction of elevated ICP. Hyperventilation should be avoided during the first 24 h after injury when CBF is often critically reduced. If hyperventilation is used, jugular venous O$_2$ sat or brain O$_2$ tension measurements are recommended. Keep PaCO$_2$ 35–40 mm Hg if the ICP is otherwise controlled.

(Continued)

Table 2.3 2007 Brain Trauma Foundation Guidelines for the Assessment of Traumatic Brain Injury *(continued)*

	Level I	Level II	Level III
Steroids	The use of steroids is not recommended for improving ICP or outcome. High-dose methylprednisolone is associated with increased mortality (MRC CRASH trial).	None	None

See Chapter 22 for descriptions of Levels of Recommendation by the Brain Trauma foundation

Abbreviations: ARDS, acute respiratory distress syndrome; BP, blood pressure; CBF, cerebral blood flow; CPP, cerebral perfusion pressure; CT, computed tomography; EEG, electroencephalogram; EVD, external ventricular drain; GCS, Glasgow Coma Scale; ICH, intracerebral hemorrhage; ICP, intracranial pressure; LMWH, low molecular weight heparin; SBP, systolic blood pressure; sat, saturation.

Data from: Murray GD, Butcher I, McHugh GS, et al. Multivariable prognostic analysis in traumatic brain injury: results from the IMPACT study. J Neurotrauma 2007;24(2):329–337.

Temkin NR, Dikmen SS, Wilensky AJ, Keihm J, Chabal S, Winn HR. A randomized, double-blind study of phenytoin for the prevention of post-traumatic seizures. N Engl J Med 1990;323(8):497–502.

Edwards P, Arango M, Balica L, et al. Final results of MRC CRASH, a randomised placebo-controlled trial of intravenous corticosteroid in adults with head injury-outcomes at 6 months. Lancet 2005;365(9475):1957–1959.

Surgical Treatment

Surgical treatment is often needed for enlarging mass lesions and refractory ICP. The neurosurgeon should consider evacuation of any symptomatic mass lesion to minimize secondary deterioration due to impaired blood flow and persistent edema. Generally, lesions in the mesiotemporal lobes and posterior fossa have less room for expansion. As a rule, tenuous ICP control tends to worsen with time, and lesions associated with refractory ICP should be removed. Decompressive hemicraniectomy or bifrontal craniectomy has been shown to be valuable in improving ICP, cerebral perfusion pressure (CPP), and cerebral oxygenation in TBI patients with intractable ICP (**Table 2.4**).[7,15–18]

Table 2.4 2006 Surgical Recommendations for the Treatment of Traumatic Brain Injury

Traumatic Parenchymal Lesions	Patients with signs of progressive neurologic deterioration referable to the lesion, medically refractory ICP, or signs of mass effect on CT should be treated operatively. Patients with GCS 6–8 with frontal or temporal contusions >20 mL in volume with midline shift ≥5 mm and/or cisternal compression on CT and any lesion >50 mL in volume should be treated operatively. Patients with parenchymal mass lesions who do not have neurologic compromise, have controlled ICP, and no signs of mass effect on CT may be managed nonoperatively with intensive monitoring and serial imaging. Decompressive procedures including bifrontal decompressive craniectomy for patients with diffuse medically refractory cerebral edema and elevated ICP within 48 h are treatment options.
Acute Subdural Hematoma	SDH with thickness >10 mm or a midline shift >5 mm on CT should be surgically evacuated regardless of GCS. All patients with GCS <9 and SDH should undergo ICP monitoring. Patients with GCS <9 and SDH <10 mm and midline shift <5 mm should undergo evacuation if the GCS score decreases by ≥2 points and/or the patient presents with asymmetric or fixed and dilated pupils and/or the ICP ≥20 mm Hg. Evacuation should be performed using a craniotomy with or without bone flap removal and duraplasty.
Acute Epidural Hematoma	EDH >30 mL should be evacuated regardless of GCS. EDH <30 mL and <15-mm thickness and <5 mm midline shift in patients with GCS >8 without focal deficit can be managed nonoperatively with serial CT. EDH in patients with GCS <9 with anisocoria should undergo immediate evacuation.
Posterior Fossa Mass Lesions	Patients with mass effect on CT (distortion, dislocation, or obliteration of the fourth ventricle or compression of basal cisterns or obstructive hydrocephalus) or neurologic dysfunction or deterioration referable to the lesion should undergo operative intervention. Patients with lesions and no significant mass effect on CT and with a normal neurologic exam may be managed with observation and serial imaging. If the decision is made to evacuate, surgery should be done immediately, as patients can rapidly deteriorate. If the decision is made to evacuate, suboccipital craniectomy is recommended.

(Continued)

Table 2.4 2006 Surgical Recommendations for the Treatment of Traumatic Brain Injury *(continued)*

Depressed Cranial Fractures	Open or compound depressed fractures (overlying scalp laceration in continuity with the fracture site and with galeal disruption) greater than the thickness of the cranium should undergo operative intervention to prevent infection.
	Patients with open depressed fractures may be treated nonoperatively if there is no clinical or radiographic evidence of dural penetration, no significant ICH, no depression >1 cm, no frontal sinus involvement, no gross cosmetic deformity, and no wound infection/contamination, or pneumocephalus.
	Nonoperative management of closed (simple) depressed fractures (no galeal disruption) is an option.
	In operative patients, early elevation and débridement to reduce infection are recommended.
	Primary bone fragment replacement is a surgical option in the absence of wound infection.
	All management strategies for open depressed fractures should include antibiotics.

Abbreviations: CT, computed tomography; EDH, epidural hematoma; GCS, Glasgow Coma Scale; ICH, intracerebral hemorrhage; ICP, intracranial pressure; SDH, subdural hemorrhage.

Data from: Bullock MR, Chesnut R, Ghajar J, et al. Surgical management of traumatic parenchymal lesions. Neurosurgery 2006; 58(3, Suppl):S25–S46; discussion Si-iv.

Bullock MR, Chesnut R, Ghajar J, et al. Surgical management of posterior fossa mass lesions. Neurosurgery 2006; 58(3, Suppl):S47–S55; discussion Si-iv.

Bullock MR, Chesnut R, Ghajar J, et al. Surgical management of depressed cranial fractures. Neurosurgery 2006; 58(3, Suppl):S56–S60; discussion Si-iv.

Bullock MR, Chesnut R, Ghajar J, et al. Surgical management of acute subdural hematomas. Neurosurgery 2006; 58(3, Suppl):S16–S24; discussion Si-iv.

Bullock MR, Chesnut R, Ghajar J, et al. Surgical management of acute epidural hematomas. Neurosurgery 2006; 58(3, Suppl):S7–S15; discussion Si-Siv.

■ Prognosis

The IMPACT study of 8686 TBI patients assessed Glasgow Outcome Score at 6 months and found GCS motor score, pupillary response, Marshall CT class, and traumatic SAH to be the strongest independent predictors of outcome. Other important predictors of outcome include age, hypotension, hypoxia, eye and verbal components of GCS, glucose level, platelet count and hemoglobin level.[9] Mortality for EDH is ~10%, whereas the mortality rate for SDH ranges from 40 to 60%. Hypotension (increases mortality rate up to 2 times) and hypoxia both negatively affect outcome after TBI and should be rigorously avoided.[19] Recovery from TBI can be prolonged, with improvement seen over a year after injury.

Pearls and Pitfalls

- Head CT is critical to diagnosis, management, and prognosis following TBI.
- Managing hypotension, hypoxia, and ICP early are critical to preventing secondary injury. Neuromonitoring techniques may guide ICP and CPP management.
- Assessment for surgical intervention should be rapid and is best performed at centers with experienced personnel.

References

1. Thurman DJ, Alverson C, Dunn KA, Guerrero J, Sniezek JE. Traumatic brain injury in the United States: a public health perspective. J Head Trauma Rehabil 1999;14:602–615
2. Haydel MJ, Preston CA, Mills TJ, Luber S, Blaudeau E, DeBlieux PM. Indications for computed tomography in patients with minor head injury. N Engl J Med 2000;343(2):100–105
3. Stiell IG, Lesiuk H, Wells GA, et al. Canadian CT head rule study for patients with minor head injury: methodology for phase II (validation and economic analysis). Ann Emerg Med 2001;38(3):317–322
4. Marshall LF, Marshall SB, Klauber MR, et al. The diagnosis of head injury requires a classification based on computed axial tomography. J Neurotrauma 1992;9(Suppl 1):S287–S292
5. van Dongen KJ, Braakman R, Gelpke GJ. The prognostic value of computerized tomography in comatose head-injured patients. J Neurosurg 1983;59(6):951–957

6. Oertel M, Boscardin WJ, Obrist WD, et al. Posttraumatic vasospasm: the epidemiology, severity, and time course of an underestimated phenomenon: a prospective study performed in 299 patients. J Neurosurg 2005;103:812–824

7. Bullock MR, Chesnut R, Ghajar J, Gordon D, Hartl R, Newell DW, Servadei F, Walters BC, Wilberger JE., Surgical management of acute epidural hematomas. Neurosurgery 58(3, Suppl):S7-15; discussion Si-iv, 2006

8. Brown CV, Zada G, Salim A, et al. Indications for routine repeat head computed tomography (CT) stratified by severity of traumatic brain injury. J Trauma 2007;62(6):1339–1344; discussion 1344–1335

9. Murray GD, Butcher I, McHugh GS, et al. Multivariable prognostic analysis in traumatic brain injury: results from the IMPACT study. J Neurotrauma 2007;24(2):329–337

10. Narayan RK, Kishore PR, Becker DP, et al. Intracranial pressure: to monitor or not to monitor? A review of our experience with severe head injury. J Neurosurg 1982;56:650–659

11. Cooper DJ, Myles PS, McDermott FT, et al. Prehospital hypertonic saline resuscitation of patients with hypotension and severe traumatic brain injury: a randomized controlled trial. JAMA 2004;291(11):1350–1357

12. Myburgh J, Cooper DJ, Finfer S, et al. Saline or albumin for fluid resuscitation in patients with traumatic brain injury. N Engl J Med 2007;357(9):874–884

13. Temkin NR, Dikmen SS, Wilensky AJ, Keihm J, Chabal S, Winn HR. A randomized, double-blind study of phenytoin for the prevention of post-traumatic seizures. N Engl J Med 1990;323(8):497–502

14. Edwards P, Arango M, Balica L, et al. Final results of MRC CRASH, a randomised placebo-controlled trial of intravenous corticosteroid in adults with head injury-outcomes at 6 months. Lancet 2005;365(9475):1957–1959

15. Bullock MR, Chesnut R, Ghajar J, et al. Surgical management of traumatic parenchymal lesions. Neurosurgery 2006; 58(3, Suppl):S25–S46; discussion Si-iv

16. Bullock MR, Chesnut R, Ghajar J, et al. Surgical management of posterior fossa mass lesions. Neurosurgery 2006; 58(3, Suppl):S47–S55; discussion Si-iv

17. Bullock MR, Chesnut R, Ghajar J, et al. Surgical management of depressed cranial fractures. Neurosurgery 2006; 58(3, Suppl):S56–S60; discussion Si-iv

18. Bullock MR, Chesnut R, Ghajar J, et al. Surgical management of acute subdural hematomas. Neurosurgery 2006; 58(3, Suppl):S16–S24; discussion Si-iv

19. Chesnut RM, Marshall LF, Klauber MR, et al. The role of secondary brain injury in determining outcome from severe head injury. J Trauma 1993;34:216–222

3 Intracerebral Hemorrhage

Stanley Tuhrim

Intracerebral hemorrhage (ICH) occurs in 12 to 31 per 100,000 people each year in the United States, accounting for 10% of all strokes.[1] It has the highest mortality rate among stroke types (30 to 50%).[2] The rate is expected to double in the next 50 years because of the increasing age of the population and the increased use of antithrombotic therapy. ICH is more common among men, the elderly, African Americans and Japanese, and people with low low-density lipoprotein (LDL) cholesterol. Hypertension is the major modifiable risk factor for ICH. Excessive alcohol consumption also markedly increases risk. Although clinical trials of specific interventions have been disappointing, rapid recognition and comprehensive management are essential to limiting mortality and long-term morbidity. Due to a variety of factors, estimates of in-hospital mortality have been halved over the past three decades.

Case Example

A 50-year-old African American woman arrives at the hospital with the abrupt onset of a left hemiparesis and right gaze preference. Initially she is alert but becomes increasingly obtunded. Her blood pressure is 220/110 mm Hg.

Questions

- What was the time of onset? (When was the patient last seen normal?)
- Was there a seizure at onset?
- What were the patient's activities at onset?
- Does the patient have a bleeding disorder?
- Was the patient taking any anticoagulant or antiplatelet medications?
- Is there physical evidence of trauma?

Urgent Orders

- Consider intubation (airway, breathing, circulation [ABCs]).
- Order noncontrast head computed tomography (CT).
- Order routine laboratories, including coagulation studies, platelet count, pregnancy test, toxicology screen.
- Neurosurgical evaluation for evacuation, ventricular drainage, or intracranial pressure (ICP) monitoring.
- If the patient has received anticoagulant or antiplatelet medication, or has abnormal coagulation or platelet studies, order appropriate reversal agents as soon as possible (see Chapter 4).

■ History and Examination

History

- Assess for history of hypertension; check for blood pressure medications and noncompliance.
- Assess for history of cancer, smoking, weight loss, or tobacco use (metastatic disease).
- Assess for history of dementia (amyloid) or trauma. Check for history of vascular abnormalities (aneurysm, arteriovenous malformation [AVM], etc.).
- Alcohol or illicit drug use should be determined, as should use of warfarin, antiplatelet, or antithrombotic therapy.
- Liver disease, renal disease (uremic platelets), and hematologic disease history should be obtained.
- Decreased mental status is more common with ICH than ischemic stroke, and vomiting is more common with ICH than with either subarachnoid hemorrhage (SAH) or ischemic stroke.

Physical Examination

Note blood pressure (BP), evidence of head or other trauma.

Neurologic Examination

- A full neurologic examination, including assessment of mental status, cranial nerves, motor skills, and reflexes, as well as a sensory and cerebellar exam, should be performed on all patients.
- Review clues to localization of an ICH (**Table 3.1**).

Table 3.1 Clues to Localization of an Intracerebral Hemorrhage

Location	Exam Findings
Subcortical white matter or putamen	Aphasia (left) or neglect (right) Contralateral motor or sensory deficits Conjugate gaze palsy, hemianopia
Thalamus	Aphasia (left) or neglect (right) Contralateral sensory ± motor deficits (from involvement of adjacent internal capsule) Wrong-way gaze (away from lesion), downward eye deviation Sectoranopia Small reactive pupils
Brainstem	Coma Quadriparesis Locked-in syndrome at the level of the pontine tegmentum (conscious and quadriparetic with preserved vertical eye movements) Horizontal gaze paresis (pontine hemorrhage) Ocular bobbing (pontine hemorrhage) Pinpoint pupils (pontine hemorrhage) Fixed midposition pupils, hippus (midbrain hemorrhage) Nystagmus Hyperthermia Abnormal breathing patterns
Cerebellum	Limb or truncal ataxia Nystagmus Skew deviation Brainstem signs from mass effect Signs of hydrocephalus and elevated ICP from compression of the fourth ventricle

Abbreviation: ICP, intracranial pressure.

■ Differential Diagnosis

Ischemic stroke, metabolic coma, hypoxic ischemic encephalopathy, and nonconvulsive status epilepticus can all mimic ICH, though the diagnosis is readily determined with CT. Below is a differential diagnosis of ICH by etiology.

1. *Chronic hypertension.* Common locations include basal ganglia (40 to 50%), lobar regions (20 to 50%), thalamus (10 to 15%), pons (5 to 12%), cerebellum (5 to 10%) (dentate nucleus is common for hypertensive ICH and vermis for coagulopathic ICH), and other brainstem sites (1 to 5%).

   • Related to rupture of Charcot-Bouchard microaneurysms, lipohyalinosis, and fibrinoid necrosis affecting penetrating arteries

   • Intraventricular hemorrhage (IVH) occurs in one-third of cases; commonly related to a thalamic or caudate ICH that ruptures into the ventricle

   • Clinical history of hypertension, especially uncontrolled, or eclampsia

   • Assess for left ventricular hypertrophy (LVH) on electrocardiogram (ECG) and hypertensive changes in retina or kidney.

2. *Amyloid angiopathy*

   • Age >60 years old

   • ß-amyloid deposition in small- and medium-sized arteries

   • Apo E2 and E4 alleles are more common with cerebral amyloid angiopathy–related ICH.

   • Lobar location, leukoariosis, multiple posteriorly located gradient echo signals on magnetic resonance imaging (MRI)

   • History of Alzheimer's dementia

   • Multicompartmental bleeds (ICH + subdural hemorrhage SDH or ICH + SAH)

   • Recurrent ICH (recurrence rate up to 10% annually)

3. *Coagulopathy*

- Clinical history, including warfarin use, hemophilia, or other clotting abnormality, liver or renal disease (uremic platelets)

- Warfarin is a risk factor for ICH expansion, with expansion continuing longer than in patients not taking warfarin, and is associated with worse outcomes.

- Multifocal bleeds more common

- Cerebellar vermis location common

4. *Arteriovenous malformation*

- Deep or superficial location

- Flow voids on imaging studies

- History of seizures or headaches

- Absence of clinical history of hypertension or coagulopathy

- Younger age

- Initial bleeding rate is 2 to 4% per year; recurrent bleeding rate is 6 to 18% per year.[3-5]

- Lifetime risk of hemorrhage is 105 minus patient's age (in years).[6]

5. *Cavernous angioma*

- Deep or superficial location

- History of headaches or seizures

- Frequently multiple "popcorn" gradient echo lesions on MRI with varying ages of blood

- Angiographically occult (may see associated developmental venous anomaly)

- Annual bleeding rate is 0.25 to 1.1% in the anterior circulation with a rebleeding rate of 4.5% per year. The annual bleeding rate for posterior fossa cavernous malformations is 2 to 3% with a 17 to 21% rebleeding rate.[7]

- Genetics—*KRIT-1* (*CCM-1*), *CCM-2*, *PDCD-10* mutations

6. *Cocaine, methamphetamine, or sympathomimetic drug use*

7. *Dural sinus thrombosis with hemorrhage*

- Seen in hypercoagulable states, dehydration, Crohn's disease
- Common cause of postpartum period ICH
- Look for signs of elevated ICP; check opening pressure with lumbar puncture.
- Requires full-dose anticoagulation, even with hemorrhage present[8]

8. *Neoplasm*

- Most common primary tumors with hemorrhage—glioblastoma multiforme (GBM), oligodendroglioma, pituitary adenoma
- Most common metastatic tumors with hemorrhage—lung, melanoma, thyroid, renal, choriocarcinoma

9. *Vasculopathy*

- Rupture of small- or medium-sized arteries produces hemorrhage.
- Typically preceded by weeks to months of headache, cognitive decline, psychiatric symptoms, and multiple strokes
- May be associated with systemic illness (polyarteritis nodosa [PAN]; Wegener's granulomatosis; Churg–Strauss syndrome; cryoglobulinemia; systemic lupus erythematosus [SLE]; rheumatoid arthritis; Sjögren's syndrome; tuberculosis [TB]; bacterial, fungal, or viral vasculitis; hepatitis; herpes; selective serotonin reuptake inhibitors [SSRIs]; postpartum; Lyme disease; sarcoidosis; Behçet's disease; syphilis; drug-induced [cocaine and methamphetamines] vasculopathy; sickle cell disease or carcinomatous vasculopathy) or limited to the central nervous system (Call-Fleming syndrome, primary CNS granulomatosis, lymphomatoid granulomatosis, MoyaMoya disease)

10. *Ischemic stroke with hemorrhagic conversion*

- Underlying vascular territory lesion with petechial hemorrhage. Hemorrhagic infarction is typically heterogeneous and conforms to an arterial distribution. Primary ICH is homogeneous and does not necessarily conform to an arterial territory.
- More common with embolic strokes with reperfusion
- Occurs in 6% of patients after intravenous (IV) tissue plasminogen activator (tPA)[9]

11. *Trauma*

- External evidence of trauma
- Multifocal hemorrhages
- Associated SDH, SAH, contusion, skull fracture

Life-Threatening Diagnoses Not to Miss

- *Coagulopathy-induced ICH* because rapid factor correction can limit ICH expansion
- *Surgical lesions or associated IVH requiring ventricular drainage*

■ Diagnostic Evaluation

- *Imaging studies*
  - CT: Assess volume by A*B*C/2 method,[10] assess location (deep, superficial, cerebellar, IVH), presence of hydrocephalus, midline shift (measured from septum pellucidum), or evidence of trauma (contusion, SAH); assess for AVM or underlying mass. CT scan remains the initial study of choice to distinguish infarction from ICH. Thirty-eight percent of patients will have a 33% increase in ICH size within 3 hours (two-thirds of cases will have expansion within 1 hour).[11] Increase in ICH volume is associated with early neurologic deterioration.[12] CT angiography may be useful for identifying an aneurysm or vascular malformation.
  - MRI is at least as sensitive for diagnosing ICH but more difficult to interpret because the appearance of ICH changes as blood products age.[13] MRI (with contrast) is superior to CT for detecting underlying structural lesions (tumors, cavernous malformations, ischemic stroke), delineating edema, and identifying venous thrombosis (MR venography). MRI may not be feasible due to impaired consciousness, hemodynamic instability, pacemaker, or agitation. MRI with gadolinium should be considered in patients with a history of cancer or risk factors for cancer, no history of hypertension, or suspicious ICH location (i.e., lobar at the gray–white junction) (**Table 3.2**).

Table 3.2 Appearance of Blood of Different Ages on Magnetic Resonance Imaging

Phase	Time	T1	T2	Hemoglobin
Hyperacute	<24 h	Gray/black	White	Oxyhemoglobin (intracellular)
Acute	1–3 d	Gray/black	Black	Deoxyhemoglobin (intracellular)
Early subacute	3–7 d	White	Black	Methemoglobin (intracellular)
Late subacute	7–14 d	White	White	Methemoglobin (extracellular)
Chronic	>14 d	Black/gray	Black	Hemosiderin (extracellular)

- ◦ Angiography is indicated for ICH with SAH, vascular abnormalities, isolated IVH, abnormal calcifications, and blood in unusual locations (i.e., sylvian fissure). Angiographic yield depends on the patient's age, location of hemorrhage, and history of hypertension. Patients with SAH, patients age <45, patients with lobar hemorrhage, and nonhypertensive patients should be considered for angiography (**Table 3.3**).[14]

Table 3.3 Angiographic Yield for an Etiologic Abnormality

| | Angiographic Yield % | | |
	Lobar Location	Deep Location	Isolated IVH
≤45 years old; history of HTN	NA	0	67
≤45 years old; no history of HTN	65	48	67
>45 years old; history of HTN	10	0	63
>45 years old; no history of HTN	NA	7	63

Abbreviations: HTN, hypertension; IVH, intraventricular hemorrhage; NA, not available.

Data from: Zhu XL, Chan MS, Poon WS. Spontaneous intracranial hemorrhage: which patients need diagnostic cerebral angiography? A prospective study of 206 cases and review of the literature. Stroke 1997;28(7):1406–1409.

- *ICP monitoring* may be helpful in patients with decreased level of consciousness or IVH (particularly IVH in the third or fourth ventricle).

- *Continuous blood pressure and cardiac rhythm* monitoring should be performed at least for the initial 24 hours because of the high rate of cardiovascular instability.

- *Laboratory studies.* Review prothrombin time/partial thromboplastin time/international normalized ratio (PT/PTT/INR), complete blood count (CBC), type and hold, troponin, chemistry panel, magnesium, liver function test, D-dimer test, fibrinogen, and toxicology screen.

■ Treatment

Medical Treatment

- See 2007 AHA/ASA guidelines in **Table 3.4**.

Table 3.4 2007 AHA/ASA Guidelines for the Management of Spontaneous Intracerebral Hemorrhage in Adults

Category	Guidelines
Class I Level A	ICH is a medical emergency with early bleeding, deterioration, and high morbidity and mortality, and should be promptly recognized and diagnosed.
Class I Level A	CT and MRI are each first-choice initial imaging modalities. In patients with contraindications to MRI, CT should be performed.
Class I Level B	Monitoring and management of ICH should take place in an ICU setting.
Class I Level B	Appropriate antiepileptic medications should be used for treatment of clinical seizures in patients with ICH.
Class I Level C	Sources of fever should be treated, and antipyretic medications should be administered to lower temperature.
Class I Level C	Early mobilization and rehabilitation are recommended.
Class I Level B	Patients with acute ICH and hemiparesis/hemiplegia should have intermittent pneumatic compression for VTE prevention.

(Continued)

Table 3.4 2007 AHA/ASA Guidelines for the Management of Spontaneous Intracerebral Hemorrhage in Adults *(continued)*

Category	Guidelines
Class I Level B	Treatment of HTN for long-term therapy is indicated because this decreases the risk of recurrent ICH.
Class IIa Level B	Treat ICP in a graded fashion, beginning with simple measures such as elevation of head of bed, analgesia, and sedation. More aggressive therapies such as osmotic agents (mannitol and hypertonic saline), CSF drainage, neuromuscular blockade, or hyperventilation generally require concomitant ICP and blood pressure monitoring to maintain a CPP goal >70 mm Hg.
Class IIa Level C	Persistent hyperglycemia (>140–185 mg/dL) during the first 24 h is associated with poor outcomes and should be treated.
Class IIb Level B	Treatment with rFVIIa within the first 3–4 h after onset has shown promise, but efficacy and safety have not been shown in phase III trials.
Class IIb Level C	A brief period of prophylactic antiepileptic therapy soon after ICH onset may reduce the risk of early seizures in patients with lobar ICH.
Class IIb Level B	After cessation of bleeding, low-dose subcutaneous LMWH or UFH may be considered in patients with hemiplegia after 3–4 days from onset.
Class IIb Level C	Patients with clinical or subclinical PE or with acute proximal VTE should be considered for acute IVC filter.
Class IIb Level C	The decision for long-term antithrombotic therapy several weeks or more after placement of an IVC filter should take into consideration the likely cause of ICH (amyloid—higher risk of rebleed compared with hypertensive ICH), associated conditions with increased arterial thrombotic risk (atrial fibrillation), and the overall health and mobility of the patient.
Class I Level B	Patients with cerebellar ICH >3 cm who are deteriorating neurologically or have brainstem compression and/or hydrocephalus from ventricular obstruction should have surgical removal as soon as possible.
Class IIb Level B	Stereotactic infusion of urokinase into clot cavity within 72 h reduces clot burden and risk of death, but functional outcome is not improved.
Class IIb Level B	Minimally invasive clot evacuation utilizing a variety of mechanical devices and/or endoscopy awaits further testing.

(Continued on next page)

Table 3.4 2007 AHA/ASA Guidelines for the Management of Spontaneous Intracerebral Hemorrhage in Adults *(continued)*

Category	Guidelines
Class IIb Level B	Patients with supratentorial lobar clots within 1 cm of the cortical surface may be considered for evacuation.
Class IIb Level B	Ultra-early craniotomy is not proven to improve functional outcome or mortality. Operative removal within 12 h, particularly when performed by less invasive methods, has the most evidence. Very early craniotomy may be associated with an increased risk of recurrent bleeding.
Class IIb Level C	Too few data currently exist to comment on the potential of decompressive craniectomy to improve outcome after ICH.
Class III Level A	Routine evacuation of supratentorial ICH by standard craniotomy within 96 h is not recommended (except lobar ICH within 1 cm of surface).
Class III Level A	Delayed evacuation by craniotomy offers little benefit. In patients with coma and deep ICH, removal by craniotomy may worsen outcomes and is not recommended.

Abbreviations: AHA, American Heart Association; ASA, American Stroke Association; CPP, cerebral perfusion pressure; CSF, cerebral spinal fluid; CT, computed tomography; HTN, hypertension; ICH, intracerebral hemorrhage; ICP, intracranial pressure; ICU, intensive care unit; IVC ; inferior vena cava; IVH, intraventricular hemorrhage; LMWH, low molecular weight heparin; MRI, magnetic resonance imaging; PE, pulmonary embolism; rFVIIa, recombinant factor VII a; UFH, unfractionated heparin; VTE, venous thromboembolism.

Data from: Broderick J, Connolly S, Feldmann E, et al. Guidelines for the management of spontaneous intracerebral hemorrhage in adults: 2007 update: a guideline from the American Heart Association/American Stroke Association Stroke Council, High Blood Pressure Research Council, and the Quality of Care and Outcomes in Research Interdisciplinary Working Group. Stroke 2007;38(6):2001–2023.

- *Blood pressure control.*[15] PET (positron emission tomography) studies have shown that autoregulation is likely intact in the penumbra surrounding the ICH (**Table 3.5, Table 3.6**).
- *ICP management.* Comatose (noncommand following) patients and patients with intraventricular hemorrhage should be considered for ICP monitoring (see Chapter 15).
- *Glucose management.* Hyperglycemia predicts mortality after ICH, and efforts to control glucose early are crucial (see Chapter 19).

Table 3.5 2007 AHA/ASA Recommendations for Blood Pressure Control

Blood Pressure	Suggested Management
SBP > 200 mm Hg or MAP > 150 mm Hg	Aggressive reduction of BP with cIV infusion, monitoring BP every 5 min
SBP > 180 mm Hg or MAP > 130 mm Hg and evidence of elevated ICP	Consider ICP monitoring Reduce BP using intermittent or cIV medications targeting CPP >60–80 mm Hg
SBP > 180 mm Hg or MAP > 130 mm Hg no evidence of elevated ICP	Reduce BP with intermittent or cIV medications targeting BP 160/90 mm Hg or MAP 110 mm Hg, monitoring BP every 15 min

Abbreviations: AHA, American Heart Association; ASA, American Stroke Association; BP, blood pressure; cIV, continuous intravenous; CPP, cerebral perfusion pressure; ICP, intracranial pressure; MAP, mean arterial pressure; SBP, systolic blood pressure.

Data from: Broderick J, et al. Guidelines for the management of spontaneous intracerebral hemorrhage in adults: 2007 update: a guideline from the American Heart Association/American Stroke Association Stroke Council, High Blood Pressure Research Council, and the Quality of Care and Outcomes in Research Interdisciplinary Working Group. Stroke 2007;38(6):2001–2023.

Table 3.6 Suggested Medications for Blood Pressure Control

Drug	Intravenous Bolus Dose	Continuous Infusion Rate
Labetalol	5–20 mg every 15 min	2 mg/min (max 300 mg/d)
Nicardipine	NA	5–15 mg/h
Esmolol	250 µg/kg IVP loading dose	25–300 µg/kg/min
Enalapril	1.35–5 mg IVP every 6 h	NA
Hydralazine	5–20 mg IVP every 30 min	1.5–5 µg/kg/min
Nitroprusside*	NA	0.1–10 µg/kg/min
Nitroglycerin	NA	20–400 µg/min

*Not recommended—can raise intracranial pressure, cyanide toxicity.

Abbreviations: IVP, intraventricular pressure; NA, not applicable.

Data from: Broderick J, et al. Guidelines for the management of spontaneous intracerebral hemorrhage in adults: 2007 update: a guideline from the American Heart Association/American Stroke Association Stroke Council, High Blood Pressure Research Council, and the Quality of Care and Outcomes in Research Interdisciplinary Working Group. Stroke 2007;38(6):2001–2023.

- *Recombinant factor VIIa.* In a phase IIb trial,[16] rFVIIa administered within 4 hours of ictus limited ICH expansion and improved outcomes compared with placebo; however, these results were not supported by a larger phase III trial.[17] Recombinant factor VIIa is not currently recommended for early ICH treatment.

- *Antiepileptic drugs.* Up to 28% of patients with ICH have seizures, which are often nonconvulsive. Seven days of prophylactic antiepileptics may be reasonable for patients with ICH (particularly lobar ICH, noncommand following patients and patients with evidence of elevated ICP). All patients with seizures should receive antiepileptics. There should be a low threshold for continuous electroencephalogram (EEG) monitoring in comatose ICH patients.

- *Temperature management.* Fever worsens outcome after ICH and should be aggressively treated.

Surgical Treatment

The STICH trial[18] randomized 1033 patients with supratentorial ICH to craniotomy or medical management within 96 hours.[18] Clinical equipoise was necessary prior to randomization, and 26% of patients crossed over from the medical arm to the surgical arm. On intention to treat analysis, there was no difference in 6-month outcomes including death, modified Rankin Scale, and Barthel Index. Subgroup analysis found a trend toward benefit in patients with a Glasgow Coma Scale (GCS) of 9 to 12, lobar clots, and clots <1 cm from the surface. Patients with GCS 5 to 8 did better with medical management.

◼ Prognosis

Mortality rates vary by location of ICH: 57% for lobar ICH, 51% for deep ICH, 42% for cerebellar, and 65% for brainstem ICH.[15] The overall prognosis depends on the patient's age, hematoma size, level of consciousness, the location of the ICH, and general medical health. A simple grading scale, the ICH Score, is a useful tool for stratifying patients at presentation (**Table 3.7**).[19] Recurrence rates for ICH depend on the initial etiology of ICH: 2%/year for hypertensive ICH, 10%/year for amyloid angiopathy, 6 to 18%/year for arteriovenous malformation (AVM), 4.5%/year for cavernous angioma, and 0.15%/year for developmental venous anomaly.[20]

Table 3.7 The ICH Score

	ICH Points		ICH Points
GCS Score		Infratentorial location	
3–4	2	Yes	1
5–12	1	No	0
13–15	0	Age	
ICH volume		≥80 years old	1
≥30 cm^3	1	<80 years old	0
<30 cm^3	0	Total score	
IVH			
Yes	1		
No	0		

Note: Total score = % mortality: 0 = 0%; 1 = 13%; 2 = 26%; 3 = 72%; 4 = 97%; 5 = 100%.

Abbreviations: GCS, Glasgow Coma Score; ICH, intracerebral hemorrhage; IVH, intravetricular hemorrhage.

Data from: Hemphill JC III, et al. The ICH score: a simple, reliable grading scale for intracerebral hemorrhage. Stroke 2001;32(4):891–897.

Pearls and Pitfalls

- Evaluate early for possible surgical intervention (cerebellar or lobar ICH) or ventricular drainage (IVH).
- Reverse coagulopathy as soon as possible (see Chapter 4).
- Consider angiography in young patients, those without a history of HTN, lobar ICH, or isolated IVH.
- Consider MRI with gadolinium in patients with lobar hemorrhages to look for underlying tumor or vascular abnormality.

References

1. Gebel JM, Broderick JP. Intracerebral hemorrhage. Neurol Clin 2000; 18(2):419–438
2. Flaherty ML, et al. Long-term mortality after intracerebral hemorrhage. Neurology 2006;66(8):1182–1186

3. Mast H, et al. Risk of spontaneous haemorrhage after diagnosis of cerebral arteriovenous malformation. Lancet 1997;350(9084):1065–1068

4. Stapf C, et al. Predictors of hemorrhage in patients with untreated brain arteriovenous malformation. Neurology 2006;66(9):1350–1355

5. Yamada S, et al. Risk factors for subsequent hemorrhage in patients with cerebral arteriovenous malformations. J Neurosurg 2007;107(5):965–972

6. Brown RD Jr. Simple risk predictions for arteriovenous malformation hemorrhage. Neurosurgery 2000;46(4):1024

7. Fritschi JA, Reulen HJ, Spetzler RF, Zabramski JM. Cavernous malformations of the brain stem: a review of 139 cases. Acta Neurochir (Wien) 1994;130(1–4):35–46

8. Sacco RL, Adams R, Albers G, et al. Guidelines for prevention of stroke in patients with ischemic stroke or transient ischemic attack: a statement for healthcare professionals from the American Heart Association/American Stroke Association Council on Stroke: co-sponsored by the Council on Cardiovascular Radiology and Intervention: the American Academy of Neurology affirms the value of this guideline. Stroke 2006;37(2):577–617

9. Tissue plasminogen activator for acute ischemic stroke: the National Institute of Neurological Disorders and Stroke rt-PA Stroke Study Group. N Engl J Med 1995;333(24):1581–1587

10. Gebel JM, et al. Comparison of the ABC/2 estimation technique to computer-assisted volumetric analysis of intraparenchymal and subdural hematomas complicating the GUSTO-1 trial. Stroke 1998;29(9):1799–1801

11. Brott T, et al. Early hemorrhage growth in patients with intracerebral hemorrhage. Stroke 1997;28(1):1–5

12. Brott T, Broderick J, Kothari R, et al. Early hemorrhage growth in patients with intracerebral hemorrhage. Stroke 1997;28(1):1–5

13. Kidwell CS, et al. Comparison of MRI and CT for detection of acute intracerebral hemorrhage. JAMA 2004;292(15):1823–1830

14. Zhu XL, Chan MS, Poon WS. Spontaneous intracranial hemorrhage: which patients need diagnostic cerebral angiography? A prospective study of 206 cases and review of the literature. Stroke 1997;28(7):1406–1409

15. Broderick J, Connolly S, Feldmann E, et al. Guidelines for the management of spontaneous intracerebral hemorrhage in adults: 2007 update: a guideline from the American Heart Association/American Stroke Association Stroke Council, High Blood Pressure Research Council, and the Quality of Care and Outcomes in Research Interdisciplinary Working Group. Stroke 2007;38(6):2001–2023

16. Mayer SA, Brun NC, Begtrup K, et al. Recombinant activated factor VII for acute intracerebral hemorrhage. N Engl J Med 2005;352(8):777–785

17. Mayer SA, Brun NC, Begtrup K, et al. Efficacy and safety of recombinant activated factor VII for acute intracerebral hemorrhage. N Engl J Med 2008;358(20):2127–2137

18. Mendelow AD, Gregson BA, Fernandes HM, et al. Early surgery versus initial conservative treatment in patients with spontaneous supratentorial intracerebral haematomas in the International Surgical Trial in Intracerebral Haemorrhage (STICH): a randomised trial. Lancet 2005;365(9457):387–397

19. Hemphill JC III, Bonovich DC, Besmertis L, Manley GT, Johnston SC. The ICH score: a simple, reliable grading scale for intracerebral hemorrhage. Stroke 2001;32(4):891–897

20. Qureshi AI, Tuhrim S, Broderick JP, Batjer HH, Hondo H, Hanley DF. Spontaneous intracerebral hemorrhage. N Engl J Med 2001;344(19):1450–1460

21. Broderick J, et al. Guidelines for the management of spontaneous intracerebral hemorrhage in adults: 2007 update: a guideline from the American Heart Association/American Stroke Association Stroke Council, High Blood Pressure Research Council, and the Quality of Care and Outcomes in Research Interdisciplinary Working Group. Stroke 2007;38(6):2001–2023

22. Hemphill JC III, et al. The ICH score: a simple, reliable grading scale for intracerebral hemorrhage. Stroke 2001;32(4):891–897

4 Antiplatelet- and Anticoagulation-Associated Intracranial Hemorrhage

Fred Rincon, Andres Fernandez,
and Stephan A. Mayer

Antiplatelet- and anticoagulation-associated intracranial hemorrhages are a neurologic emergency. As the population ages, anticoagulation-associated intracranial hemorrhage is expected to increase in frequency.

Case Example

A 39-year-old right-handed Hispanic man with a history of recent mechanical aortic valve replacement (AVR) was admitted to the hospital for an evaluation of his chest wound infection. The day after admission his mental status worsened, and the physical examination revealed a new right hemiparesis with left-gaze deviation.

Questions

- What was the time of onset? (When was the patient last seen normal?)
- Is the patient on antiplatelet or anticoagulant medications?
- If the patient is having an ischemic stroke, should we administer intravenous (IV) tissue plasminogen activator (tPA) or consider any other intervention?
- In case of coagulopathic ICH, when can we restart anticoagulation in this patient with a mechanical aortic valve?

Urgent Orders

- Assess for intubation (airway, breathing, circulation [ABCs]).
- Perform head computed tomography (CT) without contrast.
- Check coagulation and platelet profiles.
- Order appropriate reversal agents as soon as possible if the patient has received anticoagulant or antiplatelet medication, or has abnormal coagulation or platelet studies.

■ History and Examination

History

- Assess antiplatelet use (aspirin, clopidogrel, dipyridamole, ketorolac, ticlopidine, GPIIb/IIIa medications), anticoagulation medications (low molecular weight heparin, unfractionated heparin, direct thrombin inhibitors, or warfarin), as well as when each medication was last administered.

- Assess for previous stroke, baseline functional status, history of hypertension (HTN), dementia, liver disease, or renal failure.

- Check for history of tobacco, cocaine, amphetamine, and over-the-counter drug use.

- Assess for dysfunctional platelets (renal disease) or intrinsic coagulopathy (hemophilia, von Willebrand disease).

Physical Examination

Note blood pressure (BP); fever should be aggressively treated.

Neurologic Examination

- A full neurologic examination, including assessment of mental status, cranial nerves, motor skills, and reflexes, as well as a sensory and cerebellar exam, should be performed on all patients.

- Decreased mental status is more common with ICH than ischemic stroke, and vomiting is more common with ICH than with either subarachnoid hemorrhage (SAH) or ischemic stroke (see Chapter 3).

■ Differential Diagnosis

1. *Intracranial hemorrhage (intracerebral hemorrhage [ICH], subarachnoid hemorrhage [SAH], subdural hematoma [SDH], or epidural hematoma [EDH]).* Although SAH is often accompanied by "the worst headache in my life" and SDH/EDH by history of head trauma, they may occur spontaneously, especially in the setting of coagulopathy. A growing source of ICH is vitamin K inhibitor use, which accounts for ~10 to 15% of ICH.[1] Coagulopathic bleeds are often multifocal. Common sites include the cerebellar vermis and hemorrhage into previously ischemic tissue. Patients with warfarin-

or antiplatelet-associated ICH have increased mortality and increased risk of ICH expansion compared with noncoagulopathic ICH.

- *Long-term anticoagulation* may increase the risk of ICH by 10-fold, and the annual rate of ICH for patients on warfarin is ~1%.[2] The main risk factors for warfarin-associated ICH include age, hypertension, intensity of anticoagulation, concomitant aspirin use, cerebral amyloid angiopathy, and leukoaraiosis.[3] The risk of ICH increases with international normalized ratio (INR) values over 3.5 to 4.5 and nearly doubles for each increase of 0.5 point over 4.5.[1] Despite this increased risk with increasing INR, most anticoagulation-associated bleeds occur with an INR in the recommended therapeutic range.

- *Antiplatelet agent use* has a risk of symptomatic bleeding complications, but there is meager evidence implicating the use of a single antiplatelet agent as a risk factor for ICH.[4,5] However, the combination of antiplatelet agents such as aspirin (ASA) and ADP-receptor blockers such as clopidogrel carries a higher incidence of ICH. Other antiplatelet agents such as the glycoprotein receptor blocking agents (GPIIb/IIIa) produce hematologic abnormalities that may put the patient at risk of bleeding as well.

2. *Ischemic stroke.* In patients with a history of a cardiac disease (recent open heart surgery and mechanic AVR) or atrial fibrillation (AF), ischemic stroke is a plausible diagnosis. The etiology of ischemic stroke in these settings is usually embolic (thrombus or septic emboli). Hemorrhage into an area of ischemic infarction occurs when vessel walls are damaged by ischemia, and blood then extravasates into the brain parenchyma. The transformation requires sufficient time for an ischemic lesion to develop and then partial or total reperfusion with restoration of blood flow through the vessel or by collateralization. Large infarct size, older age, hyperglycemia, sustained hypertension, thromboembolic mechanism (as opposed to penetrator occlusion), and preexisting microhemorrhages on magnetic resonance imaging (MRI) have been identified as risk factors for hemorrhagic conversion of an infarct. Small asymptomatic petechiae are less important than frank hematomas, which may be associated with neurologic decline. In general, spontaneous hemorrhagic conversion after ischemic stroke occurs in 0.6 to 5% of patients admitted to the hospital. Management of spontaneous hemorrhagic transformations depends on the amount of blood and clinical symptoms. According to the Euro-

Table 4.1 Hemorrhagic Conversion of an Infarct

HI 1	Small petechial hemorrhage
HI 2	Confluent petechial hemorrhage
PH 1	Hematoma in <30% of the infarcted area with minimal mass effect
PH 2	Hematoma in >30% of the infarcted area with significant space occupying effect

Abbreviations: HI, hemorrhagic infarct; PH, parenchymal hematoma.

Data from: Molina CA, Alvarez-Sabin J, Montaner J, et al. Thrombolysis-related hemorrhagic infarction: a marker of early reperfusion, reduced infarct size, and improved outcome in patients with proximal middle cerebral artery occlusion. Stroke 2002;33(6):1551–1556.

pean Cooperative Acute Stroke Study (ECASS) criteria, hemorrhagic conversion of an infarct is graded as seen in **Table 4.1**.[6] Patients exposed to recombinant tissue plasminogen activating factor (rtPA) for ischemic stroke or myocardial infarction have a risk of symptomatic ICH of 6 to 7% and 0.2 to 1.4%, respectively. ICH following fibrinolysis has a 30-day mortality rate of 60%.[2]

- *Seizures.* New onset seizures with focal neurologic deficits (Todd's paralysis) may be considered as part of the differential diagnosis. It is important to mention that seizures may accompany some stroke types, especially hemorrhagic ones.

Life-Threatening Diagnoses Not to Miss

- Coagulopathy associated hemorrhage as urgent reversal can improve outcome.
- Ischemic stroke that may qualify for thrombolysis (see Chapter 6).

◼ Diagnostic Evaluation

- *Laboratory studies.* Review prothrombin time/partial thromboplastin time/international normalized ratio (PT/PTT/INR), complete blood count (CBC), type and hold, troponin, chemistry panel, magnesium, calcium, phosphorus, and liver function test for all patients. In selected patients check D-dimer, fibrinogen, toxicology screen, and bleeding time.

- *Imaging studies.* Order head CT without contrast, consider CT angiogram, MRI, MR angiogram (see Chapter 3).
- *ICP monitoring* may be helpful in patients with decreased level of consciousness or IVH.
- *Continuous blood pressure and cardiac rhythm monitoring* should be performed at least for the initial 24 hours because of the high rate of cardiovascular instability.

■ Treatment

Reversal Suggestions[7] (Table 4.2)

Table 4.2 Reversal of Coagulopathy

Coagulopathy	Reversal Agent	Timing	Comments
Warfarin	Vitamin K 10 mg IV over 10 min (monitor for hypotension/anaphylaxis) *and* 50 units/kg IV of PCC (also known as factor IX concentrates, Bebulin or Profilnine: contains factors II, VII, IX, and X in varying amounts). If PCC is unavailable, give 15 cc/kg of FFP IV.	ASAP Fast reversal is linked to less rebleeding and better outcome. Vitamin K requires 6–24 h for full reversal effect. Half-life of PCC 6–12 h	Warfarin is an inhibitor of vitamin K–dependent coagulation factors II, VII, IX, and X (as well as Protein C and S) at the hepatic level. Patients with a history of recent warfarin use, regardless of INR or PT, should have urgent reversal. PCC does not require thawing and can reverse coagulopathy more quickly and with less volume than FFP. PCC or FFP should be used with caution in patients with recent thrombotic events or DIC.
Warfarin and emergency neurosurgical intervention	*Above plus:* Consider recombinant factor VIIa 20–80 µg/kg IV	ASAP Half-life 2.6 h May require repeat doses	Contraindicated in acute thromboembolic disease Thromboembolic complications in 7% (primarily arterial)

(Continued)

Table 4.2 Reversal of Coagulopathy *(continued)*

Coagulopathy	Reversal Agent	Timing	Comments
Liver failure	Vitamin K 10 mg IV over 10 min (monitor for hypotension/ anaphylaxis) *and* 50 IU/kg of PCC. If INR ≥2.0, give an additional 15 ml/kg of FFP. If PCC is unavailable, give 15 cc/kg of FFP total.	ASAP	For patients with known coagulopathy or elevated PT or INR ≥1.5
Unfractionated heparin	Stop infusion, no further action for minor bleeding. For severe or intracranial bleeding, use protamine. Dosage of protamine based on time from last heparin dose. Protamine maximum dose 50 mg, max infusion rate 5 mg/min	Half-life of heparin is 2 h. 0–30 minutes; 1.0 mg protamine IV per 100 units heparin. 31–60 min; 0.75 mg protamine IV per 100 units heparin. 61–120 min; 0.5 mg protamine IV per 100 units heparin. >2 h; 0.4 mg protamine IV per 100 units heparin	Heparin produces an anticoagulant effect by attaching to and upregulating the activity of the plasma protein antithrombin-III (AT-III). The AT-III-heparin complex rapidly interacts with circulating thrombin, inhibiting several other circulating coagulation proteases. Monitor for anaphylaxis/ hypotension/bradycardia/flushing with protamine.
Low molecular weight heparin	1 mg protamine IV per 1 mg of LMWH given in last 8 h; if bleeding continues, give an additional 0.5 mg protamine IV per 1 mg of LMWH in last 8 h.	No protamine if >8 h from dose	The mechanism of action of LMWH involves inhibition of activated factor X (Xa) during clot formation. Effect may last for up to 4–12 h for single dose of LMWH. Suggestions for reversal apply to enoxaparin, and timing may vary based on type of LWMH. Protamine reverses only 60–75% of the effect of enoxaparin. Protamine has minimal efficacy against danaparoid or fondaparinux.

(Continued on next page)

Table 4.2 Reversal of Coagulopathy *(continued)*

Coagulopathy	Reversal Agent	Timing	Comments
Direct thrombin inhibitor	No direct reversal agent. Reduce plasma concentration with hemodialysis or modified ultrafiltration. Increase other factors with rFVIIa or PCC/FFP.	Argatroban half-life 39–51 min Lepirudin half-life 1.3 h Bivalirudin half-life 25 min	Agents directly inhibit plasma thrombin.
Aspirin, NSAID, or platelet aggregation inhibitors (clopiogrel/ ticlopidine)	DDAVP 0.3 µg/kg IV x 1 (20 µg in 50 mL NS over 15–30 min) *and* transfuse 5–6 units platelets	ASAP For any antiplatelet use in the last 7 d	ASA and NSAIDs irreversibly block platelet cyclooxygenase, inhibiting production of thromboxane A2, resulting in inhibition of platelet aggregation for up to 7–10 d. Clopidogrel and ticlopidine alter platelet aggregability by irreversibly inhibiting the surface ADP binding site and by reducing ADP release from activated platelets.
GPIIb/IIIa inhibitors	D/C medication DDAVP 0.3 µg/kg IV x 1 (20 µg in 50 mL NS over 15–30 min) *and* transfuse 5–6 units platelets	ASAP Abciximab half-life 30 min Eptifibatide half-life 2.5 h Tirofiban half-life 2 h	Reversibly bind to the GPIIb/IIIa receptor, inhibiting platelet aggregation
Uremic platelets	DDAVP 0.3 µg/kg IV x 1 (20 µg in 50 mL NS over 15–30 min) *and* 6 units of cryoprecipitate or FFP for clinical deterioration	ASAP	Generally for patients on renal replacement therapy, but can be considered in any patient with elevated creatinine
Thrombocytopenia	Transfuse platelets for platelet count <50,000 in ICH	ASAP	Threshold for platelet transfusion widely debated

(Continued)

Table 4.2 Reversal of Coagulopathy *(continued)*

Coagulopathy	Reversal Agent	Timing	Comments
Thrombolytic-induced coagulo-pathy	Stop medication 12 units of cryoprecipitate (to replace fibrinogen and factor VIII) 6–8 units of platelets	ASAP	Anticoagulation effect by directly increasing fibri-nolytic activity Draw PT/PTT/platelet count and fibrino-gen Obtain STAT noncon-trast head CT
Hemophilia without inhibitor	Factor 8: Adults—40 units/kg, then 20 units/kg every 12 h Children—50 units/kg, then 25 units/kg every 12 h Factor 9: Adults—80 units/kg then 40 units/kg every 24 h Children—100 units/kg then 50 units/kg every 24 h	ASAP	Consult hematology
Hemophilia with inhibitor	Factor 8 Inhibitor bypassing activity (FEIBA) give 75 units/kg IV every 12 h If ICH worsens, give recombinant factor VIIa 90 units/kg IV every 2 h	ASAP	Consult hematology

Abbreviations: ASA, aspirin; ASAP, as soon as possible; CT, computed tomography; DDAVP, desmopressin acetate; DIC, disseminated intravascular coagulation; FFP, fresh frozen plasma; ICH, intracranial hemorrhage; INR, international normalized ratio; IV, in-travenous; LMWH, low molecular weight heparin; NS, normal saline; NSAIDs, nons-teroidal antiinflammatory drugs; PCC, prothrombin complex concentrate; PT, prothrombin time; STAT, immediately.

Timing of Reinstitution of Anticoagulation

Patients with ICH receiving long-term anticoagulation for atrial fibrillation (AF) or mechanical valve replacement present a challenging therapeutic scenario, as normalization of INR increases the risk of embolic stroke. The risk of embolization is increased with mitral valve prostheses, caged-ball valves, and multiple prosthetic valves. Nonetheless, in the context of intracranial hemorrhage, these patients should all be acutely reversed. In all of these patients, there is a compelling argument to resume anticoagulation fairly soon after stabilization of a central nervous system (CNS) bleed. Eckman et al[8] developed a decision model for reinstituting anticoagulation after ICH in patients with atrial fibrillation. For patients with prior lobar ICH suggestive of amyloid angiopathy, withholding anticoagulation therapy indefinitely was the most beneficial strategy for improving quality-adjusted life expectancy. In sensitivity analyses for patients with deep ICH and atrial fibrillation, anticoagulation could be considered if the risk of thromboembolic stroke is particularly high (>7%/year).[8] A recent retrospective review investigated the risk of thromboembolism after withholding or reversing the effect of warfarin therapy following a major hemorrhage in patients with prosthetic heart valves. In total, 27 patients were included, two patients suffered ICH. The mean time of warfarin withholding was 15 ± 4 days, and none of these patients had thromboembolic events during this period.[9] When warfarin is restarted after a major ICH, it can usually safely be started between 7 and 10 days after onset (**Table 4.3**).

Table 4.3 2007 AHA/ASA Guidelines for the Management of Spontaneous Intracerebral Hemorrhage in Adults

Category	Guidelines
Class I Level B	Protamine sulfate should be used to reverse heparin-associated ICH, with dosing depending on the time from cessation of heparin.
Class I Level B	Patients with warfarin-associated ICH should be treated with intravenous vitamin K.
Class IIb Level B	Prothrombin complex concentrates, factor IX complex concentrates, and rFVIIa normalize INR rapidly with less volume than FFP, but with greater potential of thromboembolism. FFP is another potential choice, but it is associated with greater volumes and much longer infusion times.

(Continued)

Table 4.3 2007 AHA/ASA Guidelines for the Management of Spontaneous Intracerebral Hemorrhage in Adults *(continued)*

Category	Guidelines
Class IIb Level B	The decision to restart antithrombotic therapy after ICH related to antithrombotic therapy depends on the risk of subsequent arterial or venous thromboembolism, the risk of recurrent ICH, and the overall state of the patient. For patients with a comparatively lower risk of cerebral infarction and a higher risk of amyloid angiopathy or with very poor overall neurologic function, an antiplatelet agent may be an overall better choice for prevention of ischemic stroke. In patients with a very high risk of thromboembolism in whom restarting warfarin is considered, warfarin therapy may be restarted at 7–10 days after onset of the original ICH.
Class IIb Level B	Treatment of patients with ICH related to thrombolytic therapy includes urgent empirical therapies to replace clotting factors and platelets.

Abbreviations: AHA, American Heart Association; ASA, American Stroke Association; FFP, fresh frozen plasma; ICH, intracerebral hemorrhage; INR, international normalized ratio; rFVIIa, recombinant factor VIIa.

Data from: Broderick J, Connolly S, Feldmann E, et al. Guidelines for the management of spontaneous intracerebral hemorrhage in adults: 2007 update: a guideline from the American Heart Association/American Stroke Association Stroke Council, High Blood Pressure Research Council, and the Quality of Care and Outcomes in Research Interdisciplinary Working Group. Stroke 2007;38(6):2001–2023.

■ Prognosis

Among ICH patients, warfarin doubles the risk of death and increases the risk of progressive bleeding and clinical deterioration. Failure to rapidly normalize the INR to below 1.4 further increases these risks.[10]

Pearls and Pitfalls

- Recognition of the type of stroke (ICH, SAH, SDH, or hemorrhagic conversion of ischemic stroke) in the context of coagulopathy is of utmost importance, as this will dictate further management.
- Failure to rapidly normalize the INR to below 1.4 in patients with coagulopathic ICH increases the risk of complications and death.

References

1. The Stroke Prevention in Reversible Ischemia Trial (SPIRIT) Study Group. A randomized trial of anticoagulants versus aspirin after cerebral ischemia of presumed arterial origin. Ann Neurol 1997;42(6):857–865

2. Cavallini A, Fanucchi S, Persico A. Warfarin-associated intracerebral hemorrhage. Neurol Sci 2008;29(Suppl 2):S266–S268

3. Broderick J, Connolly S, Feldmann E, et al. Guidelines for the management of spontaneous intracerebral hemorrhage in adults: 2007 update: a guideline from the American Heart Association/American Stroke Association Stroke Council, High Blood Pressure Research Council, and the Quality of Care and Outcomes in Research Interdisciplinary Working Group. Stroke 2007;38(6):2001–2023

4. Johnsen SP, Pedersen L, Friis S, et al. Nonaspirin nonsteroidal anti-inflammatory drugs and risk of hospitalization for intracerebral hemorrhage: a population-based case-control study. Stroke 2003;34(2):387–391

5. Saloheimo P, Juvela S, Hillbom M. Use of aspirin, epistaxis, and untreated hypertension as risk factors for primary intracerebral hemorrhage in middle-aged and elderly people. Stroke 2001;32(2):399–404

6. Hacke W, Kaste M, Fieschi C, et al. Intravenous thrombolysis with recombinant tissue plasminogen activator for acute hemispheric stroke. The European Cooperative Acute Stroke Study (ECASS). JAMA 1995;274(13):1017–1025

7. Mayer SA, Brun NC, Begtrup K, et al. Recombinant activated factor VII for acute intracerebral hemorrhage. N Engl J Med 2005;352(8):777–785

8. Eckman MH, Rosand J, Knudsen KA, Singer DE, Greenberg SM. Can patients be anticoagulated after intracerebral hemorrhage? A decision analysis. Stroke 2003;34(7):1710–1716

9. Ananthasubramaniam K, Beattie JN, Rosman HS, Jayam V, Borzak S. How safely and for how long can warfarin therapy be withheld in prosthetic heart valve patients hospitalized with a major hemorrhage? Chest 2001;119(2):478–484

10. Fredriksson K, Norrving B, Stromblad LG. Emergency reversal of anticoagulation after intracerebral hemorrhage. Stroke 1992;23(7):972–977

11. Molina CA, Alvarez-Sabin J, Montaner J, et al. Thrombolysis-related hemorrhagic infarction: a marker of early reperfusion, reduced infarct size, and improved outcome in patients with proximal middle cerebral artery occlusion. Stroke 2002;33(6):1551–1556

5 Status Epilepticus

Jan Claassen and Lawrence J. Hirsch

Status epilepticus (SE) is a life-threatening medical and neurological emergency and requires prompt diagnosis and treatment. Every hour delay in treatment increases mortality. Traditionally, SE has been defined as continuous or repetitive seizure activity persisting for at least 30 minutes without recovery of consciousness between attacks. Nowadays, patients should be considered to be in SE if seizures persist for more than 5 minutes.[1] SE may be classified into convulsive and nonconvulsive based on the clinical presence of seizure-like activity.

In neuroscience intensive care units, up to a third of patients will have nonconvulsive seizures (and most of these patients will be in nonconvulsive status epilepticus [NCSE]).[2] In the medical intensive care unit, up to 10% of patients undergoing continuous electroencephalogram (EEG) monitoring have nonconvulsive seizures.[3] Up to 50% of patients with generalized tonic-clonic seizures will have nonconvulsive seizures after convulsions have subsided. The annual incidence of SE is 100,000 to 200,000 cases in the United States. Refractory status epilepticus (RSE) is defined by failure to respond to two intravenous drugs and occurs in up to 43% of patients with SE.[4,5]

The most common cause of SE is a prior history of epilepsy (22 to 34%). Other causes include remote brain lesion (stroke, tumor, or subdural hemorrhage [SDH], etc., 24%), new stroke (22%), anoxia/hypoxia (10%), metabolic (10%), and ethyl alcohol (EtOH) withdrawal (10%).[6]

Case Example

A 63-year-old healthy woman presented with viral symptoms, including fever, for a few days followed by a generalized tonic-clonic seizure lasting ~6 minutes associated with eye deviation. Two hours later she is not following commands and has left hemiparesis.

Questions

- Is the patient still seizing, even if only subtly?
- What is the level of consciousness?
- Is the patient already intubated?
- Is there a seizure history, and is the patient on any antiepileptic medications?
- What are the antiepileptic doses and levels?
- Is the patient diabetic, and what is the finger stick?

Urgent Orders

- Immediately address airway, breathing, circulation (ABCs; intubate).
- Obtain intravenous (IV) access; administer thiamine 100 mg IV and 50 mL of D50 IV unless hypoglycemia is excluded, followed by lorazepam (0.1 mg/kg IV total in 2–4 mg aliquots over 2 minutes).
- Load with 20 mg/kg of fosphenytoin IV.

■ History and Examination

History

- *Seizure semiology.* Obtain a detailed description of the seizure (gaze deviation, face or extremity jerking, automatisms, altered mental status, etc.).
- *Seizure duration.* Attempt to establish when the patient was last seen normal as an onset time. Determine duration of convulsive component of seizure and duration of postictal or potentially nonconvulsive period of altered mentation.
- *Past medical history* of epilepsy or epilepsy risk factors (history of head trauma with loss of consciousness, meningitis/encephalitis, or febrile seizures); history of hypoglycemia or diabetes, history of structural brain lesion (stroke, tumor, subdural, etc.)
- *If epileptic,* determine what antiepileptic drugs (AEDs) the patient was taking and if there is a history of noncompliance.
- *Medication history* (review medications that reduce seizure threshold)
- *Social history,* with particular attention to illicit drug use or EtOH use

■ Physical and Neurologic Examinations

- A full neurologic examination, including assessment of mental status, cranial nerves, motor skills, and reflexes, as well as a sensory and cerebellar exam, should be performed in all patients.

- *Mental status.* Typically, patients who present with generalized convulsive SE are expected to awaken gradually after the motor features of seizures disappear. If the level of consciousness is not improving by 20 minutes after cessation of movements, or if mental status remains abnormal 30 to 60 minutes after the convulsions cease, NCSE must be considered, and urgent EEG monitoring is advised.

- *Symptoms may include:*
  - Negative symptoms such as coma, lethargy, confusion, aphasia, amnesia, speech arrest, and staring
  - Positive symptoms such as automatisms, blinking, facial twitching, agitation, nystagmus, eye deviation, and perseveration
  - It is crucial to recognize and treat NCSE early because prognosis worsens with increasing duration of seizure activity.

- *Focal exam findings.* Todd's paralysis and Todd's-equivalents, such as aphasia, numbness, etc. Any focal finding indicates a potential focal brain lesion.

■ Differential Diagnosis

1. *Status epilepticus and/or NCSE*
2. *Postictal state*—if mental status remains abnormal 30 to 60 minutes after the convulsions cease, NCSE must be considered, and urgent EEG is advised.
3. *Movement disorders* (myoclonus, asterixis, tremor, chorea, tics, dystonia)
4. *Herniation* (decerebrate or decorticate posturing)
5. *Limb-shaking transient ischemic attacks (TIAs),* most commonly associated with perfusion failure due to severe carotid stenosis
6. *Psychiatric disorders* (psychogenic nonepileptic seizures, conversion disorder, acute psychosis, catatonia)

7. *Any condition that may lead to decreased level of consciousness* (e.g., toxic-metabolic encephalopathies, including hypoglycemia and delirium, anoxia, and central nervous system [CNS] infections), transient global amnesia, sleep disorders (e.g., parasomnias), syncope

Life-Threatening Diagnoses Not to Miss

• *Status epilepticus and NCSE*

■ Diagnostic Evaluation

• *EEG.* Urgent EEG is indicated in any patient with fluctuating or unexplained alteration of behavior or mental status, and after convulsive seizures or SE if the patient does not rapidly awaken.

  ◦ Spot EEG (30-minute recording) picks up about one-third of nonconvulsive seizures (using 24-hour EEG as a gold standard), and about half of clinical events.

  ◦ Limited montage (6-channel or hairline EEG) is not sensitive for seizures or epileptiform discharges.

  ◦ Continuous EEG (cEEG) is preferred. Twenty-four hours of monitoring detects 95% of seizures in noncomatose patients and 80% in comatose patients (comatose patients should have cEEG for 48 hours before nonconvulsive seizure is ruled out).[7]

  ◦ Video EEG monitoring is helpful to distinguish true electrographic activity from common ICU artifact (ventilator, continuous venovenous hemofiltration [CVVH], nursing-related artifact).

  ◦ EEG findings in the aftermath of SE may include generalized periodic epileptiform discharges (GPEDs), periodic lateralized epileptiform discharges (PLEDs) or bilateral but independent periodic discharges (BiPLEDs). These controversial EEG findings in the setting of SE may be considered on an ictal/interictal continuum because they do not meet formal seizure criteria, and their exact nature and significance are not well understood.

• *Benzodiazepine trial.* May help to make the diagnosis of NCSE. Administer sequential small doses of rapidly acting, short-duration benzodiazepines (e.g., midazolam 1 mg). Resolution of the potentially ictal EEG pattern and either an improvement in the clinical state or the appearance of previously absent normal EEG patterns would be considered a positive response. If EEG improves but the patient does not (e.g., due to marked sedation), the result is equivocal.

- *Imaging studies*
  - ○ MRI: Seizure focus may show up as a bright signal on diffusion-weighted imaging (DWI) and dark signal on apparent diffusion coefficient imaging (ADC) in a nonvascular territory possibly with leptomeningeal enhancement. Gyral increased signal and gyral thickening are sometimes seen on fluid attenuated inversion recovery (FLAIR) and is a reversible change. This pattern may mimic acute infarction.

■ Treatment

General Concepts

- *Treat quickly.* Eighty percent of patients will respond to first line medications if treatment is begun within 30 minutes, but <40% respond if treated within 2 hours. Mortality doubles with a 24 hour delay in treatment of nonconvulsive status epilepticus.[8]
- *Do not withhold seizure medications* because of fear of respiratory suppression leading to intubation. When given by paramedics for out-of-hospital SE in adults, the rate of respiratory depression or circulatory complications was lower with lorazepam and diazepam than with placebo.[9] These, as well as other studies, confirm that not giving benzodiazepines is riskier than giving them for prolonged convulsive seizures.

First-Line Antiepileptic Medications

Lorazepam is superior to phenytoin or diazepam as a first line agent.[10] In a trial comparing four treatments for generalized convulsive status epilepticus, lorazepam aborted 65% of seizures, phenobarbital 58%, phenytoin + diazepam 56%, and phenytoin alone 44%.[11] A randomized trial comparing lorazepam, diazepam, and placebo for the treatment of out-of-hospital status epilepticus found status epilepticus was terminated more frequently with lorazepam or diazepam compared with placebo. There was a trend for more seizure termination with lorazepam compared with diazepam, but this was not statistically significant.[9] Lorazepam is preferred as first line over diazepam because it has a longer duration of action (4 to 6 hours) and less fat distribution. If no IV access is available, diazepam is available in a rectal form, and midazolam can be given buccally or intranasally.

Second-Line Antiepileptic Medications

Due to the time-dependent loss of potency of lorazepam and the need for a maintenance antiepileptic drug (AED), phenytoin or fosphenytoin is typically administered even if seizure activity has stopped after lorazepam is given. Fosphenytoin is usually used as a loading agent, particularly when a patient is still seizing. Because of its cheaper cost, phenytoin is used as a maintenance agent (**Table 5.1**).

Table 5.1 Medications for Second-Line Treatment of Seizures

Medication	Dosing	Pros	Cons
Phenytoin	20 mg/kg IV, max infusion rate 50 mg/min; after SE, target-free phenytoin level 2–3 µg/mL	500 mg = $2	28–50% hypotension when infused at 50 mg/min due mostly to propylene glycol carrier, arrhythmias, hepatotoxicity; not compatible w/ dextrose solutions
Fosphenytoin	20 mg/kg IV, max infusion rate 150 mg/min (3 times rate of phenytoin), target-free phenytoin level 2–3 µg/mL	Can be given IM, less hypotension; fosphenytoin displaces phenytoin from albumin binding and rapidly increases free phenytoin levels in patients chronically on phenytoin	500 mg = $60 Requires refrigeration

Abbreviations: IM, intramuscular; IV, intravenous; SE, status epilepticus.

Third-Line Antiepileptic Medications (for Refractory Status)

Although agreement may be reached on the early steps of SE treatment, the later steps especially for refractory SE (RSE) remain very controversial. A systematic review of the literature on treatment of RSE found no difference in mortality (48%) comparing 193 RSE patients treated with continuous IV propofol, continuous IV midazolam, or continuous IV pentobarbital.[12] The review also showed no differences between propofol and midazolam for clinical end points such as acute treatment failure, breakthrough seizures, and post-treatment seizures. By contrast, pentobarbital had a lower frequency of acute treatment failure and breakthrough seizures but also the highest rates of hypotension. Because the vast majority of patients treated with a goal of EEG background suppression were given pentobarbital (79 of 87), it is difficult to conclude whether pentobarbital or the titration goal per se might be responsible for the improved treatment response observed in the pentobarbital group (**Table 5.2**).

Fourth-Line Seizure Medications

Pentobarbital is reserved for those refractory to third-line agents. It provides excellent seizure control at the expense of hypotension, cardiosuppression, immunosuppression, and prolonged sedation due to its half-life of 15 to 60 hours.

Treatment of Seizures Due to Metabolic Derangements

Correcting the metabolic problem is more effective than administering AEDs. Fever, hypoxia, and hypotension should also be treated concurrently, as these can exacerbate seizures and the associated neuronal injury. Patients should not be pharmacologically paralyzed unless absolutely necessary, and continuous EEG should be recorded. Use of medications that can lower the seizure threshold should be identified and minimized (**Table 5.3**).

Table 5.2 Medications for Third-Line Treatment of Seizures

Medication	Dosing	Pros	Cons
Midazolam (cIV infusion)	Load 0.2 mg/kg. Repeat 0.2–0.4 mg/kg boluses every 5 min until seizures stop, up to a max total loading dose of 2 mg/kg. cIV: 0.05–2.0 mg/kg/h	Effective in minutes; minimal cardiovascular side effects; easy to titrate	Same class as other benzodiazepines, can argue for trying another class; short $t^1/_2$; should use cIV; tachyphylaxis in 24–48 h requiring increased dosing
Propofol (cIV infusion)	Load: 1 mg/kg; repeat 1–2 mg/kg boluses every 35 min until seizures stop, up to max loading dose of 10 mg/kg. cIV: 1–15 mg/kg/h	Different mechanism for seizure control; easy to titrate; rapid onset	PRIS—lactic acidosis, rhabdomyolysis, renal failure, and death; more in children but reported in adults, worse when combined with steroids/catecholamines. Caution with >5 mg/kg/h for >24–48 h; Risk of refractory acidosis with carbonic anhydrase inhibitors (topiramate, zonisamide); immunosuppression; cardiosuppression; lipid load, pancreatitis
IV valproic acid	Load: 40 mg/kg in patients exposed to phenytoin or 20 mg/kg in phenytoin naive patients. Maximum bolus rate: approved for rates up to 3 mg/kg/min. Faster rates (5–6 mg/kg/min) have been well tolerated. Target serum level: 70–140 µg/mL	Minimal hypotensive, sedative, or respiratory effect, may avoid intubation	Competes for albumin binding with phenytoin; metabolic interaction with phenytoin, hepatotoxicity (including fatal); thrombocytopenia; pancreatitis; hyperammonemic encephalopathy
IV phenobarbital	Load: 20 mg/kg IV at 50–100 mg/min. Target serum level: 30–45 µg/mL	Well-established drug; physician familiarity	Most patients require intubation; hypotension common; interacts with phenytoin; Long $t^1/_2$ 87–100 h, prolonged sedation; allergy including Stevens-Johnson syndrome; blood dyscrasia

Abbreviations: cIV, continuous intravenous; IV, intravenous; PRIS, propofol infusion syndrome; $t^1/_2$, half-life.

Table 5.3 Algorithm for Treatment of Status Epilepticus

Time (minutes)	Action
0–5	Diagnose. Consider toxicology, trauma (immobilization), and infection (isolation); ABCs; begin ECG monitoring; obtain IV access; draw blood chemistry, magnesium, calcium, phosphate, CBC, liver function tests, coagulation studies, antiepileptic drug levels, troponin, ABG; toxicology screen (urine and blood), salicylates, EtOH, head CT, pregnancy test
6–10	Thiamine: 100 mg IV; 50 mL of D50 IV unless adequate glucose known. *Lorazepam*: Begin with *4 mg IV over 2 min*; if still seizing, repeat at 5 min *4 mg IV over 2 min (for a total of 0.1 mg/kg)*. Monitor blood pressure during administration If no rapid IV access, give diazepam 20 mg PR or midazolam 10 mg intranasally, buccally, or IM*
10–20	1. *Begin fosphenytoin* 20 mg/kg IV at a maximum rate of 150 mg/min, with blood pressure and ECG monitoring. If seizures persist: fosphenytoin additional 10 mg/kg IV at 150 mg/min *OR* 2. *IV valproate: 20 mg/kg over ~10 min*. If still seizing, additional 20 mg/kg over ~5 min. *OR* 3. *In patients with known seizure disorder (taking either Depakote [valproate], Keppra [levetiracetam], or phenobarbital at home), reload with the home medication as follows:* *IV valproate:* 20 mg/kg over ~10 min. If still seizing, additional 20 mg/kg over ~5 min *IV Keppra:* 1000–4000 mg IV *IV phenobarbital:* 20 mg/kg IV at 50–100 mg/min This step may initially be skipped, especially if proceeding to midazolam or propofol. If seizures are stopped after benzodiazepines, this step is usually needed anyway, but it can be done more slowly and after obtaining additional history as long as seizures were stopped with lorazepam.
20–60	If seizures persist, intubation typically necessary, begin third-line agent. *cIV midazolam:* load—0.2 mg/kg; repeat 0.2–0.4 mg/kg boluses every 5 min until seizures stop, up to a maximum total loading dose of 2 mg/kg. Initial cIV rate: 0.1 mg/kg/h. cIV dose range: 0.05–2.0 mg/kg/h (up to 200 mg/h for 70 kg person). If still seizing, proceed to or add IV pentobarbital or propofol. *Mix* 50 mg midazolam in 50 cc NS (1 mg = 1 cc). *OR* *IV valproate:* 40 mg/kg over ~10 min if previously received phenytion or fosphenytoin; otherwise load with 20 mg/kg. If still seizing, additional 20 mg/kg over ~5 min. If still seizing, proceed to or add cIV midazolam or propofol.

(Continued on next page)

Table 5.3 Algorithm for Treatment of Status Epilepticus *(continued)*

Time (minutes)	Action
	OR
	IV propofol: load—1 mg/kg; repeat 1–2 mg/kg boluses every 3–5 min until seizures stop, up to maximum total loading dose of 10 mg/kg. Initial cIV rate: 2 mg/kg/h. cIV dose range: 1–15 mg/kg/h (do not exceed > 5 mg/kg/h for >24 h). If still seizing, proceed to or add cIV midazolam or pentobarbital.
	OR
	IV phenobarbital: 20 mg/kg IV at 50–100 mg/min. If still seizing, proceed to cIV midazolam, propofol, or pentobarbital.
>60	If seizures persist, begin fourth-line agent.
	cIV pentobarbital: Load—5 mg/kg at up to 50 mg/min; repeat 5 mg/kg boluses until seizures stop. Initial cIV rate: 1 mg/kg/h. cIV dose range: 0.5–10 mg/kg/h; traditionally titrated to suppression burst. Begin continuous EEG monitoring ASAP if patient does not rapidly awaken, or if any cIV treatment is used.

*The IV solution of diazepam can be given rectally if Diastat is not available. The IV solution of midazolam can be given by any of these routes.

Abbreviations: ABCs, stabilize airway, breathing, and circulation; ABG, arterial blood gas; ASAP, as soon as possible; CBC, complete blood count; cIV, continuous intravenous infusion; CT, computed tomography; ECG, electrocardiogram; EEG, electroencephalogram; EKG, electrocardiogram; EtOH, ethyl alcohol; IM, intramuscular; IV, intravenous; NS, normal saline; PR, per rectum.

Tapering Off Continuous Infusions of AEDs

In all patients treated with continuous infusions of an AED, the effective dose should be continued for 12 to 24 hours after seizures are stopped before a gradual taper is started. This taper should occur slowly over ~24 hours. If seizures recurred with a prior taper, it may be necessary to treat longer and taper more slowly the next time while maintaining high therapeutic levels of other AEDs.

Aggressiveness of Seizure Treatment

No studies have demonstrated a convincing difference in outcome based on the goal of treatment (seizure suppression vs burst suppression vs flat-line) independent of etiology.

Seizure Prophylaxis

- *Postcraniotomy.* In a double-blind trial Phenytoin versus placebo in 203 patients with supratentorial craniotomy, 8% of those on Dilantin experienced seizures compared with 17% of those in the placebo group.[13] Seventy-five percent of seizures occurred in the first month after craniotomy. Adding Dilantin on top of preexisting seizure medications for prophylaxis has not proved efficacious. In many centers, patients who undergo supratentorial craniotomy and have no history of seizure receive 7 days of antiepileptic prophylaxis.

- *Traumatic brain injury (TBI).* In a randomized controlled trial, 404 patients with significant TBI (cortical contusion, SDH, epidural hematoma [EDH], intracranial hemorrhage [ICH], subarachnoid hemorrhage [SAH], depressed skull fracture, penetrating head wound, and Glasgow Coma Score [GCS] <11) were randomized to Dilantin versus placebo for 1 year. Between day 0 and 7 after TBI, 4% of the Dilantin group and 14% of the placebo group experienced a seizure ($p < .001$). Between day 8 and 1 year, 22% of the Dilantin group and 16% of the placebo group had a seizure ($p = .2$). Between 1 and 2 years, 28% of the Dilantin group and 21% of the placebo group had a seizure ($p = .2$).[14] Based on these data, many practitioners will administer prophylactic antiepileptics for 7 days to patients with TBI to limit early seizure occurrence.

- *Intracerebral hemorrhage (ICH).* Among patients receiving continuous EEG monitoring, 28% had seizures during the first 72 hours after ICH, and 18 to 20% of these patients seize even if already treated with Dilantin.[15] Although there are no large studies, many practitioners will administer prophylactic anticpileptics to patients who are not following commands, patients with lobar ICH, or patients with evidence of elevated ICP.

- *Subarachnoid hemorrhage (SAH).* Ten percent of SAH patients seize at onset, 4% seize during hospital stay, and 7% have late seizures. Risk factors for seizure include ICH, middle cerebral artery (MCA) aneurysms, infarcts, and hypertension. Because seizures may increase rebleeding risk prior to securement of a ruptured aneurysm, it is recommended that all SAH patients receive antiepileptic prophylaxis prior to aneurysm repair. Although conventionally many practitioners have extrapolated data from randomized trials of TBI to spontaneous SAH patients and have treated patients with medication for 7 days, data suggest that antiepileptics such as Dilantin, phenobarbital, and carbamazepine retard cognitive recovery.[16] After aneurysm exclusion, command-following patients and patients undergoing continuous EEG monitoring for seizure detection may be managed without antiepileptic prophylaxis at the treating physician's discretion. All patients who have experienced a seizure should continue with antiepileptic treatment.

■ Prognosis

Overall, mortality in SE is ~17 to 26% and higher for patients with NCSE or RSE. An additional 10 to 23% of survivors are left with disabling neurologic deficits.

Important predictors of death include old age, acute symptomatic etiology (outcomes are worse if SE follows anoxic brain injury or stroke), impairment of consciousness, and duration of SE. In a study of NCSE in ICU patients, seizure duration was the single major predictor of mortality on multivariate analysis: if duration was less than 10 hours, 60% returned home, and 10% died; if duration was greater than 20 hours, none returned home, and 85% died.[9-11] Patients with SE due to antiepileptic withdrawal or alcohol tend to do better.

Pearls and Pitfalls

- A patient should be considered to be in status epilepticus (SE) if a seizure persists for more than 5 minutes.

- Early recognition of SE allows for prompt treatment and increases the likelihood of treatment success and prevention of further neuronal damage.

- If the level of consciousness is not improving by 20 minutes after cessation of movements, or the mental status remains abnormal 30 to 60 minutes after the convulsions cease, nonconvulsive SE must be considered.

- In the ICU, most seizures are nonconvulsive and would be missed without continuous EEG monitoring.

References

1. Lowenstein DH. Status epilepticus: an overview of the clinical problem. Epilepsia 1999;40(Suppl 1):S3–S8; discussion S21–22
2. Jordan KG. Status epilepticus. A perspective from the neuroscience intensive care unit. Neurosurg Clin N Am. 1994;5:671–686
3. Towne AR, Waterhouse EJ, Boggs JG, Garnett LK, Brown AJ, Smith JR, Jr., DeLorenzo RJ. Prevalence of nonconvulsive status epilepticus in comatose patients. Neurology 2000;54:340–345
4. DeLorenzo RJ, Pellock JM, Towne AR, Boggs JG. Epidemiology of status epilepticus. J Clin Neurophysiol 1995 Jul;12(4):316-25
5. Holtkamp M, Othman J, Buchheim K, Meierkord H. Predictors and prognosis of refractory status epilepticus treated in a neurological intensive care unit. J Neurol Neurosurg Psychiatr. 2005;76(4):534-539.
6. Chen JW, Wasterlain CG. Status epilepticus: pathophysiology and management in adults. Lancet Neurol 2006;5(3):246–256
7. Claassen J, Mayer SA, Kowalski RG, Emerson RG, Hirsch LJ. Detection of electrographic seizures with continuous eeg monitoring in critically ill patients. Neurology 2004;62:1743–1748
8. Young GB, Jordan KG, Doig GS. An assessment of nonconvulsive seizures in the intensive care unit using continuous EEG monitoring: an investigation of variables associated with mortality. Neurology 1996;47(1):83–89
9. Alldredge BK, Gelb AM, Isaacs SM, et al. A comparison of lorazepam, diazepam, and placebo for the treatment of out-of-hospital status epilepticus. N Engl J Med 2001;345(9):631–637
10. Prasad K, Al-Roomi K, Krishnan PR, Sequeira R. Anticonvulsant therapy for status epilepticus. Cochrane Database of Systematic Reviews (Online) 2005(4):CD003723
11. Treiman DM, Meyers PD, Walton NY, et al. A comparison of four treatments for generalized convulsive status epilepticus. Veterans Affairs Status Epilepticus Cooperative Study Group. N Engl J Med 1998;339(12):792–798
12. Claassen J, Hirsch LJ, Emerson RG, Mayer SA. Treatment of refractory status epilepticus with pentobarbital, propofol, or midazolam: a systematic review. Epilepsia 2002;43(2):146–153
13. North JB, Penhall RK, Hanieh A, Hann CS, Challen RG, Frewin DB. Postoperative epilepsy: a double-blind trial of phenytoin after craniotomy. Lancet 1980;1(8165):384–386
14. Temkin NR, Dikmen SS, Wilensky AJ, Keihm J, Chabal S, Winn HR. A randomized, double-blind study of phenytoin for the prevention of post-traumatic seizures. N Engl J Med 1990;323(8):497–502
15. Vespa PM, O'Phelan K, Shah M, et al. Acute seizures after intracerebral hemorrhage: a factor in progressive midline shift and outcome. Neurology 2003;60(9):1441–1446
16. Naidech AM, Kreiter KT, Janjua N, et al. Phenytoin exposure is associated with functional and cognitive disability after subarachnoid hemorrhage. Stroke 2005;36(3):583–587

6 Malignant Ischemic Stroke

Katja E. Wartenberg

Malignant strokes are large strokes with edema and swelling that cause secondary injury due to mass effect. Neurologic deterioration occurs as a consequence of cytotoxic edema that causes an early rise in intracranial pressure and subsequent herniation and death. Large anterior circulation (proximal middle cerebral artery [MCA] or internal carotid artery [ICA] territory strokes) or large cerebellar infarcts are an important cause of morbidity and mortality in the neurologic intensive care unit. Malignant infarcts constitute ~10% of all ischemic strokes.[1] The typical etiology of these infarcts is either cardioembolic or due to large vessel occlusion. Malignant edema is more common in women and is classically described as developing within 24 hours, although edema often develops after 3 to 4 days. Early swelling can be attributed to reperfusion edema or possibly the effects of tissue plasminogen activator (tPA).

Though not all patients with massive stroke deteriorate, sensitive predictors of decompensation include high NIH Stroke Scale scores (NIHSS) (**Table 6.1**), depressed level of consciousness, history of hypertension (HTN) or heart failure, asymmetric pupil size, early nausea and vomiting, younger age (mean age 56 years), coma on the day of admission, poor collateral circulation, and carotid dissection.[2] Radiographic predictors include computed tomography (CT) hypodensity of >50% of the affected MCA territory, large magnetic resonance imaging (MRI) diffusion weighted and apparent diffusion coefficient volume, and small perfusion to diffusion mismatch.

Case Example

A 45-year-old butcher suddenly collapsed in his store. Emergency services was called right away and brought him to the nearest emergency department, where he was found with his eyes open, unresponsive to verbal stimuli, with left gaze deviation and right hemiplegia. A CT scan of the head did not show any bleeding or hypodensity. He received 0.9 mg/kg intravenous (IV) recombinant tissue plasminogen activator (rtPA) 1.5 hours after symptom onset and was admitted to the intensive care unit. Fifteen hours later the nurse calls, as she noticed labored breathing and unresponsiveness to painful stimuli.

Questions

- What was the time of onset? (When was the patient last seen normal?)
- What are the blood pressure, heart rate, oxygen saturation, temperature, and glucose levels?
- Did the patient receive any sedating drugs recently?
- Are there any signs of bleeding after thrombolysis?
- Could the patient be seizing (convulsive or nonconvulsive)?

Urgent Orders

- Consider intubation (airway, breathing, circulation [ABCs]).
- Order noncontrast head CT.
- Institute treatment of intracranial pressure if appropriate.
- Check coagulation tests, including fibrinogen and electrolytes.
- Check glucose level, sodium level, and chemistry panel immediately; avoid 5% dextrose in water (D5W) or any hypotonic fluids.

■ History and Examination

History

- Obtain a timeline for onset of the stroke: establish time to thrombolysis, initial NIHSS, and time of decompensation.
- Check for history of rhythmic movement or subtle twitching that might point to seizure activity.

Physical Examination

Look for signs of neurologic deterioration from cerebral edema and impending herniation after large hemispheric stroke or brainstem compression and/or hydrocephalus after large cerebellar infarction, including:

- *Vital signs.* Cushing's triad (hypertension, bradycardia, respiratory irregularity)—classic signs of elevated intracranial pressure (ICP)
- Assess for nausea, vomiting.
- Assess for hyperventilation or hypoventilation, Cheyne–Stokes breathing, and apneustic, cluster, or ataxic respirations.
- Assess for arrhythmia, bradycardia, sustained hypertension, or blood pressure lability.

■ Neurologic Examination

- With large, anterior circulation malignant strokes, the neurologic examination typically reveals depressed mental status, forced gaze deviation, aphasia or neglect, visual field defects, and/or hemiparesis.
- In posterior circulation strokes, look for crossed cranial nerve and long track signs, quadriparesis, depressed mental status, multiple cranial neuropathies, abnormal pupils, ataxia, dysarthria, abnormal brainstem reflexes (corneal, oculocephalics, gag), nausea/ vomiting (due to either elevated ICP or irritation of the area postrema at the floor of the fourth ventricle), downward gaze deviation (sign of hydrocephalus due to enlarged third ventricle and compression of the rostral intermedial longitudinal fasciculus), and/or elevated tone in the lower extremities (early indication of hydrocephalus).
- Assess for subtle twitching or eye deviation away from the side of the lesion that might indicate seizure activity.
- Assess for impending herniation:
  - First sign is usually drowsiness, followed by progressive obtundation to stupor or coma.
  - Pupillary asymmetry, ocular deviation (unilateral oculomotor palsy from uncal herniation or traction on the third nerve)
  - Contralateral motor posturing (decorticate = flexor posturing, decerebrate = extensor posturing) or Kernohan's notch phenomenon (long track signs/weakness ipsilateral to the lesion due to herniation and compression of the contralateral cerebral peduncle)
  - Bilateral motor posturing and lower extremity rigidity
- The NIH Stroke Scale is commonly used to follow the neurological exam (**Table 6.1**).

Table 6.1 NIH Stroke Scale

1a	Level of consciousness 0 = alert, 1 = drowsy, 2 = stuporous, 3 = comatose
1b	Level of consciousness questions 0 = answers both correctly, 1 = answers one correctly, 2 = both incorrect
1c	Level of consciousness commands 0 = obeys both correctly, 1 = obeys one correctly, 2 = both incorrect
2	Best gaze 0 = normal, 1 = partial gaze palsy, 2 = forced deviation
3	Visual fields 0 = no visual loss, 1 = partial hemianopsia, 2 = complete hemianopsia, 3 = bilateral hemianopsia
4	Facial paresis 0 = normal movement, 1 = minor paresis, 2 = partial paresis, 3 = complete palsy
5–8	Right/left arm/leg motor 0 = no drift, 1 = drift, 2 = some effort v gravity, 3 = no effort v gravity, 4 = no movement
9	Limb ataxia 0 = absent, 1 = present in 1 limb, 2 = present in 2 or more limbs
10	Sensory 0 = normal, 1 = partial loss, 2 = dense loss
11	Best language 0 = no aphasia, 1 = mild–moderate aphasia, 2 = severe aphasia, 3 = mute
12	Dysarthria 0 = normal articulation, 1 = mild–moderate dysarthria, 2 = unintelligible or worse
13	Neglect/inattention 0 = no neglect, 1 = partial neglect, 2 = complete neglect

*Total score 0–42; 0 = best, 42 = worst, v = versus

Data from: www.NIHSS.com.

■ Differential Diagnosis

1. *Development of cerebral edema* with tissue shifts, eventually resulting in herniation

2. *Intracranial bleeding* (e.g., after thrombolytic therapy)

3. *Hydrocephalus after cerebellar infarction*

4. *Ongoing ischemia.* Exclude hypoperfusion in large artery stenosis/occlusion, ongoing embolization from a cardiac or vessel source (i.e., dissection—look for headache; neck, eye, or face pain; recent stress on neck; cranial neuropathies), progression of posterior circulation thrombosis (lethargy/coma, top of the basilar syndrome, cranial neuropathies with crossed long track signs, cortical blindness, cerebellar findings), or vascular compression of the anterior and posterior cerebral arteries against the falx or tentorium (rare; due to swelling and mass effect).

5. *Seizure.* Perform continuous electroencephalogram (EEG) monitoring; consider antiepileptic drugs

6. *Sedating drugs*—discontinue

7. *Fever* (see Chapter 20)

8. *Hypo- or hyperglycemia.* Correct and maintain strict normoglycemia.

9. *Hypoxia, hypercarbia.* Check arterial blood gas (ABG), intubate if necessary, adjust ventilator settings

10. *Metabolic causes.* Renal or hepatic insufficiency → check laboratories, including electrolytes, determine underlying cause, and treat accordingly.

11. *Infection.* Pneumonia, urinary tract infection, meningitis/ventriculitis (after neurosurgical procedures), line infection, sinusitis, intra-abdominal abscess → check complete blood count (CBC), C-reactive protein (CRP), procalcitonin, chest radiograph (CXR), urine analysis, blood-, urine-, and deep tracheal aspiration cultures. Treat ventilator-associated pneumonia and sepsis with a combination of broad-spectrum antibiotics. Change central lines if appropriate.

Life-Threatening Diagnoses Not to Miss

- *Herniation*
- *Obstructive hydrocephalus from edema*
- *Intracranial hemorrhage/hemorrhagic conversion*
- *Ongoing ischemia*
- *Status epilepticus*

■ Diagnostic Evaluation

- *Laboratory studies*
  - ○ Evaluate CBC, electrolytes, liver function, glucose level, coagulation studies, urine toxicology screening if appropriate, antiepileptic drug (AED) levels if on AED and suspicion of seizure, ABG.
  - ○ In febrile patients, check urine analysis; blood-, urine-, and deep tracheal aspiration cultures; CXR; CRP; procalcitonin; further detailed search for infection focus if appropriate.
- *Imaging studies*
  - ○ Immediate noncontrast CT scan: mass effect on CT such as compression of the frontal horn, shift of the septum pellucidum, and later shift of pineal gland are worrisome features for impending clinical deterioration or herniation.[3]
  - ○ CT perfusion, CT angiogram, and/or MRI, MR angiogram, MR perfusion are useful if the CT scan does not reveal the cause of neurologic deterioration and/or ongoing ischemia is suspected.
  - ○ Digital subtraction angiography can be useful to assess the etiology of stroke and collateral circulation, particularly if ongoing ischemia or hypoperfusion is suspected.
- *Other diagnostic studies*
  - ○ Consider continuous EEG monitoring.
  - ○ Transcranial Doppler ultrasound to determine if the ICA, MCA, or basilar artery is open.
  - ○ ICP, brain oxygen monitoring, or microdialysis may be considered to monitor treatment of cerebral edema in large hemispheric strokes.

■ Treatment

Initial Management

Revascularization should be considered at presentation for patients with large ischemic strokes. This constitutes intravenous (IV) rtPA/alteplase (0.9 mg/kg IV, 10% as an initial bolus over 1 minute, and the rest as an infusion over the remaining hour, maximum dose: 90 mg) in patients who present within a 3-hour time window of ischemia onset (American Heart Association/American Stroke Association [AHA/ASA] class I, level A)[4,5] and do not have any contraindications (**Table 6.2**).[4]

- There is no upper size limit, age limit, or NIHSS limit for the administration of IV thrombolysis. Patients with seizure at the time of onset of stroke may be eligible for IV tPA treatment if the physician is convinced that the residual impairments are due to stroke and not a postictal phenomenon (AHA/ASA class IIa, level C).[5] Blood pressure should be controlled prior to and after tPA administration according to **Table 6.3**.[5]

- In patients who do not receive thrombolysis, the treatment threshold for lowering blood pressure (BP) acutely after ischemic stroke is 220/120 mm Hg (AHA/ASA class I, level C).[5]

- In patients who receive IV tPA, if the patient develops severe headache, acute hypertension, nausea, or vomiting, IV tPA should be discontinued and an emergency CT scan obtained and emergent reversal should be given (see Chapter 4). Physicians should be aware of the complication of angioedema that can cause partial airway obstruction. After tPA administration, BP should be measured every 15 minutes for the first 2 hours and then every 30 minutes for the next 6 hours. Placement of nasogastric tubes, indwelling bladder catheters, or intra-arterial catheters should be deferred. A follow-up CT scan should be obtained at 24 hours before starting anticoagulants or antiplatelet agents.[5]

- Patients who are not within the time window or are not eligible for IV tPA (i.e., recent surgery) may be eligible for intra-arterial thrombolysis (within 6 hours for the anterior circulation [AHA/ASA class I, level B][5,6] and up to 24 hours in the posterior circulation) or mechanical thrombectomy within 8 hours (class IIb, level B)[5,7,8] in selected centers for patients without contraindications. The availability of intra-arterial treatment should not preclude the use of IV tPA in eligible patients (class III, level C).[5]

Table 6.2 AHA/ASA Contraindications to IV tPA

Onset of symptoms >3 h before beginning treatment
Head trauma or prior stroke in previous 3 months
Myocardial infarction in previous 3 months
GI or urinary tract hemorrhage in previous 21 d
Major surgery in previous 14 d
Arterial puncture at noncompressible site in previous 7 d
History of previous ICH
Blood pressure >185/110 mm Hg after attempted BP treatment
Evidence of active bleeding or acute trauma (fracture)
Anticoagulant use or INR >1.7
Received heparin in last 48 h and PTT elevated
Platelet count <100,000
Blood glucose <50 mg/dL (new guidelines have no upper glucose limit)
Seizure with postictal residual neurologic impairments (relative contraindication)
Neurologic signs clearing spontaneously (relative contraindication)
Neurologic signs minor or isolated (relative contraindication)
Symptoms suggestive of SAH
CT with hemorrhage
Caution in patients with major deficits
Caution if CT shows multilobar infarction with major hypodensity > one-third cerebral hemisphere (check time of onset)

Abbreviations: AHA, American Heart Association; ASA, American Stroke Association; BP, blood pressure; CT, computed tomography; GI, gastrointestinal; ICH, intracranial hemorrhage; INR, international normalized ratio; IV, intravenous; PTT, partial thromboplastin time; SAH, subarachnoid hemorrhage; tPA, tissue plasminogen activator.

Data from: Adams HP Jr, del Zoppo G, Alberts MJ, et al. Guidelines for the early management of adults with ischemic stroke: a guideline from the American Heart Association/American Stroke Association Stroke Council, Clinical Cardiology Council, Cardiovascular Radiology and Intervention Council, and the Atherosclerotic Peripheral Vascular Disease and Quality of Care Outcomes in Research Interdisciplinary Working Groups: the American Academy of Neurology affirms the value of this guideline as an educational tool for neurologists. Stroke 2007;38(5):1655–1711.

Manno EM, Nichols DA, Fulgham JR, Wijdicks EF. Computed tomographic determinants of neurologic deterioration in patients with large middle cerebral artery infarctions. Mayo Clin Proc 2003;78(2):156–160.

Table 6.3 Controlling Blood Pressure Prior to and After tPA Administration

Timing	Blood Pressure	Treatment
Eligible for tPA or other acute reperfusion intervention	SBP >185 mm Hg *or* DBP >110 mm Hg	Labetalol 10–20 mg IV over 1–2 min, may repeat × 1 *or* Nitropaste 1–2 inches *or* Nicardipine infusion, 5 mg/h, titrate up by 0.25 mg/h at 5–15 min intervals (maximum 15 mg/h); when desired BP attained, reduce to 3 mg/h If BP does not decline and remains >185/110 mm Hg, do not administer rtPA
After tPA given	SBP 180–230 mm Hg *or* DBP 105–120 mm Hg	Labetalol 10 mg IV over 1–2 min, may repeat every 10–20 min (maximum 300 mg) *or* Labetalol 10 mg IV followed by an infusion at 2–8 mg/min
	SBP >230 mm Hg *or* DBP 121–140 mm Hg	Labetalol 10 mg IV over 1–2 min, may repeat every 10–20 min (maximum 300 mg) *or* Labetalol 10 mg IV followed by an infusion at 2–8 mg/min. *or* Nicardipine infusion, 5 mg/h, titrate up by 2.5 mg/h at 5–15 min intervals (maximum 15 mg/h)
	If BP not controlled	Consider sodium nitroprusside*

Abbreviations: BP, blood pressure; DBP, diastolic blood pressure; IV, intravenous; SBP, systolic blood pressure; tPA, tissue plasminogen activator.

Data from: Adams HP Jr, del Zoppo G, Alberts MJ, et al. Guidelines for the early management of adults with ischemic stroke: a guideline from the American Heart Association/American Stroke Association Stroke Council, Clinical Cardiology Council, Cardiovascular Radiology and Intervention Council, and the Atherosclerotic Peripheral Vascular Disease and Quality of Care Outcomes in Research Interdisciplinary Working Groups: the American Academy of Neurology affirms the value of this guideline as an educational tool for neurologists. Stroke 2007;38(5):1655–1711.

*Nitroprusside can raise ICP and cause cyanide toxicity

- In the ECASS III trial, a randomized, placebo controlled trial of IV tPA versus placebo administered in a 3–4.5 hour time window, patients receiving IV tPA had significantly improved clinical outcome at 3 months. Currently, IV tPA is not FDA approved for a 3–4.5 hour time window.[9]

Medical Management

- *Mechanical ventilation* is recommended for patients with acute stroke who have a decreased level of consciousness or bulbar dysfunction causing airway compromise (AHA/ASA class I, level C).[5]
- *Cerebral edema and elevated ICP or shift* should be treated (see Chapter 15). It should be noted that many patients with malignant stroke herniate with normal ICP values.[10] This occurs due to pressure gradients. Aggressive management of edema should occur in deteriorating patients, even if the ICP is "normal." The AHA/ASA recommends measures to lessen the risk of edema and close monitoring for neurologic deterioration during the first few days after stroke (class I, level B). There is limited evidence to show that aggressive medical management of edema improves outcomes (class IIa, level C),[5] but such treatment is reasonable, particularly as a bridge to decompressive hemicraniectomy. Hyperventilation should be used only for a short period of time or during frank herniation. Steroids have not been shown to be useful for edema related to ischemic stroke and are not recommended (class III, level A).[5]
- *Anticonvulsants.* Prophylactic anticonvulsants are not recommended in large hemispheric or cerebellar stroke (class III, level C).[5] However, seizures (incidence 2 to 33% after large hemispheric stroke) may worsen cerebral edema, increase ICP, and induce neurologic deterioration. Treatment with phenytoin, fosphenytoin, or levetiracetam can be considered in these cases. Continuous electroencephalographic monitoring (cEEG) may be helpful in patients in persistent stupor or coma to enable detection and treatment of nonconvulsive seizures or status epilepticus. Patients who have experienced a seizure should be treated with anticonvulsants.
- *Fever.* Persistent fever after stroke impacts mortality and outcome. Even small temperature elevations have been shown to worsen neuronal injury and increase mortality. Therefore, fever should be treated aggressively (see Chapter 20). According to the AHA/ASA

guidelines,[5] sources of fever should be treated and antipyretic medications should be administered to lower temperature in febrile patients with stroke (class I, level C). Prophylactic antibiotics are not recommended (class III, level B).[5] At this time, insufficient evidence exists to recommend induced hypothermia for the treatment of patients with acute stroke (class III, level B).[5] Induced hypothermia may be considered as part of an ICP management algorithm (see Chapter 15).

- *Cardiac monitoring* should be performed during at least the first 24 hours after ischemic stroke (AHA/ASA class I, level B).[5]

- *Nutrition and glucose control.* Patients who cannot consume food orally should receive nasogastric, nasoduodenal, or percutaneous endoscopic gastrostomy tube (PEG) feedings. The timing of PEG placement is uncertain (class IIa, level B).[5] Small-bore nasoduodenal feeding tubes are preferred to lower the risk of aspiration. Nutritional supplements are not needed (class III, level B).[5] As hyperglycemia may worsen outcome after brain injury, glucose- or dextrose-containing solutions should be avoided. Persistent hyperglycemia should be treated vigorously by means of an insulin protocol utilizing continuous insulin infusions. The ideal glucose target is currently an area of investigation (see Chapter 19). The AHA recommends that glucose control be initiated for serum glucose levels of "possibly 140–185 mg/dL" (class IIa, level C).[5]

- *Deep venous thrombosis prophylaxis.* Subcutaneous anticoagulants are recommended in immobilized patients (class I, level A). The use of intermittent compression devices is recommended in patients who cannot receive subcutaneous anticoagulants (class IIa, level B)[5] (see Chapter 18).[5]

Surgical Management

Cerebellar Stroke

Large cerebellar strokes can develop not only surrounding edema leading to brainstem compression, but can also cause obstructive hydrocephalus due to compression of the fourth ventricle. Suboccipital craniectomy, cerebellectomy, or external ventricular drainage (EVD) are indicated for:

- Deterioration of mental status or development of new brainstem signs
- Surgical decompression should occur expediently prior to herniation.

CT criteria:

- Effacement of the fourth ventricle
- Hydrocephalus
- Compression of the brainstem
- Compression of the basal cisterns
- Median cerebellar infarction

In a series of 50 patients with cerebellar stroke,[10] the indication for selected surgical procedures was stratified as follows:

- Complete effacement of the fourth ventricle → decompression and EVD
- Fourth ventricle open, not completely effaced, Glasgow Coma Score (GCS) normal → medical management of cerebral edema
- Fourth ventricle open, not completely effaced, GCS deteriorating:
  - With hydrocephalus → EVD
  - No hydrocephalus → decompression

According to ASA/AHA guidelines, patients with acute hydrocephalus after cerebellar stroke can be treated with an EVD, though upward herniation is a concern (class I, level B). Decompressive evacuation of a space-occupying cerebellar infarction is potentially life saving, can treat both hydrocephalus and brainstem compression, and is recommended for patients with major cerebellar infarctions (class I, level B).[5]

Decompressive Surgery for Large Hemispheric Stroke

Hemicraniectomy for large hemispheric infarction has been performed for decades. Horizontal and vertical tissue shifts and ventricular and vascular compression by massive brain edema are relieved by removal of the bone flap over the frontal, temporal, and parietal lobe at the infarct site. This allows the edematous brain to expand extracranially, improves cerebral perfusion pressure (CPP) and retrograde flow in the MCA, preserves cerebral blood flow (CBF), and may prevent further ongoing ischemia. The diameter of the

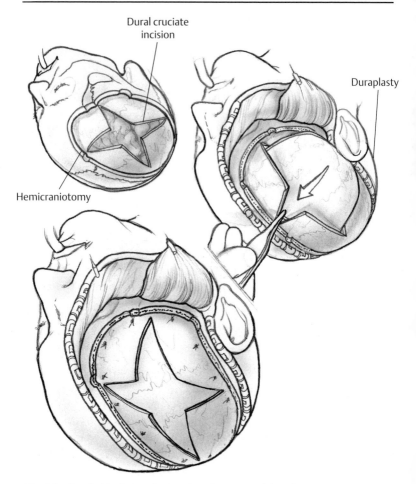

Dural cruciate incision

Duraplasty

Hemicraniotomy

Fig. 6.1 Surgical technique for hemicraniectomy and duraplasty.

craniectomy should be at least 12 cm (14 to 15 cm anterior-posterior, and 10 to 12 cm from the temporal base to the vertex is recommended). A small diameter hemicraniectomy can result in compression and kinking of bridging veins, or mushroom-like herniation of the brain with shearing distortion and additional ischemic injury (**Fig. 6.1**). Resection of the infarction is not advisable, as the margins between infarct and penumbra are poorly defined, however tissue resection is occasionally required in cases of extreme swelling when skin closure is difficult. The bone flap can be conserved in the abdominal subcutaneous tissue or in a cooled sterile isotonic solution. Synthetic bone flaps can be constructed as an alternative. Reimplantation of the bone flap is possible 6 to 12 weeks after removal, once the sweiling has resolved. Potential complications include intracranial, wound, and bone flap infection, subdural and epidural hematoma, subdural cerebral spinal fluid (CSF) hygroma, paradoxical herniation after the swelling period, and persistent hydrocephalus linked to delayed replacement of the bone flap.

- *Timing.* Early surgery (<24 to 48 hours) has a greater impact on reduction of mortality.

- *Size.* Fifty to 66% infarction of the MCA territory is typical for decompression.

- *Age.* Young patients (<50 to 60 years old) tend to have a better outcome.

- *Dominance.* A meta-analysis found no difference in functional outcome comparing left- versus right-sided hemicraniectomy for malignant stroke.[11,12] The side of the stroke should not be an exclusion criterion for hemicraniectomy. The characteristics and results of the three completed randomized, controlled trials of hemicraniectomy to date and two meta-analyses are listed in **Table 6.4**.[10,12-15]

Table 6.4 Characteristics and Results of the Three Completed Randomized, Controlled Trials of Hemicraniectomy and Two Meta-analyses

| Study | Design | Outcome | |
		Medical Arm	Surgical Arm
HeaDDFIRST (Hemi-craniectomy and Duro-tomy for Deterioration From Infarction-Related Swelling Trial)	26 patients Age 18–75 years Complete MCA/ICA infarction (>50% MCA territory, >90 mL volume by CT) Surgery within 4 h of randomization versus medical management Randomization at time of septal shift > 7.5 mm, pineal shift > 4 mm	Mortality at 21 d: 40% 90 d: 40% 180 d: 40%	Mortality at 21 d: 20% 90 d: 36% 180 d: 35.5%

(Continued on next page)

Table 6.4 Characteristics and Results of the Three Completed Randomized, Controlled Trials of Hemicraniectomy and Two Meta-analyses *(continued)*

Study	Design	Outcome	
		Medical Arm	Surgical Arm
DESTINY (Decompressive Surgery for the Treatment of Malignant Infarction of the Middle Cerebral Artery)	32 patients Age 18–60 years NIHSS 18 for nondominant, 20 for dominant strokes CT criteria: 2/3 MCA territory and at least part of the basal ganglia involved Randomized controlled trial of surgery within 12–36 h versus medical management Sequential design: assumed 40% mortality difference between the groups—study stopped when mortality significantly different	Mortality at 1 year: 53% mRS 2–3 at 180 d: 27% mRS 2–3 at 1 year: 27%	Mortality at 1 year: 18% $p = .03$ mRS 2–3 at 180 d: 47% $p = $ NS mRS 2–3 at 1 year: 48% $p = $ NS
DECIMAL (Sequential-design, multicenter, randomized, controlled trial of early decompressive craniectomy in malignant middle cerebral artery infarction)	38 patients Age <55 years NIHSS > 16 altered level of consciousness DWI volume > 145 cm³ Randomized controlled trial of surgery within 24 h versus medical management	Mortality at 30 d: 78% mRS 2–3 at 6 mo: 5.6% mRS 2–3 at 1 year: 22.2%	Mortality at 30 d: 25% $p < .0001$ mRS 2–3 at 6 mo: 25% $p = .01$ mRS 2–3 at 12 mo: 50% $p = .0024$
Meta-analysis of DESTINY, DECIMAL, and HAMLET (Hemicraniectomy after Middle Cerebral Artery Infarction with Life-Threatening Edema Trial)	93 patients Age 18–60 years NIHSS >15 CT: >2/3 of the MCA territory or DWI volume > 145 cm³	Survival at 12 mo: 29% mRS 0–4 at 12 mo: 24%	Survival at 12 mo: 78% $p < .0001$ mRS 0–4 at 12 mo: 75% $p < .0001$

(Continued)

Table 6.4 Characteristics and Results of the Three Completed Randomized, Controlled Trials of Hemicraniectomy and Two Meta-analyses *(continued)*

Study	Design	Outcome	
		Medical Arm	**Surgical Arm**
	Meta-analysis of randomized controlled trials of surgery within 48 h versus medical management	mRS 0–3 at 12 mo: 23%	mRS 0–3 at 12 mo: 43% $p = .014$ NNT = 2 for survival and mRS ≤4 NNT = 4 for survival and mRS ≤3
Hemicraniectomy for massive middle cerebral artery territory infarction: a systematic review	138 patients Mean age 50 years (11–76 years old) All underwent hemicraniectomy and durotomy for infarction of MCA or MCA plus another territory Mean time to surgery 60 h (8–456)	Overall mortality 24% Mortality in age > 50 = 32%, age < 50 = 14% Functional independence or mild-moderated disability in 42% Death or severe disability in 58% Death or severe disability in age > 50 = 80%, age < 50 = 32%	

Abbreviations: CT, computed tomography; DWI, diffusion-weighted image; ICA, internal carotid artery; MCA, middle carotid artery; mRS, modified Rankin Scale; NIHSS, NIH Stroke Scale Scores; NNT, number needed to treat; NS, not significant.

Data from: Frank JI. Large hemispheric infarction, deterioration, and intracranial pressure. Neurology 1995;45(7):1286–1290.

Juttler E, Schwab S, Schmiedek P, et al. Decompressive Surgery for the Treatment of Malignant Infarction of the Middle Cerebral Artery (DESTINY): a randomized, controlled trial. Stroke 2007;38(9):2518–2525.

Vahedi K, Vicaut E, Mateo J, et al. Sequential-design, multicenter, randomized, controlled trial of early decompressive craniectomy in malignant middle cerebral artery infarction (DECIMAL Trial). Stroke 2007;38(9):2506–2517.

Vahedi K, Hofmeijer J, Juettler E, et al. Early decompressive surgery in malignant infarction of the middle cerebral artery: a pooled analysis of three randomised controlled trials. Lancet Neurol 2007;6(3):215–222.

Gupta R, Connolly ES, Mayer S, Elkind MS. Hemicraniectomy for massive middle cerebral artery territory infarction: a systematic review. Stroke 2004;35(2): 539–543.

Please see Table 6.5 for a description of the modified Rankin Scale.

- *Decompressive hemicraniectomy* has received a class IIa, level B recommendation from the AHA/ASA. A discussion of the risks, benefits, and potential outcomes with the family is recommended prior to proceeding with surgical intervention.[5]

■ Prognosis

The reported mortality rate for malignant stroke varies between 42 and 80% by natural history.[10,12,13] For cerebellar stroke, the death rate is ~20 % at 3 months, and 80% of the survivors have a good outcome.[16-17] Outcome after cerebellar stroke is correlated with the degree of effacement of the fourth ventricle and preoperative GCS. Neurosurgical procedures and improvement in intensive care management have improved mortality and functional outcome for patients with malignant ischemic stroke.

Pearls and Pitfalls

- Attempts at revascularization following AHA/ASA guidelines should be preeminent early after ischemic stroke.
- Patients with malignant cerebellar stroke may experience neurologic deterioration from brainstem effacement and development of hydrocephalus. Early suboccipital decompression and external ventricular drainage are life-saving procedures in these cases.
- Younger patients (<50 to 60 years old) with malignant MCA or ICA infarction should be considered for decompressive hemicraniectomy within 48 hours of symptom onset.[13]

References
1. Aiyagari V, Diringer MN. Management of large hemispheric strokes in the neurological intensive care unit. Neurologist 2002;8(3):152–162
2. Krieger DW, Demchuk AM, Kasner SE, Jauss M, Hantson L. Early clinical and radiological predictors of fatal brain swelling in ischemic stroke. Stroke 1999;30(2):287–292

3. Manno EM, Nichols DA, Fulgham JR, Wijdicks EF. Computed tomographic determinants of neurologic deterioration in patients with large middle cerebral artery infarctions. Mayo Clin Proc 2003;78(2):156–160

4. The National Institute of Neurological Disorders and Stroke rt-PA Stroke Study Group. Tissue plasminogen activator for acute ischemic stroke. N Engl J Med 1995;333(24):1581–1587

5. Adams HP Jr, del Zoppo G, Alberts MJ, et al. Guidelines for the early management of adults with ischemic stroke: a guideline from the American Heart Association/American Stroke Association Stroke Council, Clinical Cardiology Council, Cardiovascular Radiology and Intervention Council, and the Atherosclerotic Peripheral Vascular Disease and Quality of Care Outcomes in Research Interdisciplinary Working Groups: the American Academy of Neurology affirms the value of this guideline as an educational tool for neurologists. Stroke 2007;38(5):1655–1711

6. del Zoppo GJ, Higashida RT, Furlan AJ, Pessin MS, Rowley HA, Gent M. PROACT: a phase II randomized trial of recombinant pro-urokinase by direct arterial delivery in acute middle cerebral artery stroke. PROACT Investigators. Prolyse in Acute Cerebral Thromboembolism. Stroke 1998;29(1):4–11

7. Smith WS, Sung G, Saver J, et al. Mechanical thrombectomy for acute ischemic stroke: final results of the Multi MERCI trial. Stroke 2008;39(4):1205–1212

8. Smith WS, Sung G, Starkman S, et al. Safety and efficacy of mechanical embolectomy in acute ischemic stroke: results of the MERCI trial. Stroke 2005;36(7):1432–1438

9. Hacke W, Kaste M, Bluhmki E, Brozman M, Davalos A, Guidetti D, Larrue V, Lees KR, Medeghri Z, Machnig T, et al. Thrombolysis with alteplase 3 to 4.5 hours after acute ischemic stroke. The New England Journal of Medicine 2008, 359(13):1317–1329

10. Frank JI. Large hemispheric infarction, deterioration, and intracranial pressure. Neurology 1995;45(7):1286–1290

11. Kirollos RW, Tyagi AK, Ross SA, van Hille PT, Marks PV. Management of spontaneous cerebellar hematomas: a prospective treatment protocol. Neurosurgery 2001;49(6):1378–1386 discussion 1386–1377

12. Gupta R, Connolly ES, Mayer S, Elkind MS. Hemicraniectomy for massive middle cerebral artery territory infarction: a systematic review. Stroke 2004;35(2):539–543

13. Vahedi K, Hofmeijer J, Juettler E, et al. Early decompressive surgery in malignant infarction of the middle cerebral artery: a pooled analysis of three randomised controlled trials. Lancet Neurol 2007;6(3):215–222

14. Juttler E, Schwab S, Schmiedek P, et al. Decompressive Surgery for the Treatment of Malignant Infarction of the Middle Cerebral Artery (DESTINY): a randomized, controlled trial. Stroke 2007;38(9):2518–2525

15. Vahedi K, Vicaut E, Mateo J, et al. Sequential-design, multicenter, randomized, controlled trial of early decompressive craniectomy in malignant middle cerebral artery infarction (DECIMAL Trial). Stroke 2007;38(9):2506–2517

16. Kase CS, Norrving B, Levine SR, et al. Cerebellar infarction: clinical and anatomic observations in 66 cases. Stroke 1993;24(1):76–83

17. Macdonell RA, Kalnins RM, Donnan GA. Cerebellar infarction: natural history, prognosis, and pathology. Stroke 1987;18(5):849–855

7 Cerebral Sinus Thrombosis

Isabel Fragata and Aman Patel

Thrombosis of cerebral veins and dural sinuses is an uncommon clinical entity, representing less than 1% of all stroke cases in adults. Cerebral sinus venous thrombosis (CVT) is more common in neonates and children than in adults; among adults, it is more common in women.[1] The mean age of onset is 39 years, and 75% of cases involve multiple veins and/or sinuses.[1] Obstruction of cerebral venous drainage can lead to increased venous and capillary pressure with subsequent blood–brain barrier breakdown and vasogenic cerebral edema, venous hemorrhage, and/or ischemia or cytotoxic edema. Cerebrospinal fluid (CSF) absorption is also impaired, further contributing to elevated intracranial pressure (ICP). Elevated ICP is most common with superior sagittal sinus obstruction, but it can occur with jugular or transverse sinus thrombosis. A high index of clinical suspicion and neuroimaging techniques are the key to diagnosis.[2]

Case Example

A 35-year-old woman on oral contraceptives has complained of headache for the last few days. She had been admitted for a focal seizure and is now stuporous, with a right-sided hemiparesis. On funduscopic examination, papilledema is noted.

Questions

- Is the patient protecting her airway?
- Is the patient pregnant?
- Is there any history of malignancy?
- Is the patient still seizing?
- Is there any sign of brain herniation?

Urgent Orders

- Assess airway, breathing, circulation (ABCs); consider intubation and follow seizure protocol, including administration of lorazepam and phenytoin (see Chapter 5).

- Elevate head to 30 degrees; initiate mannitol if there are signs of elevated ICP (see Chapter 15).

- Order urgent computed tomography (CT) scan followed by CT venography (CTV) or magnetic resonance venography (MRV).

■ History and Examination

History

- Assess for a history of hypercoagulable state, pregnancy/puerperium, malignancy, recent infection, inflammatory disease, dehydration (common with Crohn's disease), or drug use (particularly oral contraceptives + smoking and hormone replacement therapy).

- Variability in the clinical presentation of CVT is common. Headache is the most common complaint (90% of patients) and can sometimes resemble migraine with aura. Persistent postlumbar puncture headache should raise concern for CVT, as lumbar puncture can rarely precipitate CVT.

- Onset can be acute (<48 hours; typically with infectious etiology or during pregnancy/puerperium), subacute, or chronic (>30 days).

- Most frequent symptoms are headache, seizures (frequently associated with Todd's paresis), vision loss, encephalopathy, and motor/sensory deficits.

- Symptoms may fluctuate, which may reflect ongoing thrombosis and endogenous fibrinolysis.

■ Physical and Neurologic Examination

- Mental status: decreased alertness to coma; aphasia can occur with left transverse sinus thrombosis

- Fundoscopic exam: papilledema initially presents as an enlarging blind spot followed by color desaturation. Visual acuity loss is a late sign

- Visual field defects: hemianopsia (with vein of Labbé thrombosis)

- Cranial nerves: sixth (VI) nerve palsy (nonlocalizing sign, suggests intracranial hypertension); III, IV, V1, V2, or VI nerve palsy isolated or in combination suggests cavernous sinus thrombosis. VI nerve palsy is most common since this nerve is suspended in the middle of the cavernous sinus

- Motor/sensory deficits: depending on affected venous territory; can be bilateral and alternating in the case of superior sagittal sinus thrombosis

- Common syndromes are listed in **Table 7.1**.[3]

Table 7.1 Common Cerebral Sinus Thrombosis Syndromes

Location of CVT	Frequency%	Presenting Symptoms
Superior sagittal sinus	62	Motor deficits (predominantly affecting lower limbs); possible bilateral deficits Seizures Psychiatric symptoms
Transverse sinus	86	Intracranial hypertension, aphasia when left transverse sinus occluded
Cerebral cortical vein	17	Motor/sensory deficits according to territory Focal seizures
Deep venous system	11	Coma, alteration of mental status Bilateral motor deficits
Cavernous sinus	Rare	III, IV, V1, V2, or VI nerve palsy Orbital pain, chemosis, proptosis

Frequency column data from: Ferro JM, Canhão P, Stam J, et al. Prognosis of cerebral vein and dural sinus thrombosis: results of the International Study on Cerebral Vein and Dural Sinus Thrombosis (ISCVT). Stroke 2004;35(3):664–670.

Stam J. Thrombosis of the cerebral veins and sinuses. N Engl J Med 2005;352(17):1791–1798.

■ Differential Diagnosis

1. *Cerebral sinus thrombosis.* The most common causes are pregnancy and puerperium, oral contraceptives, local infections, and thrombophilia. Most often CVT is multifactorial: more than one cause can be found in 44% of patients. In 15% of patients, no inciting cause is found[1] (**Table 7.2**).

Table 7.2 Common Causes of Cerebral Sinus Thrombosis

Category	Causes
Hypercoagulable state (most common etiology found in 34% of patients)	Protein C, S, or antithrombin III deficiency; factor V Leiden mutation; prothrombin gene mutation; antiphospholipid syndrome (lupus anticoagulant/anticardiolipin antibody); nephrotic syndrome; hyperhomocysteinemia
Infectious (found in 10% of patients)	Encephalitis; cerebritis; meningitis; mastoiditis; otitis; sinusitis; mouth, face, and neck infections
Obstetric	Pregnancy and puerperium
Malignancy	CNS tumors with invasion of the venous sinus, hematologic cancers, hypercoagulable state due to malignancy
Inflammatory diseases	Vasculitis, lupus, Wegener's granulomatosis, inflammatory bowel disease (Crohn's and ulcerative colitis), Behçet's disease, thromboangiitis obliterans, sarcoidosis
Hematologic diseases	Polycythemia, thrombocythemia, paroxysmal nocturnal hemoglobinuria
Drugs	Oral contraceptives (particularly when combined with tobacco use or prothrombotic disease), hormone replacement therapy, asparaginase, tamoxifen, steroids, androgens
Trauma (including iatrogenic)	Head injury, lumbar puncture, neurosurgical procedures, jugular catheter occlusion
Other	Dehydration, congenital heart disease, thyroid disease

Abbreviation: CNS, central nervous system.

2. *Dural arteriovenous fistula (DAVF)*. DAVFs are characterized by a direct connection between meningeal arteries and dural venous sinuses or meningeal veins. DAVFs can be associated with sinus thrombosis or trauma. They are classified as type I—dural arterial supply drains anterograde into venous sinus; type II—dural arterial supply drains into the venous sinus, but high pressure in the sinus results in both anterograde drainage and retrograde drainage into subarachnoid veins; and type III—dural arterial supply drains retrograde into subarachnoid veins. Subarachnoid veins can form varices and aneurysms and are prone to rupture. Both type II and III DAVF should be treated endovascularly or surgically to prevent hemorrhage.[4]

3. *Stroke (ischemic or hemorrhagic)* can present with acute deficits and seizures. Headache and mental status changes are more common with hemorrhagic stroke (ICH, SAH). Venous infarct and ICH can both be caused by sinus thrombosis.

4. *Brain tumor*. A brain tumor can occasionally have strokelike sudden presentation or present with seizure, headache, and/or evidence of elevated ICP.

5. *Encephalitis/cerebritis/abscess*. Look for signs of infection, including fever, elevated white blood cell count (WBC), and lumbar puncture results. Sinus thrombosis may accompany these infections.

6. *Benign intracranial hypertension (pseudotumor cerebri)*. This can present with headache and VI nerve palsy, but encephalopathy, focal deficits, and seizure are atypical and should prompt a more thorough evaluation. Patients with suspected pseudotumor cerebri should undergo MR or CT venography (MRV or CTV) imaging to rule out sinus thrombosis.

Life-Threatening Diagnoses Not to Miss

- *Cerebral sinus thrombosis*. Expedient treatment can prevent intracranial hemorrhage.
- *Encephalitis/cerebritis/abscess* requires urgent antibiotic administration.
- *Any process that causes dangerous elevations in ICP* should be diagnosed and managed immediately.

■ Diagnostic Evaluation

- *Imaging studies*
  - ◦ Head CT:
    - Can be normal in up to 30% of CVT cases[5]
    - Noncontrast CT: The cord sign (present in 25% of cases, represents a spontaneously hyperdense thrombosed cortical vein), dense triangle sign (hyperdense torcular and/or posterior superior sagittal sinus)
    - Postcontrast CT: The empty delta sign (present in 16 to 46% of cases, represents lack of filling of the torcular and/or the posterior superior sagittal sinus)
    - Indirect/nonspecific signs of CVT include brain edema, hemorrhagic lesions, gyral enhancement, intense contrast enhancement of the falx, and tentorium.
    - CT also helps detect local infectious causes of CVT (otitis, mastoiditis, sinusitis).
  - ◦ CTV: (CT venography)
    - Increasingly and reliably used to diagnose CVT, with a reported sensitivity of 95% when compared with digital subtraction angiography (DSA)[6]
    - Fast alternative to magnetic resonance imaging (MRI), especially in patients with pacemakers or ferromagnetic implants. CTV is not subject to flow-related artifacts and pitfalls in interpretation as is MRI.
  - ◦ MRI and MRV: (MR venography)
    - Extremely sensitive for diagnosis and follow-up of CVT (**Fig. 7.1**)
    - Important pitfalls: Thrombus in the acute phase can easily be mistaken for a normal flow-void in the sinus; beware of diagnosing a nondominant transverse sinus as thrombosed; areas of slow flow in the sinuses can mimic thrombosis; time-of-flight (TOF) venography may reconstruct high signal thrombus as normal flow within the sinus (**Table 7.3**).
  - ◦ DSA:
    - Reserved for cases where a therapeutic intervention is required or when noninvasive tests are inconclusive.

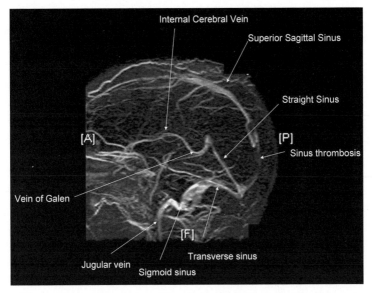

Fig. 7.1 Magnetic resonance venography demonstrating superior sagittal sinus thrombosis. A, anterior; P, posterior; F, foramen magnum

- Better for assessment of cortical vein thrombosis and dural arteriovenous fistula, which may be associated with CVT.
- Angiographic signs of CVT: Lack of filling of the venous sinuses or deep veins, "stop sign" (abrupt termination of a cortical vein), corkscrew appearance of collateral veins, or increased collateral veins draining an area of venous thrombosis.

Table 7.3 Appearance of Blood at Different Ages on Magnetic Resonance Imaging

Phase	Time	T1	T2	Hemoglobin
Hyperacute	<24 h	Gray/black	White	Oxyhemoglobin (intracellular)
Acute	1–3 d	Gray/black	Black	Deoxyhemoglobin (intracellular)
Early subacute	3–7 d	White	Black	Methemoglobin (intracellular)
Late subacute	7–14 d	White	White	Methemoglobin (extracellular)
Chronic	>14 d	Black/gray	Black	Hemosiderin (extracellular)

- Beware: Hypoplasia of the anterior portion of the sagittal sinus and hypoplasia of a nondominant transverse sinus are common normal variants.

- *Other diagnostics*
  - ○ CSF: May show raised pressure, elevated protein, and mild pleocytosis. A lumbar puncture may be therapeutic (if a large volume of 30 mL is removed) for headache or vision loss. A lumbar puncture (LP) should be performed in patients with suspected infectious etiology of sinus thrombosis.
  - ○ Electroencephalogram: Generalized or focal slow activity

- *Laboratory studies*
  - ○ Check complete blood count (CBC), chemistry panel, liver function tests, coagulation studies, urine protein (if nephrotic syndrome suspected), antinuclear antibody (ANA), homocysteine, factor V Leiden mutation, prothrombin gene mutation, antiphospholipid/anticardiolipin antibodies, lupus anticoagulant, protein C/S activity and level, antithrombin III (all hypercoagulable studies with the exception of genetic studies should be assessed before initiation of heparin or warfarin [Bristol-Myers Squibb, New York, NY]). Keep in mind that most of these studies may be positive as acute phase reactants and should be retested at 6 weeks if initially positive.

■ Treatment

1. *Anticoagulation* is important for venous recanalization to prevent thrombus propagation and to prevent systemic thrombosis in those with hypercoagulable states.

   - A randomized trial of heparin versus placebo in patients with CVT was stopped early for excess mortality in the placebo arm.[7] Another randomized trial of low molecular weight heparin versus placebo showed a nonstatistically significant benefit for the treatment group.[8] A meta-analysis of these two trials found a nonstatistically significant decrease in mortality and death or dependency with treatment.[9]

   - The 2006 American Heart Association/American Stroke Association guidelines recommend:[7]

Unfractionated heparin or low molecular weight heparin is reasonable, even in the presence of hemorrhagic infarction (class IIa, level B evidence).

Continuation of anticoagulation medication with an oral anticoagulant agent is reasonable for 3 to 6 months, followed by antiplatelet therapy (class IIa, level C evidence). According to the 2008 American College of Chest Physicians guidelines on management of ischemic stroke, patients with CVT should receive anticoagulation with unfractionated heparin or low molecular weight heparin during the acute phase, even in the presence of hemorrhage (Grade IB). Vitamin K antagonist therapy should be continued in these patients for up to 12 months (target INR 2–3) (Grade IB).[10]

- Anticoagulation medication should be continued for a longer duration in patients with thrombophilia or recurrent CVT.

2. *Thrombolysis.* When clinical deterioration occurs despite medical therapy, endovascular thrombolysis is considered an alternative. Local infusion of recombinant tissue plasminogen activator (rTPA; doses ranging between 8 and 300 mg) and/or mechanical thrombolysis can be performed, using balloons and rheolytic catheters as adjuncts to chemical thrombolysis.[11] Evidence for the use of thrombolysis in CVT was recently reviewed.[12] Although clinical outcomes are good (78% of patients had encephalopathy or coma before therapy; after treatment, 86% of patients were independent at discharge, with a total 5% mortality), they are only slightly better than those obtained with systemic anticoagulation.[13] Thrombolysis adds the risk of parenchymal and systemic bleeding, which is significantly higher than in patients treated with heparin alone. Considered altogether, endovascular thrombolysis appears to be justified only in cases of failure of medical therapy and persistent clinical deterioration.

3. Management of elevated intracranial pressure. Venous stasis, brain infarction, and hemorrhage contribute to elevated ICP in CVT. The best way to treat elevated ICP is to relieve the venous obstruction or prevent propagation with anticoagulation. Large volume lumbar puncture can be therapeutic for headache and vision loss (see Chapter 15).

4. Management of seizures. Seizures are a manifestation of CVT in 45% of adult patients.[14] All patients who seize should receive antiepileptics. In patients with elevated ICP and hemorrhage or focal deficits but no history of seizure, prophylactic antiepileptics can be considered (see Chapter 5).

■ Prognosis

CVT has a favorable prognosis if treated early in its course, with a good neurologic outcome in 80% of patients. Mortality in the acute phase is around 4% and 8% at 16-month follow-up. Main causes of death in CVT are massive intracerebral hemorrhages causing transtentorial herniation, intercurrent complications (sepsis, seizures, and pulmonary embolism), and underlying condition (systemic infection, end-stage cancer). Predictors of poor outcome are altered mental status, coma, intracerebral hemorrhage on admission, deep venous system thrombosis, central nervous system (CNS) infection, any malignancy, older age, male gender, and posterior fossa lesions.[13] Early recanalization of the sinus is a good prognostic factor and occurs in 40 to 90% of patients within the first 4 months, but clinical recovery may occur in the absence of recanalization. Recanalization is most common in deep cerebral veins and cavernous sinuses and less common in the transverse sinuses. Recurrent thromboses rates are ~1 to 2% per year.

Pearls and Pitfalls

- The key to diagnosis of CVT is keeping it in mind: always consider CVT in patients with headache, focal deficits, seizures, and altered consciousness.

- Look for local infectious causes of CVT: they are potentially serious but treatable.

- CTV and MRV are the standard studies in the diagnosis of CVT.

- Anticoagulation is the first-line treatment in CVT and can be complemented by endovascular thrombolysis in cases of treatment failure.

- Patients should receive acute anticoagulation treatment even in the context of intracerebral hemorrhage.

References

1. Ferro JM, et al. Prognosis of cerebral vein and dural sinus thrombosis: results of the International Study on Cerebral Vein and Dural Sinus Thrombosis (ISCVT). Stroke, 2004;35(3):664–70.
2. Bousser MG, Ferro JM. Cerebral venous thrombosis: an update. Lancet Neurol 2007;6(2):162–170
3. Stam J. Thrombosis of the cerebral veins and sinuses. N Engl J Med 2005;352(17):1791–1798
4. Borden JA, Wu JK, Shucart WA. A proposed classification for spinal and cranial dural arteriovenous fistulous malformations and implications for treatment. J Neurosurg 1995;82(2):166–179
5. Bousser MG, Russell RR. In: Warlow C, Van Gijn J, eds. Major Problems in Neurology. ed. C. Warlow, Van Gijn J. London: WB Saunders; 1997:27, 104.
6. Wetzel SG, et al. Cerebral veins: comparative study of CT venography with intraarterial digital subtraction angiography. AJNR Am J Neuroradiol 1999;20(2): 249–255
7. Sacco RL, Adams R, Albers G, Alberts MJ, Benavente O, Furie K, Goldstein LB, Gorelick P, Halperin J, Harbaugh R, Johnston SC, Katzan I, Kelly-Hayes M, Kenton EJ, Marks M, Schwamm LH, Tomsick T. Guidelines for prevention of stroke in patients with ischemic stroke or transient ischemic attack: A statement for healthcare professionals from the American Heart Association/American Stroke Association council on stroke: Co-sponsored by the council on cardiovascular radiology and intervention: The American academy of neurology affirms the value of this guideline. Stroke 2006;37:577–617
8. de Bruijn SF, Stam J. Randomized, placebo-controlled trial of anticoagulant treatment with low-molecular-weight heparin for cerebral sinus thrombosis. Stroke 1999;30(3):484–488
9. Stam J, De Bruijn SF, DeVeber G. Anticoagulation for cerebral sinus thrombosis. Cochrane Database Syst Rev 2002; (4):CD002005
10. Albers GW, Amarenco P, Easton JD, Sacco RL, Teal P. Antithrombotic and thrombolytic therapy for ischemic stroke: American college of chest physicians evidence-based clinical practice guidelines (8th edition). Chest 2008;133:630S–669S
11. Benveniste RJ, Patel AB, Post KD. Management of cerebral venous sinus thrombosis. Neurosurg Q 2004;14:27–35
12. Canhão P, Falcao F, Ferro JM. Thrombolytics for cerebral sinus thrombosis: a systematic review. Cerebrovasc Dis 2003;15(3):159–166
13. Canhão P, et al. Causes and predictors of death in cerebral venous thrombosis. Stroke 2005;36(8):1720–1725
14. Ferro JM, et al. Early seizures in cerebral vein and dural sinus thrombosis: risk factors and role of antiepileptics. Stroke 2008;39(4):1152–1158

8 Acute Spinal Cord Injury

Scott Meyer, Jennifer A. Frontera,
Arthur Jenkins III, and Tanvir Choudhri

Spinal cord injuries (SCIs) inflict a significant burden on patients, families, and society as a whole. The spinal cord consists of 31 segments and terminates near L1 (T10–L3) in adults. Most injuries involve not only the cord, but exiting nerves as well. SCI is most common in the young (average age 29 years) and in men (78%).[1] The most common causes of SCI are motor vehicle accidents (MVAs; 47%), falls (23%), violence (14%), sporting accidents (9%), and other causes (7%).[1] Alcohol plays a role in up to 25% of SCI and underlying spinal disease such as cervical spondylosis, atlantoaxial instability, osteoporosis, and spinal arthropathies can make patients more prone to SCI. Roughly half of all SCIs involve the cervical cord.

SCI can be divided into two separate mechanisms of action: primary and secondary SCI. Primary SCI occurs as a result of pathologic flexion, rotation, extension, compression, contusion, or shearing of the spinal cord. This can be caused by a fracture–dislocation, tearing of ligaments, or disruption and/or herniation of the intervertebral disks. Kinetic injury transmitted from bullet wounds or blasts can cause cord injury even when no foreign body has entered the spinal column. The primary SCI is irreversible, and prevention of the initial injury is the primary modifiable feature. Secondary SCI is a complex chain of events linked to ischemia, hypoxia, edema, excitotoxicity, and inflammation with changes on the cellular level. Aims of intervention and management are to limit the effects of secondary injury processes as well as prevent associated medical morbidities.

Case Example

A 19-year-old man has just arrived by ambulance after a fall from his motorcycle and is complaining of neck pain, weakness, and numbness in all four extremities.

Questions

- Are there any external signs of injury?
- Is there additional head or body trauma?
- What is the current level of consciousness?
- Is he able to move all of his extremities, and is there any change since the event?
- Is he hemodynamically stable?

Urgent Orders

- Address airway, breathing, circulation (ABCs). Up to 33% of patients with cervical spine injury will require intubation. Rapid-sequence intubation with in-line spinal immobilization is the preferred method when an airway is urgently needed. For elective intubations, use of a flexible fiberoptic laryngoscope or video-assisted intubating device may be appropriate.

- Appropriate spinal immobilization includes placement of a rigid cervical collar, barriers to lateral head movements, use of a backboard, and log-roll movements.

- Upon confirmation of neurologic deficit with suspected SCI, consider methylprednisolone for 24 to 48 hours (see below).

- Place Foley catheter to avoid harm due to bladder distention.

- Address other potential trauma. Order focused abdominal sonogram for trauma (FAST exam evaluates pericardium, right and left upper abdomen, and pelvic region for blood) if indicated; computed tomography (CT) of chest, abdomen, and pelvis when the patient is stabilized.

- Order complete blood count (CBC), chemistry panel, coagulation studies, type and cross, toxicology screen, arterial blood gas, and pregnancy test (if applicable).

- Maintain PaO_2 >60 mm Hg and systolic blood pressure (SBP) ≥90 mm Hg.

- Perform noncontrast head CT, spine CT, and/or cervical x-rays (see below).

■ History and Examination

History

- Events surrounding the accident: Use of a seatbelt or helmet, type of vehicle (motorcycle or automobile), position of the patient in the vehicle, direction from which the vehicle was hit, speed of collision, windshield or steering wheel damage (may indicate concomitant injury, aortic rupture, or other systemic injury)
- Assess for use of ethyl alcohol (EtOH) or illicit drugs, as these may confound the exam.
- Passive rewarming of hypothermic trauma patients is crucial prior to assessing the neurologic examination.

Physical Examination

- Close attention should be paid to the hemodynamic status of the patient. Because SCI may be associated with other traumatic injuries, it is important to monitor blood pressure and heart rate. In addition, neurogenic shock may result in bradycardia and hypotension. Adequate oxygen saturation and blood pressure are important to monitor to help prevent ischemic insult to the spinal cord.
- The body should be inspected for signs of external trauma. Palpation of the spinal column to assess for tenderness or step-off should be undertaken. The seventh (and occasionally even the sixth) spinous process is prominent and should not be confused with subluxation.
- Make sure that full spinal precautions are maintained throughout the examination.

Neurologic Examination

- A full neurologic examination, including assessment of mental status, cranial nerves, motor skills, and reflexes, as well as a sensory and cerebellar exam, should be performed on all patients.

- Abnormal mental status may be a sign of the need for airway protection, potential intracranial injury, or intoxication and may limit the motor and sensory portions of the initial neurologic examination.

- All muscle groups should be examined and recorded using a 5-point scale.

- A complete sensory examination should be performed, including assessment of a sensory level (using pinprick and vibration) and crossed sensory signs (indicative of a Brown-Séquard hemicord lesion).

- Reflexes should be assessed, including deep tendon reflexes, sphincter tone, and the bulbocavernosus reflex. Reflexes may be depressed acutely after injury and become hyperacute over days to weeks.

- Assessment of sacral function (perineal sensation, bulbocavernous reflex S3–S4, anal wink S5, priapism, rectal tone, and urine retention or postvoid residual) is important for prognostication.

See **Table 8.1** for the American Spinal Injury Association (ASIA) Scale and **Table 8.2** for examination findings in different types of SCI.

Table 8.1 American Spinal Injury Association Scale

Category	Description
A	Complete: No motor or sensory function is preserved below the neurologic level through sacral segments S4–S5.
B	Incomplete: Sensory but not motor function is preserved below the neurologic level and includes S4–S5.
C	Incomplete: Motor function is preserved below the neurologic level, and more than half of key muscles below the neurologic level have a muscle grade <3.
D	Incomplete: Motor function is preserved below the neurologic level, and at least half of key muscles below the neurologic level have a muscle grade ≥3.
E	Motor and sensory functions are normal.

Data from: Clinical assessment after acute cervical spinal cord injury. Neurosurgery 2002; 50(3, Suppl)S21–S29.

Table 8.2 Examination Findings in Different Types of Spinal Cord Injuries

Clinical Presentation	Motor	Sensory	Reflexes	Comments
Complete cord injury	Spared strength above the lesion, reduced at the level below the lesion, and paralysis caudal. Muscle tone is flaccid.	Spared sensation above the level of injury, reduced sensation at the level of injury, and no sensation below, including S4–S5.	Reflexes are acutely absent. Bulbocavernosus reflex is absent.	Urinary retention and bladder distention occur. Priapism may occur.
Incomplete cord injury	Partial preservation of motor function below the level of injury	Partially preserved in dermatomes below the injury. Sensation spared to a greater extent than motor function.	Reflexes are acutely absent. Bulbocavernosus reflex is often present.	Anal sensation often present.
Central cord syndrome	Upper >lower extremity motor impairment. Distal >proximal loss of function in extremity	Variable loss below the level of injury Cape-like distribution of pain and temperature loss Dysesthesias (burning sensation) common Sacral sparing	Reflexes are acutely absent.	Bladder dysfunction present. Typical in setting of mild trauma with cervical spondylosis
Anterior cord syndrome	Variable motor loss below the level of the injury	Sparing of dorsal columns: loss of pain, temperature, and variable light touch with preserved vibration and proprioception Autonomic dysfunction can occur.	Reflexes are acutely absent.	Lesions affecting anterior two-thirds of spinal cord, related to retropulsed disk or anterior spinal artery injury

(Continued)

Table 8.2 Examination Findings in Different Types of Spinal Cord Injuries *(continued)*

Clinical Presentation	Motor	Sensory	Reflexes	Comments
Brown-Séquard	Ipsilateral motor loss	Ipsilateral loss of vibration, proprioception, and light touch; contralateral pain; temperature loss	Reflexes are acutely absent.	Hemicord syndrome
Transient paralysis and spinal shock	Flaccid paralysis eventually converts to spastic paresis. Complete recovery can occur (most often in young patients with sports injuries). Spinal concussion refers to complete recovery without structural damage.	Sensory loss below the lesion	Reflexes are acutely absent.	Absent bowel and bladder control. Priapism may occur. Bradycardia and hypotension may occur—may last hours to weeks.
Conus medullaris lesion	Variable motor loss in lower limbs	Variable sensory loss in lower limbs	Initially decreased, followed by hyperreflexia	Sacral cord injury with or without injury to lumbosacral roots Bowel and bladder dysfunction
Cauda equina lesions	Variable motor loss in lower limbs	Variable sensory loss in lower limbs	Areflexia	Injury to lumbosacral nerve roots. Bowel and bladder dysfunction

■ Differential Diagnosis

Acute Presentation

1. *Spinal cord trauma*
   - *Fracture of bony elements with cord or nerve injury*
     - ◦ *Jefferson fracture* (**Fig. 8.1**): Typically a four-part fracture of the atlas (C1), with bilateral fractures to the anterior and posterior arches, usually from axial load compression (such as from a diving injury)
     - ◦ *Hangman's fracture (traumatic spondylolisthesis)* (**Fig. 8.2**): Bilateral pars fracture of axis (C2) vertebral body with various degrees of anterior subluxation and disruption of the C2/3 disk space, usually due to extension trauma from an MVA or hanging
   - *Ligamentous injury* (injury causing subluxation may only be seen on dynamic studies such as flexion-extension plain films or magnetic resonance imaging [MRI])
   - *Herniation of intervertebral disk*

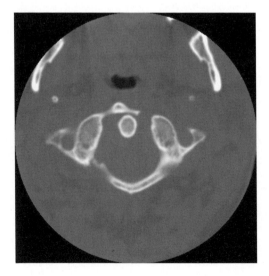

Fig. 8.1 Computed tomography scan demonstrating a C1 Jefferson fracture.

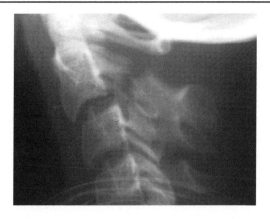

Fig. 8.2 Lateral x-ray demonstrating a C2 hangman's fracture.

- *Penetrating injury* (bullet, knife wound, etc.)
- *Kinetic injury* (blast or nearby bullet wound)
- *Spinal cord injury without radiographic abnormality (SCIWORA)*: More common in children; may be due to longitudinal distraction or transient ligamentous deformation with spontaneous reduction

2. *Vascular.* The blood supply to the cord consists of one anterior and two posterior arteries.
   - *Carotid/vertebral dissection* can occur in the setting of trauma or bony fracture. Consider arterial imaging with CT angiogram, magnetic resonance angiography (MRA), or digital subtraction angiography.
   - *Spinal cord infarction* can be *due to vessel disruption, emboli, or hypoperfusion.* T4–T8 represents the watershed territory between the anterior spinal artery and the artery of Adamkiewicz originating at T9. At any particular level, the central part of the cord is the watershed area. Cervical hyperextension injuries can cause ischemia, resulting in central cord syndrome. Minor vascular supply comes from branches of the vertebral artery and thyrocervical trunk as well, so injury to these structures may lead to ischemia.
   - *Vascular malformations*
   - *Epidural hematoma*

Subacute-Chronic Presentation

1. *Inflammatory diseases.* Transverse myelitis, sarcoid, paraneoplastic syndromes

2. *Infections.* Epidural abscess, bacterial diskitis, viral transverse myelitis, human immunodeficiency virus (HIV) myelopathy, human T-cell lymphotropic virus (HTLV-1) myelopathy, syphilis, tuberculosis, schistosomiasis

3. *Toxic/metabolic.* Subacute combined degeneration (B12 deficiency), radiation myelopathy, nitrous oxide poisoning, Vitamin E deficiency

4. *Neoplasms.* Extra-axial metastases with epidural compression, intramedullary tumors such as astrocytoma and ependymoma

5. *Inherited or degenerative.* Amyotrophic lateral sclerosis (ALS), hereditary spastic paraparesis, adrenomyeloneuropathy, Friedreich's ataxia

Life-Threatening Diagnoses Not to Miss

- *Unstable fractures* such as hangman's fracture or anterior/posterior column disruption requiring operative intervention (traction may be contraindicated)

- *Acute epidural hematoma* requiring surgical evacuation

■ Diagnostic Evaluation

- *Imaging*
  - Plain films: Three-view evaluation of the cervical spine including anteroposterior, lateral, and open-mouth odontoid views. It is crucial that all areas of the cervical spine be visualized in a true nonrotated lateral view. Oblique views are helpful for suspected lateral mass or facet injury. A swimmer's view should be performed if the C7/T1 vertebral bodies are not well visualized. The basion (anterior aspect of the foramen magnum) and opisthion (posterior aspect of the foramen magnum) must be visualized along with the remainder of the cervical spine, including the C7/T1 disk space and facet joints, as well as all seven cervical spinous processes. The odontoid view allows for assessment of the odontoid process and C1–C2 lateral mass articula-

tion. Neurologic symptoms and signs with normal plain films require further evaluation.

- CT: The speed at which a CT can be acquired and its sensitivity to delineate cervical fractures make it a viable alternative to plain films. When performed to evaluate the cervical spine, imaging should be carried caudal to T4, as the upper thoracic vertebrae are often poorly visualized on plain films. CT also provides information about the extent of a fracture, including the degree of compression and canal compromise, and whether the foramina transversarium is involved.

- MRI: MRI is superior to CT in visualization of the soft tissue, ligaments, disks, and epidural masses, whereas CT better visualizes bone. Indications for an MRI include neurologic deficit not explained by fracture, SCIWORA, surgical planning, and prognosis. MRI may detect a herniated disk or epidural hematoma not seen on other imaging studies and may demonstrate changes within the cord from injury without associated fracture. MRA and/or neck MRI with fat saturation can be useful for identifying vessel dissection.

- Clearing the cervical spine: The Canadian C-spine rule[2] was developed for adults presenting with blunt trauma to the head/neck, stable vital signs, and a Glasgow Coma Score (GCS) of 15. It states that radiography should be performed in patients with any of the following: age ≥65 years, dangerous mechanism of injury (fall >1 m or five stairs, axial load such as diving, MVA at high speed, motorized recreational vehicle accident, bicycle accident with immovable object), or paresthesias in the extremities. In patients with none of the above, low-risk factors include simple rear end MVA, sitting position in emergency room, ambulatory at any time, delayed onset of neck pain, and absence of midline cervical spine tenderness. Radiography should be performed if none of the low-risk factors are present, and active range of motion should be performed in patients with any low-risk factor. Patients who are unable to actively rotate the head 45 degrees to the left and right should undergo radiography. The NEXUS criteria[3] recommend radiography in all trauma patients unless there is no posterior midline cervical spine tenderness, no evidence of intoxication, normal level of alertness, no focal neurologic deficits, and no painful distracting injuries. If the patient has altered mental status, then the cervical spine should be immobilized until a clinical exam and three-view plain films or high-resolution CT are possible to conduct safely. The sensitivity of three-view plain films for detecting cervical spine injury is ~93%.[4]

Controversy exists over the method of clearing the C-spine in comatose patients with a normal CT and/or three-view plain films because ligamentous injury can be present in a small percentage of patients and can be devastating if not diagnosed. Options include static flexion-extension films, which carry a risk of exacerbating neurologic injury, flexion-extension fluoroscopy under the guidance of an experienced neurosurgeon, or MRI (the sensitivity of MRI decreases after 72 hours). In a recent meta-analysis of patients with normal plain films or CT and blunt injury, MRI had a negative predictive value of 100%, a 94% positive predictive value, and detected injury in 21% of patients with normal plain films and/or CT.[5]

■ Treatment

Medical Treatment

See Urgent Orders section.

- *Methylprednisolone (MPS).* There is extensive controversy surrounding the use of MPS in the acute phase of SCI. Several studies have shown its effectiveness in patients with nonpenetrating SCI, although several have questioned its benefit. The National Acute Spinal Cord Injury Studies (NASCIS III) demonstrated modest benefits, although long-term outcomes are unclear. There is a significant incidence of complications related to steroid use, including infections, poor wound healing, and psychiatric side effects, among others.[6,7] The use of steroids is considered a treatment option for nonpenetrating acute SCI by the American Association of Neurological Surgeons (AANS) and the Congress of Neurological Surgeons (CNS).[8] According to CNS guidelines, "Treatment with methylprednisolone for either 24 or 48 hours is recommended as an option in the treatment of patients with acute spinal cord injuries that should be undertaken only with the knowledge that the evidence suggesting harmful side effects is more consistent than any suggestion of clinical benefit." The following treatment suggestions can be made, if the patient does not have medical conditions that preclude the use of steroids (diabetes, active infections, etc.):

- ◦ MPS should be started within 8 hours of acute spinal cord injury, and within 3 hours if possible.
- ◦ Initially, a loading dose of 30 mg/kg over 15 minutes is given. This is followed by 5.4 mg/kg/h for either 23 hours (if initiated within 3 hours) or 47 hours (if initiated 3 to 8 hours after injury).

- *Neurogenic shock.* Autonomic function is transmitted in the anterior anteromedial tract of the spinal cord. Sympathetic fibers exit at C7/T1 to L2 and parasympathetic fibers at S2–S4. Higher level lesions cause more autonomic dysfunction. Neurogenic shock refers to hypotension, bradycardia, reflex vasodilation, and hypothermia that result from autonomic disruption after SCI. Spinal shock refers to complete loss of cord function below and sometimes even a few levels above the injury level, including reflexes and rectal tone with accompanying autonomic dysfunction. Intravenous fluid resuscitation may be required if the patient is hypovolemic. Patients may require norepinephrine to provide both α and β adrenergic stimulation. In rare cases external pacing or atropine may be necessary for symptomatic bradycardia. Neurogenic shock below T6 is uncommon, and in lesions below this level hypotension must by assumed due to hemorrhage until proven otherwise. Chronic autonomic dysreflexia can occur with episodic hypertension, bradycardia, flushing, and sweating. Hyperreflexia is usually a late (>1 week) finding, so presence in a patient with acute injury suggests antecedent spasticity, not an acute change.

- *Respiratory.* The degree of respiratory dysfunction depends on the level of injury. With C1–C2 injury, vital capacity is 5 to 10% of normal, and cough is absent. With C3–C6 injury, vital capacity is 20% of normal, and cough is ineffective. With T2–T4 injury, vital capacity is 30 to 50% of normal, and cough is weak. Below T11 respiratory dysfunction is minimal. Diaphragm function contributes to 65% of inspiratory effort; the rest is due to intercostals from T1–T11, trapezoid, sternocleidomastoid, and scalene activity.[9] Those with SCI frequently develop pulmonary complications such as atelectasis, mucous plugging, pneumonia, and pulmonary embolism.

- *Deep venous prophylaxis.* Without prophylaxis, acute SCI patients have the highest risk of deep vein thrombosis (DVT; 60 to 80%)

among all hospitalized groups. Level I evidence exists for the use of low molecular weight heparin over unfractionated heparin as soon as hemostasis is achieved for DVT prophylaxis (American College of Chest Physicians [ACCP] grade 1B). Inferior vena cava (IVC) filter placement for prophylaxis is not recommended (ACCP grade 1C).[10] DVT prophylaxis should be continued for 12 weeks in patients with complete spinal cord injuries (see Chapter 18).

- *Gastrointestinal.* SCI patients are at high risk for stress ulcers, especially if they have been treated with steroids, and should receive a proton pump inhibitor or H2 blocker.

- *Urinary catheterization is preferred* to indwelling catheters to limit urinary tract infections beyond the acute period.

Surgical Treatment

- *Closed reduction.* For cervical fracture with subluxation, traction involves using tongs or a halo headpiece. Three to 5 pounds per vertebral level is applied, taking lateral x-rays after each increment of 5 pounds is applied (maximum 35 pounds, although higher weights can be applied on a case-by-case basis).

- *Open decompression.* Indications include significant cord compression with neurologic deficits that are not amendable or do not respond to closed reduction or an unstable vertebral fracture or dislocation. There is evidence in animal studies that early decompression (within 8 hours) of spinal cord compression leads to neurologic improvement.[11,12] There exists controversy over the safety, utility, and timing of surgical intervention. If the patient does not have any other life-threatening trauma or associated medical problems, it can be recommended that urgent decompression be performed within 24 hours. In addition, there is evidence that surgery reduces the length of stay and may reduce medical complications after the SCI. Deferred surgery in ASIA A patients for stabilization is an option.

■ Prognosis

Up to 20% of SCI patients will die early after admission. The most important clinical prognostic factors are age and completeness of injury. Patients typically fare better if they are younger and have an incomplete lesion. Most recovery takes place in the first 3 to 6 months. Ten to 15% of patients with ASIA A grade injury will improve to some extent, though only 3% will improve to ASIA D level. Of ASIA B patients, 54% recover to ASIA C or D. Among ASIA C or D patients, 86% will regain some ambulatory function.[13] MRI findings including higher calculated maximum spinal cord compression, spinal cord hemorrhage, and edema are signs of a poor prognosis for neurologic recovery after SCI. **Table 8.3** shows the estimated life expectancies in years according to the National Spinal Cord Injury Statistical Center.[1] The leading cause of death was once renal failure; however, currently the most common causes of death are pneumonia, pulmonary emboli, and sepsis.[1]

Table 8.3 Life Expectancy in Years Based on Age at the Time of Injury and Degree of Initial Neurological Injury

Age at Injury	No SCI	Motor Function at Any Level	Paraplegic	Low Tetraplegic (C5–C8)	High Tetraplegic (C1–C4)	Ventilator Dependent at Any Level
20	78.4	73.3	65.6	60.6	56.1	36.6
40	79.5	74.8	68.0	63.5	63.8	60.2
60	82.2	78.3	73.1	70.2	67.9	61.4

Abbreviation: SCI, spinal cord injury.

Pearls and Pitfalls

- Observe all spinal precautions and maintain neutral alignment until verification of the absence of instability in SCI.

- Acute hypotension in the setting of SCI should trigger a search for hemorrhage before neurogenic shock is diagnosed.

- SCI is an emergency. Timely administration of appropriate medical and surgical management is crucial to achieving optimal outcomes.

References

1. The National Spinal Cord Injury Statistical Center. Home page. Available at: www.spinalcord.uab.edu. Accessed 7/08.

2. Stiell IG, Wells GA, Vandemheen KL, et al. The Canadian C-spine rule for radiography in alert and stable trauma patients. JAMA 2001;286(15):1841–1848

3. Hoffman JR, Mower WR, Wolfson AB, et al. Validity of a set of clinical criteria to rule out injury to the cervical spine in patients with blunt trauma. National Emergency X-Radiography Utilization Study Group. N Engl J Med 2000;343(2):94–99

4. Ajani AE, Cooper DJ, Scheinkestel CD, et al. Optimal assessment of cervical spine trauma in critically ill patients: a prospective evaluation. Anaesth Intensive Care 1998;26(5):487–491

5. Muchow RD, Resnick DK, Abdel MP, et al. Magnetic resonance imaging (MRI) in the clearance of the cervical spine in blunt trauma: a meta-analysis. J Trauma 2008;64(1):179–189

6. Bracken MB, Shepard MJ, Collins WF Jr, et al. A randomized, controlled trial of methylprednisolone or naloxone in the treatment of acute spinal-cord injury. Results of the Second National Acute Spinal Cord Injury Study. N Engl J Med 1990;322(20):1405–1411

7. Bracken MB, Shepard MJ, Holford TR, et al. Administration of methylprednisolone for 24 or 48 hours or tirilazad mesylate for 48 hours in the treatment of acute spinal cord injury. Results of the Third National Acute Spinal Cord Injury Randomized Controlled Trial. National Acute Spinal Cord Injury Study. JAMA 1997;277(20):1597–1604

8. Chappell ET. Pharmacological therapy after acute cervical spinal cord injury. Neurosurgery 2002;51(3):855–856, author reply 856

9. Schreiber DM. Spinal cord injuries. eMedicine. Available at: www.emedicine.com/EMERG/topic553.htm. Accessed 7/08

10. Geerts WH, Pineo GF, Heit JA, et al. Prevention of venous thromboembolism: the Seventh ACCP Conference on Antithrombotic and Thrombolytic Therapy. Chest 2004; 126(3, Suppl):338S–400S

11. Carlson GD, et al. Sustained spinal cord compression. Part 1: Time-dependent effect on long-term pathophysiology. J Bone Joint Surg Am 2003;85-A(1):86–94

12. Fehlings MG, Perrin RG. The timing of surgical intervention in the treatment of spinal cord injury: a systematic review of recent clinical evidence. Spine 2006; 31(11, Suppl):S28–S35, discussion S36

13. Waters RL, Adkins RH, Yakura JS, Sie I. Motor and sensory recovery following incomplete tetraplegia. Arch Phys Med Rehabil 1994;75(3):306–311

9 Hypoxic Ischemic Encephalopathy

Adam Webb and Owen Samuels

More than 160,000 out-of-hospital cardiac arrests occur annually. Nearly 25% of patients receive cardiopulmonary resuscitation (CPR) either from bystanders or emergency services (EMS) personnel and many regain spontaneous circulation.[1] However, despite modern improvements in CPR and critical care, less than 10 to 20% will survive to hospital discharge.[2] Of those that do survive, many will have profound neurologic injury and disability.

Hypoxic-ischemic encephalopathy is the term used to describe brain injury after cardiac arrest, severe hypoxia, or prolonged hypotension. It shares some pathophysiologic mechanisms with other causes of global cerebral injury, such as respiratory arrest, severe hypoglycemia, and carbon monoxide poisoning.

After cardiac arrest, brain oxygen supply is depleted, setting off a cascade of injury. Within minutes, adenosine triphosphate (ATP) supplies are depleted, and energy-dependent membrane ion transport begins to fail. The excitotoxic neurotransmitter glutamate is released, and intracellular calcium accumulates activating proteases and phospholipases. A second period of injury begins when spontaneous circulation is restored. Several mechanisms contribute to reperfusion injury, including the formation of damaging oxygen free radicals and impaired autoregulation of cerebral blood flow. Initially after reperfusion there is rebound hyperemia followed by hypoperfusion, which is exacerbated by impaired cerebral microcirculation.

Specific areas of the brain are selectively vulnerable to global ischemia, including CA1 neurons of the hippocampus, cerebellar Purkinje cells, and pyramidal neurons in the cerebral cortex (layers 3, 5, and 6). Watershed regions between major cerebral vascular territories are also at risk for injury.

Case Example

You are called to evaluate an unresponsive patient in the emergency room. He is a 55-year-old man with a history of coronary artery disease who collapsed at a local mall. A bystander performed CPR using an automated external defibrillator, and the patient regained spontaneous circulation.

Questions

- How long was it before CPR was initiated?
- What was the rhythm during the initial arrest?
- Did the patient lose his blood pressure?
- How long was CPR performed before he regained spontaneous circulation?
- What are the vital signs right now?
- Is the patient following commands?
- Is the patient coagulopathic or actively bleeding?
- What is the patient's baseline functional status?
- What is the patient's cardiac history?

Urgent Orders

- Address airway, breathing, circulation (ABCs)
- Hold all sedating medications.
- Begin to induce hypothermia (see Physical Examination section on next page).

■ History and Examination

History

Review the EMS record or interview any witnesses to determine how much time elapsed between the time the patient collapsed and initiation of CPR. Did the patient receive any medications during resuscitation or intubation that might influence your exam (atropine, sedatives, neuromuscular blocking agents, etc.)?

Physical Examination

- Vital signs: Assess blood pressure, temperature, heart rate and rhythm, spontaneous respirations, breathing pattern, and oxygen saturation.
- Evidence of trauma: Remember that if the patient is found down, always assume trauma is a possibility, and immobilize the cervical spine.

Neurologic Examination

- A full neurologic examination, including assessment of mental status, cranial nerves, motor skills, and reflexes, as well as a sensory and cerebellar exam, should be performed on all patients.
- Level of consciousness: Verbal responses, eye opening, response to pain
- Cranial nerves: Pupillary responses, oculomotor responses, cold water caloric responses, corneal reflex, grimace to nasal stimulus or supraorbital pressure, gag and cough reflexes
- Motor skills: Tone, motor responses to sensory stimulus, spontaneous or purposeful movements, motor posturing

---

■ Differential Diagnosis

1. *Cardiac arrest.* Review the history of the arrest and rhythm strips. It is important to determine the type of arrest (cardiac origin: ventricular fibrillation or ventricular tachycardia; metabolic or pulmonary origin: pulseless electrical activity, asystole, bradycardia).

2. *Respiratory arrest*

3. *Profound hypoglycemia.* Assess for history of liver or renal failure, iatrogenic hypoglycemia, medication overdose.

4. *Drug overdose or toxic ingestion.* Review medication access, perform a toxicology screen.

5. *Trauma* (especially if history is not well established)

6. *Nonconvulsive status epilepticus.* When in doubt, check an electroencephalogram (EEG).

7. *Stroke.* A stroke can induce cardiac arrhythmias, and cardiac arrest can cause a focal stroke, especially in a patient with underlying cerebrovascular disease. Keep a high degree of suspicion in

patients with focal findings on exam. Always test vertical eye movements to command to rule out a locked-in syndrome. Bilateral anterior cerebral artery (ACA) infarcts can produce an akinetic mute state that may mimic a persistent vegetative state.

8. *Other metabolic derangements that may cause both cardiac and cerebral dysfunction* (i.e., acute renal failure)

9. *Carbon monoxide poisoning.* Look for pallor (more common) or cherry red skin (late sign), bright red retinal veins (early sensitive sign), and a history of exposure. Typically, the PaO_2 is normal, but O_2 saturation is low. Use co-oximetry to check for elevated carboxyhemoglobin levels (levels normalize if enough time from exposure has lapsed, and chronic smokers may have levels of CO as high as 10%). Magnetic resonance imaging (MRI) may reveal bilateral globus pallidus necrosis or cerebral edema. If neurologic or cardiac dysfunction is present or CO is >40%, hyperbaric O_2 is indicated, otherwise 100% O_2 is the therapy of choice.

■ Diagnostic Evaluation

- *Laboratory studies.* Serum glucose, chemistry profile to look for reversible causes of encephalopathy, drug screen, consider serum NSE (neuron specific enolase) and S100, cerebrospinal fluid creatine kinase BB activity (CSF CKBB; if available)

- *Imaging studies*
  - ◦ Noncontrast head computed tomography (CT):
    - Used to exclude primary brain injury as a cause of both coma and cardiac arrest
    - Often normal following cardiac arrest
    - May see obscuration of gray–white junction, watershed infarcts, or abnormal appearance of deep gray matter nuclei
  - ◦ MRI:
    - Testing may take a long time, so the safety and the stability of the patient must be considered.
    - Findings are extremely variable and have not yet shown clear association with outcomes.
    - In the acute phase (<24 hours), restricted diffusion (DWI bright, ADC dark) may be seen in the basal ganglia, cerebellum, and diffusely throughout the cortex (**Fig. 9.1**).

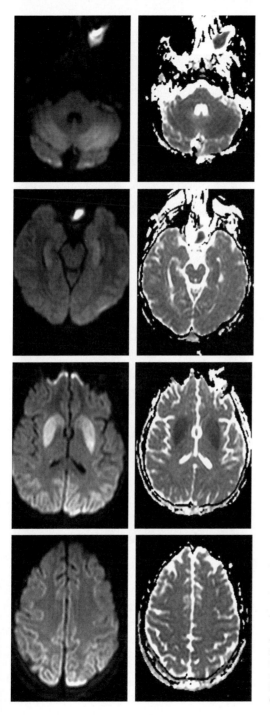

Fig. 9.1 Magnetic resonance imaging diffusion weighted image (MRI DWI) (**left**); apparent diffusion coefficient imaging (ADC) (**right**); 48 hours after tanoxic brain injury in a 21-year-old man. There is restricted diffusion in the bilateral cerebellum, medial temporal lobes, basal ganglia, and cortical ribbon.

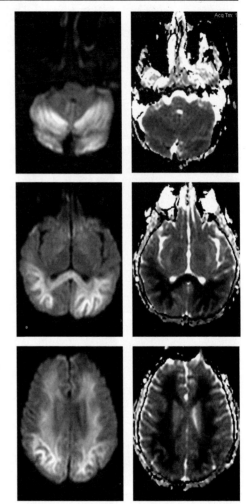

Fig. 9.2 Magnetic resonance imaging diffusion weighted image (MRI DWI) (**left**); apparent diffusion coefficient imaging (ADC) (**right**); Anoxic brain injury in the same 21-year-old man (Fig. 9.1) after 9 days. The MRI reveals restricted diffusion in the bilateral cerebellum and diffusely throughout the white matter.

- In a delayed fashion, restricted diffusion and increased T2 signal may be seen in the white matter (**Fig. 9.2**)
- *Neurophysiologic studies*
  - EEG:
    - EEG may be isoelectric or show severe suppression of background activity during and immediately after resuscitation.

- Findings may include generalized slowing, suppression of background activity, burst suppression, generalized periodic discharges, or alpha coma pattern (generally indicate poor prognosis though not invariably).
- EEG can be used to assess reactivity to various stimuli.
- The value of a single examination is limited, though serial exams may detect clinical change.
- Continuous EEG may be helpful to detect subclinical seizures.
- EEG may be difficult to interpret in the setting of drugs and concurrent metabolic derangements that affect the central nervous system (CNS).
- Electrocerebral silence (as a confirmatory exam for brain death) cannot reliably be established in an intensive care unit (ICU) setting due to artifact.

○ Somatosensory evoked potentials (SSEPs):

- Provide a bedside means of assessing brainstem and cortical function
- Less affected by medications and metabolic derangements than EEG
- Bilateral absence of N20 response with median nerve stimulation is strongly predictive of poor outcome; however, almost 50% of patients with present N20 will also have a poor outcome.[3]
- Timing is important: N20s may initially be absent and then return. Optimal timing is 1 to 3 days from arrest.
- SSEPs can be difficult to interpret in the setting of focal brain injury or peripheral neuropathy.

■ Treatment

Hypothermia

Induced moderate hypothermia (32–34°C) has been shown in multiple clinical trials to improve the probability of a good neurologic outcome as well as improve survival after ventricular fibrillation or pulseless ventricular tachycardia cardiac arrest.[4,5] Hypothermia is the only intervention shown to improve outcome after cardiac arrest and has a level IIa recommendation by the International Liaison Committee on Resuscitation (ILCOR) (see Chapter 20).[6]

Brain-Oriented Intensive Care

- Positioning: Place the head of the bed at 30 degrees, keeping the head midline to balance cerebral perfusion and venous drainage.
- Volume status: Avoid hypovolemia; use isotonic or hypertonic intravenous (IV) fluids, and avoid solutions containing glucose.
- Optimize cerebral perfusion: Avoid hypotension; maintain cerebral perfusion pressure (CPP) between 60 to 80 mm Hg.
- Cerebral edema and elevated intracranial pressure (ICP): Although global anoxia can lead to cerebral edema, frank elevation in ICP is uncommon. Patients with clinical or radiographic signs of elevated ICP should have invasive ICP monitoring and appropriate treatment. (See Chapter 15)
- Fever control: Acetaminophen, active cooling, and antibiotics to treat suspected infections
- Aggressively monitor and control serum glucose.
- Avoid hypoxia and hypercapnia.

Treatment of Seizures/Myoclonus

- Both seizures and myoclonus are common following cardiac arrest.
- Continuous EEG monitoring should be considered in patients who have undergone hypothermia therapy and are still comatose after 24 hours to determine if there is a reversible cause of coma such as subtle seizures or nonconvulsive status epilepticus.
- Prophylactic treatment with antiepileptic medications is generally not recommended.
- Seizures should be treated with appropriate anticonvulsive therapy.
- Postanoxic myoclonus is also known as Lance–Adams syndrome.
- Treatment of myoclonus (rather than myoclonic status epilepticus) has not been shown to change neurologic outcomes and is often refractory to therapy.

- Gabapentin, levetiracetam, benzodiazepines, and valproic acid are potential treatment options that have shown some success in patients with myoclonus.

Neuroprotective Medications

Many neuroprotective medications have been tested in the setting of cardiac arrest, including thiopental, corticosteroids, calcium channel blockers, glutamate antagonists, and antioxidant medications. Currently none have been found to provide significant clinical benefit.

■ Prognosis

- Survivors of cardiac arrest will have a wide range of neurologic disability. Those that regain meaningful neurologic function often will have memory dysfunction or other cognitive deficits. Less than 10% are able to return to their baseline level of function. Those that do not may progress to a minimally conscious state, vegetative state, or brain death (**Table 9.1**).[7]

- Persistent vegetative state (PVS) is a state of severe brain dysfunction with retained wakefulness but no detectable awareness of self or the environment. Sleep–wake cycles are maintained, as are complete or partial hypothalamic and brainstem functions. A persistent vegetative state can be diagnosed at 1-month posttraumatic or nontraumatic brain injury. Recovery of consciousness can occur; however, it is rare and nearly always associated with severe neurologic disability. The life expectancy of patients with PVS ranges from 2 to 5 years; survival beyond 10 years is unusual.[8] Treatment strategies have included zolpidem, levodopa, baclofen, and deep brain stimulation, but all remain speculative at this point.

- Minimally conscious state (MCS) is differentiated from PVS by discernible awareness of self and environment. It is important to make this distinction because the prognosis is better for MCS than PVS. Indicators of awareness include the ability to follow commands intermittently, gesture yes/no (regardless of accuracy), verbalize intelligibly, purposeful (nonreflexive) movement, and visual pursuit or fixation that occurs in direct response to a moving or salient stimuli. Behaviors may be intermittent but should be reproducible and/or sustained.[9]

Table 9.1 Survivors of Cardiac Arrest

Neurologic Diagnosis	Self-Awareness	Sleep—Wake Cycles	Motor Function	Eye Opening	Outcome
Coma	No	No	No purposeful movement Reflex and postural movement	No	Variable depending on etiology
Persistent vegetative state (PVS)	No self awareness No ability to interact. No sustained, purposeful, reproducible, or voluntary response to visual, auditory, tactile, or noxious stimuli	Yes	No purposeful movement. Postures or withdraws to noxious stimuli. Preserved cranial nerve function and spinal reflexes. Bowel and bladder incontinence	Yes. May briefly orient to sound or visual stimuli. Reflexive crying or smiling	Permanent if present 12 months after traumatic injury in adults and children; 3 months after nontraumatic injury in adults and children. After this time almost no chance of meaningful recovery
Minimally conscious state	Partial, intermittent command following, inconsistent but intelligible verbalization or gestures	Yes	Localizes to noxious stimuli, inconsistent command following. Purposeful movement	Yes, tracking	Better outcome at 1 year than PVS patients Better neurologic outcome in TBI than non-TBI
Locked-in syndrome	Yes, can follow commands with eyes	Yes	Quadriparetic or quadriplegic with preserved vertical eye movements	Yes, preserved vertical eye movements	Variable depending on etiology

Abbreviation: TBI, traumatic brain injury.

Data from: Giacino JT, Kalmar K. Diagnostic and prognostic guidelines for the vegetative and minimally conscious states. Neuropsychol Rehabil 2005;15(3–4):166–174.

- The main goal of prognostication is to define accurately which patients have no likelihood of meaningful neurologic recovery to justify early withdrawal or limitation of support.

- Current prognostication measures may not be valid in patients who have received hypothermic therapy. Caution is warranted when using exam findings to prognosticate in these patients at 24 and 72 hours. Prognostic guidelines in these patients is an active area of research.

The measures in **Table 9.2** have been shown to have prognostic implications after anoxic brain injury.[10]

Table 9.2 2006 American Academy of Neurology Practice Parameters

Prognostic Measure	Recommendation	Level of Recommendation
Circumstances surrounding CPR	Anoxia time, duration of CPR, and cause of cardiac arrest are all related to the likelihood of poor outcome but cannot reliably predict those patients who will have a poor outcome. Prognosis cannot be based on the circumstances of CPR.	Level B
Clinical examination	Prognosis poor: Absent pupillary or corneal responses from 24–72 hours following cardiac arrest	Level A
	Absent or extensor motor responses after 72 hours	Level A
	Development of myoclonic status epilepticus within the first 24 hours	Level B
Electroencephalogram	Generalized suppression of background (<20 μV), burst suppression, and generalized periodic patterns all suggest poor prognosis but are not sufficiently specific predictors of poor outcome.	Level C
SSEP	Bilateral absence of the N20 component on median nerve potentials performed between days 1 and 3 following cardiac arrest is a strong specific predictor of poor outcome.	Level B

(Continued on next page)

Table 9.2 2006 American Academy of Neurology Practice Parameters *(continued)*

Prognostic Measure	Recommendation	Level of Recommendation
Elevated body temperature	For each degree above 37°C, patients are 2 times more likely to have a poor outcome. However, prognosis cannot be made based on body temperature alone.	Level C
Biomarkers	Neuron specific enolase (NSE): serum level >33 µg/L 1–3 days postarrest is associated with poor outcome	Level B
	Protein S100 and CSF CKBB do not have sufficient evidence of utility in prognostication.	Level U
ICP or brain O_2 monitoring	Cytotoxic edema, elevated ICP, and poor brain oxygenation can occur postarrest. The prognostic utility of ICP and brain oxygen monitoring is unknown.	Level U
Imaging	Cerebral edema may be seen on CT or MRI, but its predictive value is not known. MRI and CT are often normal postarrest. There is insufficient evidence to indicate whether MRI or CT is indicative of poor outcome.	Level U

Abbreviations: CPR, cardio-pulmonary resuscitation; CSF CKBB, cerebrospinal fluid creatine kinase BB; CT, computed tomography; ICP, intracranial pressure; MRI, magnetic resonance imaging; SSEP, somatosensory evoked potential.

Data from: Wijdicks EF, Hijdra A, Young GB, Bassetti CL, Wiebe S. Practice parameter: prediction of outcome in comatose survivors after cardiopulmonary resuscitation (an evidence-based review): report of the Quality Standards Subcommittee of the American Academy of Neurology. Neurology 2006;67(2):203–210. These guidelines may not apply to patients who have received hypothermic theraphy.

Pearls and Pitfalls

- Neurologists should become involved in the treatment of patients early after cardiac arrest to help guide brain-oriented care with a focus on minimizing neurologic injury.
- Induced hypothermia after ventricular fibrillation and pulseless ventricular tachycardia arrest improves outcomes.
- A combination of clinical, electrophysiological, and radiographic information should be used in guiding prognosis.

References

1. Herlitz J, et al. Experiences from treatment of out-of-hospital cardiac arrest during 17 years in Goteborg. Eur Heart J 2000;21(15):1251–1258
2. de Vreede-Swagemakers JJ, et al. Out-of-hospital cardiac arrest in the 1990's: a population-based study in the Maastricht area on incidence, characteristics and survival. J Am Coll Cardiol 1997;30(6):1500–1505
3. Robinson LR, et al. Predictive value of somatosensory evoked potentials for awakening from coma. Crit Care Med 2003;31(3):960–967
4. Hypothermia After Cardiac Arrest Study Group. Mild therapeutic hypothermia to improve the neurologic outcome after cardiac arrest. N Engl J Med 2002;346(8):549–556
5. Bernard SA, Gray TW, Buist MD, et al. Treatment of comatose survivors of out-of-hospital cardiac arrest with induced hypothermia. N Engl J Med 2002;346(8):557–563
6. Nolan JP, Morley PT, Vanden Hoek TL, et al. Therapeutic hypothermia after cardiac arrest: an advisory statement by the Advanced Life Support Task Force of the International Liaison Committee on Resuscitation. Circulation 2003;108(1):118–121
7. Giacino JT, Kalmar K. Diagnostic and prognostic guidelines for the vegetative and minimally conscious states. Neuropsychol Rehabil 2005;15(3–4):166–174
8. Medical aspects of the persistent vegetative state (2). The Multi-Society Task Force on PVS. N Engl J Med 1994;330(22):1572–1579
9. Giacino JT, Ashwal S, Childs N, et al. The minimally conscious state: definition and diagnostic criteria. Neurology 2002;58(3):349–353
10. Wijdicks EF, Hijdra A, Young GB, Bassetti CL, Wiebe S. Practice parameter: prediction of outcome in comatose survivors after cardiopulmonary resuscitation (an evidence-based review): report of the Quality Standards Subcommittee of the American Academy of Neurology. Neurology 2006;67(2):203–210

10 Neurologic Infections

Stephen Krieger

Central nervous system (CNS) infections are significant causes of morbidity and mortality, and must be addressed with diagnostic and therapeutic urgency. CNS infections can be broadly categorized as meningitis, encephalitis, abscesses, and infections of the spinal cord.

Case Example

You are called to the emergency department to see a 46-year-old woman for "altered mental status." On arrival, you find an Asian woman complaining of headache, nausea, and vomiting. Her examination is notable for fever, lethargy, papilledema, and nuchal rigidity.

Questions

- Has the patient traveled outside the country recently?
- Does she have any pets?
- Any sick contacts?
- Has she had any spells that may be seizures?

Urgent Orders

- Order a head computed tomography (CT) scan without and with contrast
- Perform a lumbar puncture, optimally prior to antibiotic administration.
- Start empiric antibiotics (ceftriaxone, vancomycin, and acyclovir ± ampicillin).
- Administer Dexamethasone prior to or in conjunction with administration of antibiotics if bacterial meningitis is suspected.

■ History and Examination

History

- Time course of symptoms: Acute (<48 hour is often bacterial), subacute (often viral, can be anything), chronic/smoldering (often fungal, parasitic, or noninfectious)
- History of, risk factors for, and prior testing for human immunodeficiency virus (HIV)
- If HIV positive: CD4 count, highly active antiretroviral treatment (HAART) history, opportunistic infection history, and prophylaxis-medication compliance
- Other immunocompromised states: malignancy, malnutrition, immunosuppressive drugs, diabetes, alcoholism, renal replacement therapy, and splenectomy
- Travel history, exposures, vaccinations/inoculations
- Time of year:
  ◦ Summer/fall: Enteroviruses, arboviruses, Lyme disease, Rocky Mountain spotted fever
  ◦ Winter: Influenza
  ◦ Winter/spring: Measles, mumps, rubella, meningococcus, lymphocytic choriomeningitis

Physical Examination

- Vitals: Full set, including accurate rectal temperature
- Head, eyes, ears, nose, and throat (HEENT): Be attentive for facial rash (trigeminal zoster); ear canal vesicles (Ramsay–Hunt); thrush (HIV); parotiditis (mumps); dentition/dental abscesses; mastoid tenderness
- Evaluate carefully for nuchal rigidity, meningismus, and range of motion.
  ◦ Brudzinski's sign: neck flexion elicits flexion of hips and/or knees
  ◦ Kernig's sign: flex hip and knee with thigh against abdomen, then extend knee—note pain or resistance
  ◦ Both signs have poor sensitivity and are meaningful only in their presence and not their absence.

- Dermatologic: Examine the patient for rashes: erythema migrans (Lyme disease), petechiae (Rocky Mountain spotted fever), purpura (meningococcemia with or without meningitis), vesicles (varicella zoster virus [VZV]), maculopapular rash (measles, rubella, lymphocytic choriomeningitis), Osler nodes (red-purple, slightly raised, tender lumps on the digits), and Janeway lesions (nontender, often hemorrhagic, flat lesions mostly on the palms and soles. Both Osler nodes and Janeway lesions are clues to endocarditis).

Neurologic Examination

- A full neurologic examination, including assessment of mental status, cranial nerves, motor skills, and reflexes, as well as a sensory and cerebellar exam, should be performed on all patients.
- Mental status: Assess for encephalopathy and level of attentiveness, (Can the patient do the months backward, count 20 to 1 backward?)
  - Assess for aphasia, neglect, apraxia, or other cortical signs.
  - Be alert for ictal or postictal states.
- Cranial nerves: Cranial neuropathies are a clue to brainstem/meningeal processes (base of skull meningitis such as tuberculosis (TB) or carcinomatous meningitis, or rhombencephalitis such as caused by *Listeria*), hydrocephalus (sixth nerve palsy), or herniation syndromes (third nerve palsy). Assess the funduscopic exam for papilledema or macular star (as seen in neuroretinitis due to Lyme disease, *Bartonella*, or syphilis).
- Motor/sensory: Assess for focal deficits (epidural/parenchymal abscess, empyema, tuberculoma).
- Cerebellar: Assess for prominent cerebellar signs (consider varicella cerebellitis).

■ Differential Diagnosis

The differential diagnosis of various neurologic infections is given in **Table 10.1.**

Life-Threatening Diagnoses Not to Miss

- *Bacterial meningitis*
- *Herpes simplex virus (HSV) encephalitis*

Table 10.1 Differential Diagnosis of Various Neurologic Infections

Disease Process	Typical Organisms	Diagnostics	Clinical Clues/Comments
Acute Meningitis			
Septic	*Streptococcus pneumoniae* (47% in U.S.), *Neisseria meningitidis* (25%), Group B streptococcus (13%), *Listeria monocytogenes* (8%) *Haemophilus influenzae* (7%), TB	CSF polymorphic pleocytosis, elevated protein, low glucose, culture	No parenchymal involvement, normal mental status and nonfocal exam Mortality 25%, morbidity 60%, signs/symptoms <4 wks Consider TB particularly if recently imprisoned, coexisting cranial neuropathies. Tuberculomas in 10–20%. Look for external sources: otitis, mastoiditis, previous neuro or ENT surgery, sinusitis, dental abscess, endocarditis.
Aseptic	Enteroviruses (55–70%): Coxsackie A and B, echoviruses, poliovirus; arboviruses: St. Louis encephalitis, Eastern and Western equine encephalitis; Adenoviruses: mumps (paramyxovirus), measles (*Morbillivirus*); Herpes viruses: HSV1, HSV2, HHV-6, VZV, EBV, CMV; LCM (arenavirus); HIV seroconversion/ reconstitution with HAART; Recurrent (Mollaret's–EBV, HSV I)	CSF lymphocytic pleocytosis, elevated protein, normal glucose, culture; CSF PCR: HSV, CMV, EBV, enterovirus, VZV, arboviruses except West Nile (CSF ELISA antibody test preferred)	Mortality typically <20%, Leukopenia: LCM, Colorado tick fever, EBV, Venezuelan equine encephalitis Atypical lymphocytes: EBV, CMV Thrombocytopenia: LCM, Rocky Mountain spotted fever, Colorado tick fever, St. Louis encephalitis Anemia: mycoplasma, leptospirosis, Rocky Mountain spotted fever Renal dysfunction: leptospirosis, St. Louis encephalitis Abnormal LFTs: LCM, EBV, arboviruses, mumps leptospirosis

(Continued on next page)

Table 10.1 Differential Diagnosis of Various Neurologic Infections (continued)

Disease Process	Typical Organisms	Diagnostics	Clinical Clues/Comments
Chronic Meningitis			
Infectious	Mycobacteria: TB; Bacteria: *Listeria* (rhombencephalitis) Viral: CMV Fungal: *Cryptococcus neoformans, Coccidioides immitis, Histoplasma capsulatum, Blastomyces dermatitidis, Candida albicans, Sporothrix schenckii, Aspergillus* species, mucormycosis	TB: CSF lymphocytic pleocytosis, elevated protein, low-normal glucose, CSF TB PCR, CSF AFB, *Cryptococcus* antigen, India Ink fungal culture,	Signs/symptoms >4 wks, typically basilar predilection with continued inflammation. Most common in HIV and immunocompromised. (TB, CMV, fungal toxoplasmosis) *Cryptococcus* and toxo common with CD4<100 cells/μL. CMV with CD4 <50 cells/μL. Look for radiculomyelitis.
	Spirochetes: syphilis, Lyme	Spirochetes: CSF VDRL, serum RPR/FTA, CSF	Syphilis = the great pretender. Look also for tabes dorsalis, Argyll Robertson pupil, transverse myelitis, general paresis.
		Lyme antibody	Lyme–cranial neuropathy, erythema migrans, polyradiculoneuropathy, arthralgia/arthritis, transverse myelitis
	Parasitic: Toxoplasmosis, *Angiostrongylus cantonensis, Tania solium* (cysticercosis), *Plasmodium falciparum* (cerebral malaria), *Trichinella spiralis*	Parasites: CSF toxoplasmosis IgG, serum cysticercosis antibody, blood smear for malaria, muscle biopsy for trichinella, brain biopsy	
Non-infectious	Inflammatory/autoimmune: sarcoid, Behçet's, Wegener's granulomatosis, lupus, Sjögren's, Vogt-Koyanagi-Harada	Sarcoid: CSF and serum ACE, gallium scan, conjunctival biopsy, Wegener's, lupus, Sjögren's: serum ANA, ENA	Sarcoid: Hilar lymphadenopathy, cranial neuropathies, neuropathy, pituitary/hypothalamic dysfunction Behçet's: Aphthous and genital ulcers, uveitis Vogt-Koyanagi-Harada: Recurrent meningitis, uveitis, and white patches of hair
	Leptomeningeal carcinomatosis: breast cancer, lymphoma, leukemia, melanoma, medulloblastoma	Carcinomatosis: CSF cytology and flow cytometry (at least 10 mL), very high CSF protein, low glucose	Carcinomatous meningitis: Characteristic cerebellar meningeal enhancement on MRI, cranial neuropathies
	Drug reaction: NSAIDs, trimethoprim-sulfa...		

Disease Process	Typical Organisms	Diagnostics	Clinical Clues/Comments
Encephalitis			
Viral	Herpes viruses: HSV (up to 15% of U.S. cases), VZV, EBV, CMV, enteroviruses Arthropod borne: St. Louis encephalitis, Eastern and Western equine, West Nile, Japanese encephalitis, measles, mumps, rubella, Rocky Mountain spotted fever Rabies, lymphocytic choriomeningitis, PML Mycoplasma is a rare cause of bacterial encephalitis.	CSF HSV PCR (sens: 95%, spec: approaches 100%, less sensitive during first 72 h); Imaging (CT or MRI) showing edema and hemorrhage in anterior temporal lobes, PLEDS on EEG CSF PCR: (EBV, enterovirus, VZV, arboviruses, JC virus, *except* West Nile (CSF ELISA antibody test preferred)	HSV: Hallmark of altered mental status or focal neurologic findings. Frank meningismus is often absent. *ALL cases of encephalitis should be treated as HSV with acyclovir until proven otherwise.* Mortality of HSV encephalitis = 70% if untreated, 19% if treated. Morbidity, including seizures and cognitive/behavioral changes, seen in 97% of HSV encephalitis survivors. HSV1 (oral) more common than HSV2 (genital). Hemorrhagic encephalitis (frontal and anterior temporal lobes), seen with HSV enecephalitis SSPE: (subacute sclerosing panencephalitis) is a rare chronic encephalitis caused by persistent measles virus infection. It is more common in children.
Non-infectious	See noninfectious meningitis. Postinfectious and postvaccine encephalomyelitis, ADEM	MRI in ADEM: High T2 signal lesions and culture/PCR negative spinal fluid, IgG synthetic rate and index, oligoclonal bands are elevated	ADEM: Consider IV steroids ADEM can follow viral infections such as measles, mumps, rubella, EBV, CMV, influenza, coxsackievirus, HSV, VZV, enterovirus, and hepatitis A. ADEM can follow bacterial infections such as mycoplasma, Lyme, leptospirosis, and β hemolytic streptococcus.

(Continued on next page)

Table 10.1 Differential Diagnosis of Various Neurologic Infections *(continued)*

Disease Process	Typical Organisms	Diagnostics	Clinical Clues/Comments
Abscess	Bacteria: *Streptococcus* species (40%), notably S. milleri, S. intermedius; S. pyogenes in penetrating skull injuries. *Staphylococcus aureus:* postsurgical; shunt infections, *Proteus, Pseudomonas, Listeria monocytogenes,* anaerobes, esp. *Bacteroides* (30%) and *Fusobacterium* Fungal: *Nocardia, Candida albicans, Cryptococcus, Aspergillus* Parasitic: toxoplasmosis, cysticercosis	MRI + gadolinium: bacterial and most fungal abscesses are DWI+, ADC dark with a high sensitivity and specificity. Look for daughter abscess. Abscesses point toward the ventricle and are ring-enhancing. For toxo, look for ring-enhancing multiple lesions (difficult to differentiate from CNS lymphoma). MRS: bacterial abscess—TE 30 acetoacetate, amino acid, and succinocholine peaks	Can manifest with elevated ICP or seizures. Develop from direct spread or hematogenous dissemination. Multiple abscesses imply hematogenous spread. Check for endocarditis with TEE. Overall mortality 10%. Most hematogenously spread abscesses develop at the gray-white junction and are more common in the MCA territory.
Extra-axial infection	*Staphylococci, Streptococci,* anaerobes, subdural effusions (*H. Influenzae* meningitis); hydrocephalus (TB or fungal meningitis)	CT or MRI with evidence of epidural abscess or subdural empyema CSF may be similar to that seen with bacterial meningitis	Bacteria from superficial infections travel via valveless emissary veins into dural sinuses. Be wary in patients with previous neurosurgery or external ventricular drainage.

Abbreviations: ACE, angiotensin-converting enzyme; ADC, apparent diffusion coefficient imaging; ADEM, acute demyelinating encephalomyelitis; AFB, acid-fast bacilli; ANA, antinuclear antibody test; CMV, cytomegalovirus; CNS, central nervous system; CSF, cerebrospinal fluid; CT, computed tomography; DWI, diffusion-weighted image; EBV, Epstein-Barr virus; EEG, electroencephalogram; ELISA, enzyme-linked immunosorbent assay test; ENA, extractable nuclear antigens; ENT, ear, nose, and throat; HAART, highly active antiretroviral treatment; HHV-6, human herpesvirus 6; HIV, human immunodeficiency virus; HSV1, HSV2, herpes simplex virus 1, 2; ICP, intracranial pressure; IgG, immunogammaglobulin; IV, intravenous; IVIG, intravenous high-dose immunoglobulin; LCM, lymphocytic choriomeningitis; LFTs, liver function tests; MCA, middle cerebral artery; MRI, magnetic resonance imaging; MRS, magnetic resonance spectroscopy; NSAIDs, nonsteroidal antiinflammatory drugs; PCR, polymerase chain reaction; PLEDS, periodic lateralized epileptiform discharges; PML, progressive multifocal leukoencephalopathy; RPR/FTA, rapid plasma reagin/fluorescein test for *Treponema pallidum*; sens, sensitivity; spec, specificity; TB, tuberculosis; TEE, transesophageal echocardiogram; VDRL, venereal disease reference laboratory; VZV, varicella zoster virus.

■ Diagnostic Evaluation

- *Laboratory studies*

  - Complete blood count (CBC), chemistry panel, liver function tests (LFTs), prothrombin time/partial prothrombin time (PT/PTT), human immunodeficiency virus (HIV), RPR/FTA, Lyme antibodies, and PPD (tuberculin skin test) placement
  - Blood cultures, urinalysis (UA)/urine cultures and toxicology, sputum culture
  - Chest x-ray, electrocardiogram (ECG), cardiac/hemodynamic monitoring; consider transesophageal echocardiogram (TEE)
  - Lumbar puncture—make sure international normalized ratio (INR) <1.5, PTT<40, platelets >50; *always* check opening pressure and closing pressure (if large-volume 30 mL tap)
    - Tube #1 cells and differential
    - Tube #2 glucose and protein
    - Tube #3 gram stain and culture
      - Consider: Acid-fast and/or tuberculosis polymerase chain reaction (TB PCR), Cryptococcal antigen and India ink stains, fungal cultures, angiotensin converting enzyme (ACE), VDRL (if serum positive), Lyme antibody (if serum positive), PCR for HSV, cytomegalovirus (CMV), VZV, human herpes virus 6 (HHV-6), JC virus, and Epstein-Barr virus (EBV)
    - Tube #4 cells and differential
    - Traumatic tap: red blood cells/white blood cells (RBC: WBC) = 700:1, 1000 RBC account for 1 mg of cerebrospinal fluid (CSF) protein
    - CSF findings can be found in **Table 10.2**.

- *Imaging studies*

  - Head CT should be performed prior to lumbar puncture (LP) if the patient is >60 years old, has a history of CNS disease, has altered mental status, an inability to answer two consecutive commands, focal neurologic signs, a seizure in the past week, or a history of HIV or immunosuppression.[1] In reality, most patients will receive a head CT.

Table 10.2 Cerebral Spinal Fluid Findings

Characteristic	Normal	Bacterial meningitis	Tuberculous meningitis	Fungal meningitis	Carcinomatous meningitis	Viral ("aseptic") meningitis or encephalitis
Color	Clear may be xanthochromic if elevated serum bilirubin	May be cloudy	May be cloudy	May be cloudy	May be cloudy	May be cloudy; if HSV, may be blood-tinged
Pressure (cm H2O)	≤20–25	Increased (may be normal)	Often increased	Often increased	Normal or increased	Normal (may be slightly increased)
Cells (#/mL)	0–5 mono-nuclear	>5 to thousands PMNs > lymphs	>5–500; PMNs initially, then lymphs > PMNs	>5–800 lymphs	>5–1000 monos or atypical cells	>5–2000 mostly lymphs; RBCs indicative of HSV, may be >80% polys in first few days
Protein (mg/dL)	15–45 may be elevated in diabetes or renal failure	50–500	50–500; often elevated out of proportion with cellularity	Normal or increased	Up to 500	20–200

142

Characteristic	Normal	Bacterial meningitis	Tuberculous meningitis	Fungal meningitis	Carcinomatous meningitis	Viral ("aseptic") meningitis or encephalitis
Glucose (mg/dL)	45–80 (or 2/3 of serum glucose)	0–45 (low)	10–45 (low)	Normal or decreased	Normal or low	Normal (Reduced in 25% of cases of mumps, HSV, CMV
Microbiology studies	Negative	Gram-stain positive in 60–90%, culture in 80%; Lyme PCR positive in 70–80%	Acid-fast stain positive in 35% with first LP, up to 80% with 3 LPs; CSF cultures may take months, CSF TB PCR, PPD, Biopsy with: caseating granulomas, Langerhans' giant cells, lymphocyte and macrophage infiltrate	India Ink positive in 50–75% of Cryptococcal meningitis cases, confirm with fungal culture	Cytology sensitivity improved with large-volume tap	HSV PCR sens: 95%, spec: nearly 100%, less sensitive during first 72 hour; CMV PCR sens: 79%, spec: 95%

Abbreviations: CMV, cytomegalovirus; CSF, cerebrospinal fluid; HSV, herpes simplex virus; LP, lumbar puncture; lymphs, lymphocytes; PCR, polymerase chain reaction; PMNs, polymorphonuclear leukocytes; PPD, purified protein derivative; RBCs, red blood cells; sens, sensitivity; spec, specificity; TB, tuberculosis.

- ○ Magnetic resonance imaging/magnetic resonance angiography/magnetic resonance spectroscopy (MRI/MRA/MRS) with gadolinium is preferred to identify enhancing meninges, abscess, or possible vasculitis. Diffusion-weighted imaging (DWI) is particularly useful as it is bright with high sensitivity in bacterial and fungal abscesses.
  - ○ Digital subtraction angiography (DSA) can be considered if vasculitis is suspected.

- *Neurophysiologic testing*
  - ○ EEG: Look for temporal periodic lateralized epileptiform discharges (PLEDS) with HSV. PLEDS are nonspecific and can occur with a variety of different etiologies.

■ Treatment

- Treat immediately for bacterial meningitis (empirically with ceftriaxone, vancomycin (+ ampicillin in young, elderly, and immunocompromised patients). CSF sterilization may occur within 2 to 4 hours of initiation of intravenous (IV) antibiotics, and spinal fluid should be obtained promptly for diagnosis.

- Consider dexamethasone IV 10 mg every 6 hours for 4 days, best if begun 10 to 20 minutes prior to initiation of antibiotics. In a randomized, controlled study of dexamethasone 10 mg every 6 hours for 4 days versus placebo in patients with bacterial meningitis, use of dexamethasone 15 to 20 minutes prior to antibiotic administration reduced rates of death or unfavorable outcome.[2] Most of these results were driven by patients with pneumococcal meningitis. In a more recent randomized, double-blind study of patients with probable bacterial meningitis, dexamethasone did not reduce death or disability.[3] In a subgroup of patients with microbiologically confirmed bacterial meningitis, there was a benefit for mortality at 1 month and disability at 6 months, even when dexamethasone was administered after the initiation of antibiotics. In another randomized, placebo-controlled trial for bacterial meningitis (dexamethasone 16 mg twice daily for 4 days in a population of largely HIV-positive patients [90%]), there was no significant difference in mortality, hearing loss, or adverse events, even in patients with proven pneumococcal meningitis.[4]

In a Cochrane meta-analysis, corticosteroids for bacterial meningitis significantly reduced rates of mortality, severe hearing loss, and neurologic sequelae. Results are best if steroids are administered prior to the first antibiotic dose.[5]

- If there are any signs of encephalitis, treat ASAP with acyclovir 10 mg/kg every 8 hours intravenously for 21 days or until CSF HSV PCR is negative.

- Virulent pathogens such as gram-negative bacterial meningitis and *Staphylococcus aureus* meningitis should be treated for a minimum of 21 days and sometimes longer depending on clinical response.

- Stereotactic aspiration and drainage of intracerebral abscesses (or open surgical excision) may be warranted for abscesses that are large (>2.5 cm) or refractory to systemic antibiotics.

- Appropriate antibiotic regimens for each infection are listed in **Table 10.3**. Antibiotics should be deescalated based on culture results.

Table 10.3 Antibiotic Regimens for Infections

Streptococcus pneumoniae	Ceftriaxone 2 g q12h IV plus vancomycin 1–2 g q6h IV
Neisseria meningitides	Penicillin G 4 million U q4h IV or ceftriaxone 2 g q12h IV Note: Close contacts should be treated with rifampin 600 mg PO q12h for four doses
Listeria monocytogenes	Ampicillin 2 g q4h IV plus Gentamicin 1 mg/kg q8h IV
Helicobacter influenzae	Ceftriaxone 2 g q12h IV
Group B streptococcus	Penicillin G 50,000 U/kg q4h IV
Pseudomonas aeruginosa	Ceftazidime 2 g q8h IV plus Gentamicin 1 mg/kg q8h IV
Enterobacter cloacae	Ceftriaxone 2 g q12h IV

(Continued on next page)

Table 10.3 Antibiotic Regimens for Infections *(continued)*

***Staphylococcus aureus:* methicillin-sensitive**	Oxacillin 2 g q4h IV
***Staphylococcus aureus:* methicillin-resistant**	Vancomycin 1–2 g q6h
Cryptococcal meningitis	Amphotericin B 0.7 mg/kg/d IV x 2 wk plus 5-flucytosine 100 mg/kg/d PO x 2 wk then Fluconazole 400–800 mg PO q.d. × 8 wk then Fluconazole 200 ms PO q.d. × 6 mo, or indefinitely if HIV
Tuberculous meningitis	Rifampin 10 mg/kg/d PO Isoniazid 300 mg/d PO Pyrazinamide 30 mg/kg/d PO Ethambutol 15–25 mg/kg/d PO Pyridoxine 50 mg/d PO If clinically responding after 8 wk, stop pyrazinamide and ethambutol, and continue remaining agents for 6–12 months
HSV and VZV encephalitis	Acyclovir 10 mg/kg q8h IV x 21 d
CMV encephalitis	Ganciclovir 5 mg/kg q12h IV x 2 wk
CNS toxoplasmosis	Pyrimethamine 100–200 mg PO load × 2 d then pyrimethamine 75–100 mg q.d. PO plus sulfadiazine 1.5–2 g q 6 hours PO and folinic acid 10–50 mg/d (Continue all meds for 6 wk)
Ventriculitis	No hardware: Empiric therapy with vancomycin and cefepime/ceftazidime/or meropenem. Duration similar to meninigitis treatment. Hardware: Attempts to remove or externalize hardware are paramount. Coag negative *Staph:* antibiotics should be used for the duration that the hardware is in place and then continued for 7 d after it is replaced. The CSF should be sterile prior to shunt replacement.

(Continued)

Table 10.3 Antibiotic Regimens for Infections *(continued)*

	S. aureus or gram-negative bacilli: Antibiotics should be given for 14–21 days, and the CSF should be sterile for 7–10 days prior to hardware replacement. If hardware is not removed, antibiotics should be continued for 7–10 days after sterilization of the CSF. Longer courses of antibiotics may be needed in patients with an incomplete response. Intraventricular antibiotics can be considered in patients who fail parenteral antibiotics or who have pathogens sensitive only to antibiotics with poor CSF penetration. Prevention: A dose of antibiotics (cefazolin) should be given prior and shortly after hardware placement (see Chapter 18).
Cerebral abscess	Abscesses <2.5 cm usually respond to antimicrobial therapy. Those larger than 2.5 cm typically require surgical evacuation via aspiration or excision. Isolation of the offending microbe is essential to treatment. Antibiotic therapy is usually for 6–8 weeks. Initial coverage should be with a third generation cephalosporin (cefepime can be substituted if *Pseudomonas* is anticipated), metronidazole (to cover penicillin-resistant anaerobes), and vancomycin (if *S. aureus* is suspected). Use of steroids is controversial because they can slow the encapsulation process, reduce antibiotic penetration, increase the risk of ventricular rupture, and increase necrosis. They may be useful to treat vasogenic cerebral edema with significant mass effect related to the abscess. Most empyemas should be evacuated.

Abbreviations: CMV, cytomegalovirus; CNS, central nervous system; CSF, cerebrospinal fluid; HSV, human simplex virus; IV, intravenous; PO, by mouth; q, every; q.d., every day; VZV, varicella zoster virus.

■ Prognosis

The prognosis of neurologic infections varies widely with the type of infection, the causative organism, associated medical comorbidities, and the rapidity with which appropriate therapy is instituted. In all cases, coma and shock in the setting of CNS infection confer a poor prognosis for complete neurologic recovery.

Pearls and Pitfalls

- Treat first, ask questions later: the risk of undertreatment or delayed treatment vastly outweighs the risk of initial overtreatment.

- If you are considering/treating for meningitis, be sure to consider HSV encephalitis as well, with liberal use of acyclovir until HSV PCR is negative.

- Don't miss the big picture: search for an underlying immunocompromised state (undiagnosed HIV, leukemia/lymphoma) or a systemic source of CNS infection.

References

1. Hasbun R, Abrahams J, Jekel J, Quagliarello VJ. Computed tomography of the head before lumbar puncture in adults with suspected meningitis. N Engl J Med 2001;345(24):1727–1733
2. de Gans J, van de Beek D. Dexamethasone in adults with bacterial meningitis. N Engl J Med 2002;347(20):1549–1556
3. Nguyen TH, Tran TH, Thwaites G, et al. Dexamethasone in Vietnamese adolescents and adults with bacterial meningitis. N Engl J Med 2007;357(24): 2431–2440
4. Scarborough M, Gordon SB, Whitty CJ, et al. Corticosteroids for bacterial meningitis in adults in sub-Saharan Africa. N Engl J Med 2007;357(24):2441–2450
5. van de Beek D, de Gans J, McIntyre P, Prasad K. Corticosteroids for acute bacterial meningitis. Cochrane database of systematic reviews (Online) 2007(1):CD004405.

11 Myasthenic Crisis

Mark Sivak and
Jennifer A. Frontera

Myasthenia gravis (MG) is an autoimmune disease of the neuromuscular junction characterized by a T-cell dependent response targeted to the postsynaptic acetylcholine receptor or receptor-associated proteins. Weakness is confined to voluntary muscles (sparing smooth and cardiac muscle) and is variable in focus and degree. Breathing and swallowing may become significantly involved, with severe consequences leading to respiratory failure requiring mechanical ventilation. Respiratory insufficiency due to MG is referred to as myasthenic crisis.

Myasthenic crisis can present as a forme fruste of MG. It can begin with oropharyngeal weakness with or without appendicular symptoms and progress to crisis within hours to days, often in the context of infection or aspiration and occasionally following surgery. Half of patients with recently diagnosed MG will have a crisis within the first year and another 20% within the second year from diagnosis. Patients with long-standing MG are also at risk for crisis. Triggers include:

- Infection
- Tapering of immunosuppression
- Surgery
- Aspiration
- Worsening of other medical diseases (cardiac, renal, autoimmune, etc.)
- No apparent reason (30 to 40%)
- Certain medications can exacerbate MG or lead to crisis. (See **Table 11.1.**)

Table 11.1 Medications that Can Trigger Myasthenic Crisis

Antibiotics	Aminoglycosides, fluoroquinolones (ciprofloxacin, levofloxacin, norfloxacin), macrolides (clarithromycin, erythromycin), ampicillin, clindamycin, colistin, lincomycin, quinine, tetracyclines
Anticonvulsants	Phenytoin, gabapentin
Antipsychotics	Chlorpromazine, lithium, phenothiazines
Anesthetics	Diazepam, chloroprocaine, halothane, ketamine, lidocaine, neuromuscular blocking agents (depolarizing agents such as succinylcholine have no efficacy in myasthenic patients), procaine
Cardiovascular	Beta blockers, bretylium, procainamide, propafenone, quinidine, verapamil, and calcium channel blockers
Ophthalmologic	Betaxolol, echothiophate, timolol, tropicamide, proparacaine
Rheumatologic	Chloroquine, penicillamine
Steroids	Prednisone, methylprednisolone, corticotropin
Other	Anticholinergics, carnitine, deferoxamine, diuretics, interferon α, iodinated contrast agents, narcotics, oral contraceptives, oxytocin, ritonavir and antiretroviral protease inhibitors, thyroxine

Case Example

You are called to see a myasthenic patient with a recently diagnosed upper respiratory infection (URI). She has three- to four-word dyspnea and difficulty holding her head up. Her speech is slurred and has a nasal quality.

Questions

- What is her baseline function?
- How rapidly has she become weak?
- Has she had recent forced vital capacity (VC) or negative inspiratory force (NIF) checked?
- What is her arterial blood gas (ABG)?

Urgent Orders

- Establish airway, breathing, circulation (ABCs): consider intubation early. A myasthenic patient can deteriorate rapidly.

- Check a VC and NIF. If VC <10 to 15 mL/kg or <1 L and/or the NIF is weaker than −20 cm H_2O or rapidly worsening, the patient should be intubated. Beware that patients with bulbar dysfunction often cannot form a proper seal for respiratory testing, and results can sometimes appear worse than the patient's true respiratory status. Multiple VC/NIF measurements should be made to capture the patient's best effort.

- Pulmonary function assessment: Ask the patient to count as rapidly and as high as he or she can in one breath. Every 10 numbers counted roughly equates to 1 L of VC. If the patient cannot count to 10, intubation should be pursued.

- Check an ABG: CO_2 retention happens first, so if the patient is already hypoxic, the physician should proceed to intubation without delay.

- Patients with myasthenic crisis should be monitored in an intensive care unit (ICU) setting.

■ History and Examination

History

Does the patient have a history of MG? If so, has the patient been in crisis before? What were the triggers for the previous crises? Has the patient been intubated or had a tracheostomy (may indicate a more difficult airway) in the past? What medications is the patient taking? Have new medications been introduced or tapered? Does the patient have an infection or recent surgery?

Below are signs and symptoms of developing crisis in order of development:

- Deteriorating articulation
- Swallowing difficulty
- Accumulation of oral secretions—wet voice
- Worsening cough efficacy/reduced ability to clear secretions with cough

- Speech shift to short sentences (deteriorating length of numbers able to count aloud using a single breath)
- Patient anxiety increased due to hypoxia

Physical Examination

Concerning exam findings include:

- Increasing respiratory rate
- Use of accessory muscles of respiration
- Decreased tidal volume
- Paradoxical breathing
- Increasing pulse and blood pressure (BP)
- Diaphragmatic breathing especially at night in rapid eye movement sleep (REM). Worsening neck flexion correlates with diaphragm dysfunction.
- Unable to be supine
- In patients without a history of MG: Examine mucous membranes for evidence of diphtheria, look for ticks (particularly in children), assess for evidence of excess cholinergic stimulation (salivation, lacrimation, diarrhea, excess urination, gastrointestinal [GI] upset, emesis).

Neurologic Examination

- Mental status: normal unless CO_2 retention leads to inattentiveness
- Cranial nerves: ptosis, nasal voice, ophthalmoparesis (diplopia), facial weakness, fatigable chewing, dysarthria, hypophonic voice, difficulty swallowing with pooling of secretions, no pupillary involvement
- Motor: fatiguing proximal >distal weakness, arm >leg weakness, neck flexor weakness (C3–C5) correlates with respiratory capacity
- Sensory: normal
- Reflexes: normal to slightly decreased
- Cerebellar: normal (exam may be limited by weakness)
- Additional testing: ptosis time (have patient look up and time how long it takes for ptosis to develop), arm abduction time (duration patient can keep arms abducted), one breath counting. These measures can be used to track improvement or worsening.

■ Differential Diagnosis

1. *Myasthenic crisis*
2. *Cholinergic crisis.* Can occur from excess acetylcholine esterase inhibitor. Characterized by SLUDGE (salivation, lacrimation, urination, diarrhea, (GI) upset, and emesis), miosis, bronchospasm, and flaccid weakness. Although a Tensilon (Valeant Pharmaceuticals International, Aliso Viejo, CA) challenge can distinguish cholinergic crisis from myasthenia, this test can be dangerous and often is not necessary.
3. *Lambert–Eaton myasthenic syndrome.* Presynaptic autoimmune attack of voltage-gated calcium channels, associated with cancer in 50 to 70% (typically small cell lung cancer), limb symptoms more prominent than ocular/bulbar symptoms (5% with bulbar findings), facilitation with exercise, autonomic dysfunction, and reduced reflexes. Respiratory failure is uncommon.
4. *Botulism.* Neurotoxin produced from *Clostridium botulinum*, permanently blocks presynaptic acetylcholine release at the neuromuscular junction. Botulism causes symmetrical descending paralysis with dilated pupils (50%), and dysautonomia, but no sensory deficits. Botulism can be treated with trivalent equine antitoxin.
5. *Tick paralysis.* Ascending paralysis, ophthalmoparesis, bulbar dysfunction, ataxia, reduced reflexes. Complete cure can occur with tick removal.
6. *Organophosphate toxicity (malathion, parathion, Sarin, Soman, etc.).* Inactivates acetylcholine esterase, causing SLUDGE, miosis, bronchospasm, blurred vision, and bradycardia. Also causes confusion, optic neuropathy, extrapyramidal effects, dysautonomia, fasciculations, seizures, cranial nerve palsies, and weakness due to continued depolarization at the neuromuscular junction. Delayed polyneuropathy can occur 2 to 3 weeks after exposure. Treat with atropine, pralidoxime (2-PAM), and benzodiazepines. Avoid succinylcholine.
7. *Guillain–Barré syndrome* (see Chapter 12). Can present with areflexia and ophthalmoplegia (Miller-Fisher variant), or ascending weakness, facial weakness, diplopia, and areflexia. Often demyelinating, but can be axonal. Characterized by early loss of F waves on electromyogram (EMG). Treatable with plasmapheresis or intravenous high-dose immunoglobulin (IVIG).

8. *Neurotoxic fish poisoning.* Tetrodotoxin (pufferfish) and saxitoxin (red tide) both block neuromuscular transmission. Ciguatera toxin (red snapper, grouper, barracuda) affects voltage gated sodium channels of muscles and nerves and produces a characteristic metallic taste in the mouth and hot–cold reversal.

9. *Diphtheria, caused by Corynebacterium diphtheriae.* It is associated with a thick gray pharyngeal pseudomembrane, atrial-ventricular (AV) block, endocarditis, myocarditis, lymphadenopathy, neuropathy with craniopharyngeal involvement, proximal >distal weakness, and decreased reflexes.

10. *Myopathy.* Critical illness myopathy/neuropathy, mitochondrial myopathies (myoclonic epilepsy associated with ragged red fibers [MERRF]), acid maltase disease (adult type), polymyositis, and thyroid disease (Graves) can mimic MG.

11. *Brainstem disease with multiple cranial neuropathies* (stroke, Bickerstaff–Cloake, rhombencephalitis, basilar meningitis, carcinomatous meningitis)

Life-Threatening Diagnosis Not to Miss

- *Impending respiratory failure due to progressive neuromuscular disorder*

- *Organophosphate toxicity or botulinum toxicity,* which can be treated with an antidote if administered in a timely fashion

■ Diagnostic Evaluation

In patients diagnosed with myasthenia gravis:

- Laboratory and radiographic studies: Complete blood count (CBC); chemistry panel; liver function tests; chest radiograph (CXR); erythrocyte sedimentation rate (ESR); C-reactive protein (CRP); blood, sputum, and urine cultures should be considered in febrile patients to identify an infectious source that may have led to decompensation. Serial ABGs should be performed. The first laboratory sign of respiratory insufficiency is a rising PCO_2. By the time hypoxia is evident, respiratory failure is imminent.

- Respiratory function studies: Frequent (every 2 to 6 hours) vital capacity (VC) and negative inspiratory force (NIF) should be measured. A declining NIF or NIF worse than -20 cm H_2O and VC <10 to 15 mL/kg should prompt intubation.

In patients without a diagnosis of myasthenia gravis:

- Bedside tests: Edrophonium (Tensilon) has a rapid onset and can be used to make the diagnosis of MG in patients with obvious ptosis; 2 mg doses can be administered every 60 seconds (up to 10 mg) while looking for a clinical response. Patients should receive electrocardiogram (ECG) monitoring with atropine at the bedside while this test is being performed because of the risks of bradycardia. Because edrophonium has muscarinic effects, it can cause bronchospasm and increased secretions and is not recommended in those with crisis.

- Serologic studies: Acetylcholine receptor antibodies are present in 85% of patients with generalized MG. Rare false-positives can be seen in Lambert–Eaton myasthenic syndrome, motor neuron disease, polymyositis, primary biliary cirrhosis, lupus, thymoma without MG, and in first-degree relatives of a myasthenic patient. Fifteen to 20% of patients with MG are seronegative. Of these patients, 40 to 50% have muscle-specific tyrosine kinase (MuSK) antibodies.

- Laboratory studies: Because many patients with MG have other autoimmune diseases, testing for lupus, thyroid disease, and rheumatoid arthritis is suggested. Lumbar puncture is typically unrevealing in MG.

- EMG: Repetitive nerve stimulation can be performed by administering 2 to 3 Hz stimulation and assessing for a decremental response in compound muscle action potential (CMAP) amplitudes. An exercise protocol can be applied to increase the sensitivity of the test. Single-fiber EMG is the most sensitive test for MG. Abnormal jitter can occur in other neuromuscular disorders but is specific for a disorder of neuromuscular transmission when no other abnormalities are seen on standard EMG needle exam. EMG/nerve conduction study (NCS) can distinguish MG from other neuropathies (diphtheria, Guillain–Barré, toxic neuropathy, etc.), presynaptic neuromuscular junction disorders (Lambert–Eaton, botulism, neurotoxic fish poisoning), and myopathies.

- Imaging: Chest computed tomography (CT) or magnetic resonance imaging (MRI) to screen for thymoma should be performed on all myasthenic patients. MRI of the brain may be necessary if a central brainstem etiology is suspected.

- Serologies: Serologies specific to certain disease etiologies are listed: Lambert–Eaton—P/Q type calcium channel–binding antibodies; botulism—serum and stool botulism toxin assay;

organophosphate toxicity—measure plasma and red blood cell (RBC) cholinesterase levels; *C. diphtheriae*—culture and polymerase chain reaction (PCR) of toxin, serum diphtheria antibodies.

■ Treatment

Ventilation

MG patients with deterioration or impending crisis should be admitted to an intensive care unit because respiratory deterioration can be rapid. Although patients may be unable to handle secretions, glycopyrrolate should only be used with extreme caution as it can lead to mucous plugging. VC and NIF should be measured every 2 to 6 hours, and prompt intubation should be performed when NIF is steadily declining or worse than −20 cm H_2O and/or VC <10 to 15 mL/kg. The initial ventilator mode is typically "assist control/volume control."

After the insult triggering the crisis has been addressed and the patient has received adequate disease modifying therapy, considerations for ventilator weaning can begin. The patient should meet weaning criteria delineated in Chapter 17. A bedside measure of the patients' readiness for extubation is the ability to lift the head off the bed against resistance.

Pressure support can be used as a weaning mode, but a myasthenic patient should also undergo a T-piece or tube compensation trial prior to extubation. An example of a weaning protocol is below:

1. Check NIF/VC early on the day of trial.
   - If NIF is better than −20 cm H_2O and VC > 900 mL without cholinesterase inhibitors (AchI), begin pyridostigmine at 0.5 mg IV every 3 hours.
   - Place patient on T piece or tube compensation mode for 40 minutes, after the dose of pyridostigmine.

2. Continue to monitor patient (blood pressure [BP], pulse rate, respiratory rate).
   - Repeat NIF, VC, at 1.5 to 2 hours following the dose of acetylcholine esterase inhibitor.
   - NIF and VC should be better than initial values (NIF better than −30 cm H_2O and VC >1 L).
   - The patient should be comfortable with stable vital signs. If the patient fails to maintain the above parameters or fatigues, discontinue the weaning trial and place the patient back on a resting mode and discontinue acetylcholine esterase inhibitor.

3. Preparation for extubation:
   - At the end of the second dose of AchI, check that the patient remains stable.
   - Confirm that NIF and VC remain as above.
   - At 1 hour into the third dose of AchI, extubate the patient after good suctioning.
   - Continue to monitor the patient.

Myasthenic-Specific Treatment

- Early in a crisis, pyridostigmine is typically held since it can increase secretions.
- Underlying diseases that may have triggered a crisis should be addressed (infection, tapering of immunosuppression etc.).
- Rapid treatment is initiated early with either plasmapheresis (plasma exchange) or intravenous immunoglobulin (IVIG). Neither has been compared directly to placebo in a randomized clinical trial. Because plasmapheresis has a shorter onset of action, it is often the initial therapy used. In a prospective, randomized trial of plasmapheresis versus IVIG, 50% of patients reached a target improvement in the myasthenia muscle score by day 9 in the plasmapheresis group and by day 12 in the IVIG group, though there were no functional or strength differences by day 15, and there were fewer adverse events in the IVIG group.[1]
- Steroids are often begun concomitantly with rapid acting therapy because rapid therapy has a short duration of action. Steroids can seriously worsen weakness 5 to 10 days after initiation in up to 50% of patients and lead to respiratory failure requiring mechanical ventilation in 10%. However, the weakness produced by steroids typically lasts only 5 to 6 days and is blunted by concomitant rapid acting therapy.
- Acetylcholinesterase inhibitors (pyridostigmine) can be restarted once a patient begins to show improvement from rapid therapy.
- Long-term steroid-sparing immunomodulating therapies are typically begun in the outpatient setting, though they may be started early, particularly in patients with a contraindication to steroids. These medications have a delayed onset of action (**Table 11.2**).

Table 11.2 Treatments for Myasthenic Crisis

Type of Treatment	Dose	Onset of Effect	Maximal Effect	Pros	Cons
Rapid Therapies					
Plasmapheresis	250 mL/kg total divided every other day × 5 treatments (3–5 L per treatment)	1–7 d	1–3 wk	Directly removes acetylcholine receptor antibodies from the circulation. Clinical efficacy correlates with reduction in antibody levels. Faster onset of action than IVIG; improvement in 75% of cases after 2–3 exchanges	Requires invasive line placement: risk of line infection, hypocalcemia, hypofibrinogenemia, hypotension, dysautonomia, hypothermia, thrombocytopenia, thromboembolism; should not be performed the day before surgery. Benefits last only a few weeks.
IVIG	400 mg/kg daily for 5 d (2 g/kg total)	1–2 wk	1–3 wk	No central line is needed. Pretreatment with 250 mL of NS; Tylenol and Benadryl can mitigate complications.	Risk of hypersensitivity with IgA deficiency (should check IgA levels before starting), aseptic meningitis, headache, fluid overload, renal failure (ATN), hyperviscosity syndrome (stroke, MI—care with patients with cryoglobulinemia, monoclonal gammopathy, high lipoproteins, or preexisting vascular disease). Benefits last only a few weeks.

Type of Treatment	Dose	Onset of Effect	Maximal Effect	Pros	Cons
Symptomatic Therapy					
Pyridostigmine	60–120 mg PO q3–8 h	10–15 min	2 h	Acetylcholinesterase inhibitor; can be restarted after patient shows a response to rapid therapy	Not given acutely during a crisis due to increased secretions. Can cause cholinergic crisis, bradycardia, AV block, hypotension, diarrhea, nausea, vomiting, fasciculations, bronchospasm
Chronic Immunotherapy					
Prednisone	60–80 mg/d	2–3 wk	5–6 mo	Can help prevent rebound in acetylcholine antibody levels; faster immunosuppression than other drugs	Can cause early worsening, hyperglycemia, steroid psychosis, glaucoma, immunosuppression, ulcer, osteoporosis, weight gain
Azathioprine	1–3 mg/kg PO divided q.d. or b.i.d. (protocols vary)	4–10 mo	1–2 y	Steroid-sparing immunosuppression	Neoplasia risk, immunosuppression, pancytopenia, pancreatitis, hepatotoxicity

(Continued on next page)

Table 11.2 Treatments for Myasthenic Crisis (*continued*)

Type of Treatment	Dose	Onset of Effect	Maximal Effect	Pros	Cons
Mycophenolate mofetil	1 g PO b.i.d. (protocols vary)	2–4 mo	5–6 mo	Steroid-sparing immunosuppression	Increased risk of lymphoma, immunosuppression, teratogenicity risk, pancytopenia, GI bleed risk, renal failure, acute interstitial lung disease, HTN
Cyclosporine	2.5–4 mg/kg/day divided b.i.d. (protocols vary)	2–4 mo	7 mo	Steroid-sparing immunosuppression	Neoplasia risk, skin malignancy risk, HTN, renal failure, immunosuppression, hepatotoxicity, seizures, posterior reversible leukoencephalopathy, increased ICP, tremor
Surgery					
Thymectomy	Once 10–15% of patients with MG have thymoma.	1–10 y	1–10 y	Potential benefit to all patients with a life expectancy >10 y; can produce long-lasting improvement and liberation from medical therapy; no known chronic side effects	Operative morbidity and mortality, long delay before improvement; total remission in 35%

Abbreviations: ATN, acute tubercular necrosis; AV, Atrial-ventricular; b.i.d., twice a day; GI, gastrointestinal; HTN, hypertension; ICP, intracranial pressure; IgA, immunoglobulin A; IVIG, intravenous high-dose immunoglobulin; MG, myasthenia gravis; MI, myocardial infarction; NS, normal saline; PO, by mouth; q, every; q.d., every day.

■ Prognosis

Mortality from myasthenic crisis is <5%; however, the mean duration of mechanical ventilation is 2 weeks. Predictors for prolonged mechanical ventilation and ICU/hospital length of stay include preintubation $HCO_3 \geq 30$ mL/dL, peak VC on days 1 to 6 post-intubation of < 25 mL/kg, and age >50. The need for >2 weeks of mechanical ventilation per number of risk factors is 0/3 = 0%, 1/3 = 21%, 2/3 = 46%, 3/3 = 88%.[2]

Pearls and Pitfalls

- A myasthenic patient can deteriorate very rapidly and should be closely observed.

- Close monitoring for intubation depends on the clinical exam, VCs, and NIFs.

- Rise in PCO_2 is an early sign of respiratory insufficiency. Myasthenic crisis is advanced once a patient becomes hypoxic.

- Elective intubation is recommended for a VC <10 to 15 mL/kg and NIF worse than −20 cm H_2O or steadily declining VC and NIF.

- Crisis is treated with rapid acting agents (plasmapheresis, IVIG) and longer acting immunomodulatory agents, including steroids and immunosuppressants.

References

1. Gajdos P, Chevret S, Clair B, Tranchant C, Chastang C. Clinical trial of plasma exchange and high-dose intravenous immunoglobulin in myasthenia gravis. Myasthenia Gravis Clinical Study Group. Ann Neurol 1997;41(6):789–796
2. Thomas CE, Mayer SA, Gungor Y, et al. Myasthenic crisis: clinical features, mortality, complications, and risk factors for prolonged intubation. Neurology 1997;48(5):1253–1260

12 Guillain-Barré Syndrome

Jennifer A. Frontera

Guillain-Barré syndrome (GBS) is a heterogeneous group of immune-mediated polyneuropathies with motor, sensory, and dysautonomic features. It is the most common cause of acute flaccid paralysis in the United States, with a frequency of 1 to 3 per 100,000 people, and occurs in all age groups.[1] The pathophysiology of GBS is thought to be related to molecular mimicry triggered by recent infection producing an autoimmune humeral and cell-mediated response against the ganglioside surface molecules of peripheral nerves (**Table 12.1**). There are several clinical subtypes of GBS (**Table 12.2**).

Table 12.1 Factors Associated with Guillain-Barré Syndrome

Bacterial infection	*Campylobacter jejuni* *Haemophilus influenzae* *Mycoplasma pneumoniae* *Borrelia burgdorferi*
Viral infection	CMV EBV HIV (seroconversion)
Vaccines	Influenza vaccine Oral polio vaccine Menactra (Sanofi Pasteur, Lyon, France) meningococcal conjugate vaccine
Medications	Case reports related to streptokinase, isotretinoin, danazol, captopril, gold, heroin, and epidural anesthesia

Abbreviations: CMV, cytomegalovirus; EBV, Epstein-Barr virus; HIV, human immunodeficiency virus.

Table 12.2 The Subtypes of Guillain-Barré Syndrome

Subtype	Comments
Acute inflammatory demyelinating polyradiculoneuropathy (AIDP)	Most common subtype in the U.S. (85–90% of cases) 40% seropositive for *Campylobacter jejuni* Primarily demyelinating Progressive, symmetric weakness, absent/depressed deep tendon reflexes
Acute motor axonal neuropathy (AMAN) Acute sensorimotor axonal neuropathy (AMSAN)	Primary axonal injury 5–10% of U.S. cases 70–75% associated with preceding *Campylobacter jejuni* infection/diarrhea Up to 1/3 may be hyperreflexic Common in China, Japan, and Mexico GM1, GD1a, GalNac-GD1a, and GD1b antibodies
Miller Fisher syndrome	Triad of ataxia, ophthalmoplegia, and areflexia 1/3 develop extremity weakness GQ1b antibodies in 90% 5% of cases in U.S. and 25% of cases in Japan Bickerstaff–Cloake encephalitis—brainstem encephalitis with ophthalmoplegia, ataxia, encephalopathy, and hyperreflexia associated with GQ1b antibodies may be a related entity. It responds to IVIG and plasma exchange.
Pharyngeal-cervical-brachial	Acute arm weakness and swallowing dysfunction May have facial weakness Leg strength and reflexes preserved
Paraparesis	Involvement limited to the lower extremities
Acute pandysautonomia	Sympathetic and parasympathetic involvement Orthostatic hypotension Urinary retention Diarrhea, abdominal pain, ileus, vomiting Pupillary abnormalities Variable heart rate Decreased sweating, salivation, and lacrimation Reflexes diminished Sensory symptoms
Pure sensory	Sensory ataxia Reflexes absent GD1b antibody

Abbreviation: IVIG, intravenous high-dose immunoglobulin.

Case Example

You are called to assess a 42-year-old man with a recent diarrheal illness who complains of severe lower back pain and 5 days of tingling in his feet. He has been unable to climb stairs for the last 2 days and now finds it difficult to walk.

Questions

- Any facial involvement (i.e., diplopia, difficulty swallowing)?
- Any shortness of breath, neck or upper extremity weakness?

Urgent Orders

- Establish airway, breathing, circulation (ABCs). Check vital capacity and negative inspiratory force.
- Intubate for forced vital capacity (VC) <10 to 15 mL/kg or negative inspiratory force (NIF) worse than −20 cm H_2O or steadily declining NIF and/or VC. Beware that patients with bulbar dysfunction often cannot form a proper seal for respiratory testing, and results can sometimes appear worse than the patient's true respiratory status. Multiple VC/NIF measurements should be made to capture the patient's best effort.
- Pulmonary function assessment: Ask the patient to count as rapidly and as high as he or she can in one breath. Every 10 numbers counted roughly equates to 1 L of VC. If the patient cannot count to 10, intubation should be pursued.
- Check an arterial blood gas (ABG): CO_2 retention happens first, so if the patient is already hypoxic, the physician should proceed to intubation without delay. Monitor for arrhythmias and dysautonomia (the leading cause of death in the elderly with GBS is arrhythmia). Admit the patient to an intensive care unit (ICU) or monitored unit.

■ History and Examination

History

A typical history involves acute symmetric ascending weakness, often beginning in the proximal legs. Weakness beginning in the arms or face occurs in 10%, but eventually 50% of patients have facial or oropharyngeal weakness. Paresthesias in the hands and feet are reported in 80% of patients, as is lower back pain. Diplopia occurs in 15% due to oculomotor weakness. Dysautonomia occurs in 70% (tachycardia/bradycardia, wide swings in blood pressure, orthostasis, tonic pupils, urinary retention, ileus/constipation, hypersalivation, and anhidrosis). Respiratory failure requiring intubation occurs in 30%.[2,3]

- Assess for history of recent travel, viral illness, vaccine, or diarrhea.

Physical Examination

- Vital signs: Monitor for dysrhythmia, fluctuating blood pressure, hyperthermia, or hypothermia.
- Frequent checks of VC and NIF (every 2 to 6 hours)

Neurologic Examination

- Mental status: Normal unless CO_2 retention leads to inattentiveness; delirium/hallucination/delusions have been reported in ICU GBS patients.
- Cranial nerves: Ptosis, ophthalmoparesis (diplopia), facial weakness, dysarthria, difficulty swallowing with pooling of secretions, tonic pupils can occur in patients with dysautonomia; rare papilledema has been reported.
- Motor: Ascending symmetric proximal >distal weakness, neck flexor weakness (C3–C5) correlates with respiratory capacity, hypotonia.
- Sensory: Can have abnormal proprioception, typically sensory <motor signs, sensory ataxia can occur
- Reflexes: Absent to reduced reflexes
- Cerebellar: Sensory ataxia may be confused for cerebellar ataxia.

■ Differential Diagnosis

1. *GBS*
2. *Other polyneuropathies*
   - *Acute motor neuropathies due to arsenic, lead poisoning, and porphyria*

- *Tick paralysis:* Can mimic GBS closely with ascending paralysis, ophthalmoparesis, bulbar dysfunction, and reduced reflexes, but has a faster course of progression (hours to days) and is accompanied by ataxia, but no sensory symptoms.[4] Complete cure can occur with tick removal.

- *N-hexane (glue sniffing)*

- *Peripheral nerve vasculitis* (presents as mononeuritis multiplex and can be due to polyarteritis nodosa, Churg–Strauss, rheumatoid arthritis, lupus, etc.)

- *Diphtheria*: Caused by *Corynebacterium diphtheriae,* associated with a thick gray pharyngeal pseudomembrane, atrial-ventricular (AV) block, endocarditis, myocarditis, lymphadenopathy, neuropathy with craniopharyngeal involvement, proximal >distal weakness, and decreased reflexes

- *Ciguatera toxin (red snapper, grouper, barracuda)* affects voltage gated sodium channels of muscles and nerves and produces a characteristic metallic taste in the mouth and hot–cold reversal.

- *Neuropathy due to Lyme disease, sarcoidosis, paraneoplastic disease, and critical illness polyneuropathy*

3. *Neuromuscular junction disease.* There is no sensory involvement in any disorder of neuromuscular transmission.

   - *Myasthenia gravis:* Fatigable weakness, ptosis, nasal voice, ophthalmoparesis (diplopia), facial weakness, no pupillary involvement, fatiguing proximal >distal weakness, arm >leg weakness, normal reflexes.

   - *Lambert–Eaton myasthenic syndrome:* Presynaptic autoimmune attack of voltage gated calcium channels, associated with cancer in 50 to 70% (typically small cell lung cancer), limb symptoms more prominent than ocular/bulbar symptoms at presentation, facilitation with exercise, autonomic dysfunction, and reduced reflexes. Respiratory failure is uncommon.

   - *Botulism:* Neurotoxin produced from *Clostridium botulinum,* permanently blocks presynaptic acetylcholine release at the neuromuscular junction; causes symmetrical descending paralysis with dilated pupils (50%), no sensory deficit, and dysautonomia. Can be treated with trivalent equine antitoxin.

   - *Organophosphate toxicity (malathion, parathion, Sarin, Soman, etc.):* Inactivates acetylcholine esterase, causing SLUDGE (salivation, lacrimation, urinary incontinence, diarrhea, gastrointestinal [GI] upset, emesis), miosis, bronchospasm, blurred vision, and bradycardia. Also causes confusion, optic neuropathy, extrapyramidal effects, dysautonomia, fasciculations, seizures, cranial nerve palsies, and weakness due to continued depolarization at the neuromuscular junction. Delayed polyneuropathy can occur 2 to 3 weeks after exposure. Treat with atropine, pralidoxime (2-PAM), and benzodiazepines. Avoid succinylcholine.

- *Neurotoxic fish poisoning:* Tetrodotoxin (pufferfish) and saxitoxin (red tide) both block neuromuscular transmission.

4. *Muscle disorder:* Critical illness myopathy and acute polymyositis can mimic GBS. Can differentiate with electromyography/nerve conduction study (EMG/NCS).

5. *Spinal cord disorder:* Acute myelopathy can cause weakness, numbness, and acutely depressed deep tendon reflexes, along with bowel and bladder dysfunction. Back pain is common in GBS and spinal cord disorders. Magnetic resonance imaging (MRI) can easily distinguish between the two (enhancement of nerve roots can occur with GBS).

6. *Brainstem disease with multiple cranial neuropathies* (stroke, Bickerstaff–Cloake, rhombencephalitis, basilar meningitis, carcinomatous meningitis, Wernicke's encephalopathy)

Life-Threatening Diagnosis Not to Miss

- *Impending respiratory failure* due to progressive neuromuscular disorder
- *Spinal cord compression* requiring surgical intervention

■ Diagnostic Evaluation

Clinical Criteria

National Institute of Neurological Disorders and Stroke (NINDS) criteria for diagnosis typically apply to acute inflammatory demyelinating polyneuropathy (AIDP); patients with variants may not meet the criteria found in **Table 12.3**.[5]

Table 12.3 National Institute of Neurological Disorders and Stroke Criteria for Diagnosis of Acute Inflammatory Demyelinating Polyneuropathy

Required features	Progressive weakness of >1 limb, ranging from minimal weakness to quadriplegia, and variable trunk, bulbar, facial involvement or ophthalmoplegia Areflexia; distal areflexia with hyporeflexia at the knees and biceps is still consistent with the diagnosis of GBS

Supportive features	Progression of symptoms over days to 4 weeks and recovery starting 2–4 weeks after a plateau in symptoms
	Symmetrical involvement
	Mild sensory signs or symptoms
	CN involvement, bilateral facial weakness
	Autonomic dysfunction
	No fever at onset
	Elevated CSF protein with white cell count <10 mm^3
	EMG/NCS consistent with GBS:
	   80% have NCV slowing/conduction block
	   Patchy reduction in NCV to <60% normal
	   Distal motor latency increase up to 3x normal
	   F waves prolonged
	   15–20% of patients have normal nerve conduction studies

Diagnosis less likely	Sensory level Asymmetry in exam Severe and persistent bowel and bladder dysfunction CSF with >50 white cells or polys

Abbreviations: CN, cranial nerve; CSF, cerebrospinal fluid; EMG, electromyography; GBS, Guillain-Barré syndrome; NCS, nerve conduction studies; NCV, nerve conduction velocity.

Laboratory Findings

- Cerebrospinal fluid (CSF): Albuminocytologic dissociation (elevated CSF protein with normal white blood cells <10 cell/mm^3) appears in 80 to 90% of patients within 1 week. CSF pleocytosis can occur with human immunodeficiency virus (HIV-) associated AIDP.

- Antibodies: GQ1b (85 to 90% of patients with Miller Fisher variant); GM1, GD1a, GalNac-GD1a, and GD1b (associated with axonal variants); GT1a (associated with swallowing difficulty); GD1b (associated with pure sensory variant). Antibodies to *Campylobacter jejuni,* cytomegalovirus (CMV), HIV, Epstein-Barr virus (EBV), and *Mycoplasma pneumoniae* can be tested. Antibody tests are expensive and are not routinely used.

- EMG/NCS: AIDP begins with demyelination at the nerve roots, and nerve conduction studies (NCS) reveal early prolonged F waves and absent H reflexes. Increased distal latencies, conduction block, and temporal dispersion can also be found, but significant slowing of conduction velocities is not seen until the third to fourth week. Sural sparing is typical, while median and ulnar sensory responses are affected. There is relative preservation of compound muscle action potential (CMAP) amplitudes and sensory nerve action potential (SNAP) amplitudes. Needle exam has the highest yield if performed at least 3 weeks after symptom onset. In axonal variants, nerve conduction velocities are normal, distal latencies are not prolonged, and there is no temporal dispersion. CMAP amplitudes are reduced. Very low CMAP amplitude (<20% of normal) portends a poor prognosis (**Table 12.4**).

- MRI: Useful for ruling out cord compression, cauda equina syndrome, and other conditions. Spinal root enhancement can be seen in GBS (cauda equina nerve roots enhance in up to 83% of patients) and is due to disruption of the blood–CNS barrier.

Table 12.4 Electromyography/Nerve Conduction Study

EMG/NCS confirms AIDP	Multifocal demyelination
EMG/NCS highly suggestive of AIDP	Abnormal median SNAP and normal sural SNAP Rapid recovery of low distal CMAPs and SNAPs on subsequent studies
EMG/NCS suggestive of AIDP	Absent F waves with normal nerve conduction studies

Abbreviations: AIDP, acute inflammatory demyelinating polyneuropathy; CMAP, compound muscle action potential; EMG, electromyography; NCS, nerve conduction studies; SNAP, sensory nerve action potential.

■ Treatment

Ventilation

Acute respiratory failure occurs in 30% of GBS patients. GBS patients with deterioration or impending crisis should be admitted to an intensive care unit because respiratory deterioration can be rapid. Although patients may be unable to handle secretions, glycopyrrolate should only be used with extreme caution, as it can lead to mucous plugging. VC and NIF should be measured every 2 to 6 hours, and prompt intubation should be pursued when NIF is worse than -20 cm H_2O and/or VC <10 to 15 mL/kg or if there is a steadily declining NIF and/or VC. Succinylcholine should be avoided during intubation. The initial ventilator mode is typically "assist control/volume control."

Patients should meet weaning criteria delineated in Chapter 17 prior to extubation. A bedside measure of the patient's readiness for extubation is the ability to lift the head off the bed against resistance. Pressure support can be used as a weaning mode, but GBS patients should also undergo a T-piece or tube compensation trial prior to extubation.

Guillain-Barré Syndrome

Specific treatment for Guillain-Barré syndrome is given in **Table 12.5**.[6,7]

American Association of Neurologists' Practice Parameters[8]

- Treatment with IVIG or plasma exchange speeds recovery.
- IVIG and plasma exchange are equivalent.
- Plasma exchange is recommended for GBS patients unable to walk who start treatment within 4 weeks of onset of symptoms. Plasma exchange is also recommended for ambulatory patients who start treatment within 2 weeks of symptom onset.
- IVIG is recommended for nonambulatory GBS patients who start treatment within 2 or possibly 4 weeks from symptom onset.
- The time to onset of recovery is shortened by 40 to 50% by plasma exchange or IVIG.
- Combining IVIG and plasma exchange is not beneficial.
- Steroids alone are not beneficial.[9]

Table 12.5 Guillain-Barré Syndrome Treatments

Type of Treatment	Dose	Pros	Cons
PE	250 mL/kg total divided every other day × 5 treatments (3–5 L per treatment)	PE is believed to remove circulating complement, antibodies, and soluble biological response modifiers. In a meta-analysis of 6 randomized controlled trials: Compared with supportive care, PE reduced the median time to recover walking, the time to onset of motor recovery, the percentage of patients requiring mechanical ventilation, and the duration of mechanical ventilation. PE also increased the proportion of patients who improved one disability grade at 4 weeks. PE is most effective if started within 7 days of symptom onset.	Requires invasive line placement; risk of line infection, hypocalcemia, hypofibrinogenemia, hypotension, dysautonomia, hypothermia, thrombocytopenia, thromboembolism
IVIG	400 mg/kg daily for 5 days (2 g/kg total)	IVIG is believed to interfere with the activation and function of T and B cells, to reduce the activation of complement, and reduce the production of cytokines. No central line is needed. Pretreatment with 250 mL of NS, Tylenol, and Benadryl can mitigate complications. In a meta-analysis no difference in clinical outcome as measured by disability scale was found between IVIG and PE.	Risk of hypersensitivity with IgA deficiency (should check IgA levels before starting), aseptic meningitis, headache, fluid overload, renal failure (ATN), hyperviscosity syndrome (stroke, MI—care with patients with cryoglobulinemia, monoclonal gammopathy, high lipoproteins, or preexisting vascular disease)

Abbreviations: ATN, acute tubercular necrosis; IgA, immunoglobulin A; IVIG, intravenous high-dose immunoglobulin; MI, myocardial Ischemia; NS, normal saline; PE, plasma exchange.

Data from: Raphael JC, Chevret S, Hughes RA, Annane D. Plasma exchange for Guillain-Barré syndrome. Cochrane Database Syst Rev 2002; (2):CD001798.

Hughes RA, Raphaël JC, Swan AV, et al. Intravenous immunoglobulin for Guillain-Barré syndrome. Cochrane Database Syst Rev 2006; (1):CD002063.

- Recommendations for vaccination are as follows:[8]
  - ◦ Vaccinations are not recommended during the acute phase of GBS and are not suggested for at least 1 year after GBS onset.
  - ◦ Future avoidance of a particular vaccine is suggested if it was administered within 6 weeks from the onset of GBS.
  - ◦ For patients with GBS not provoked by influenza vaccine, the benefits of yearly vaccine outweigh the risks of recurrent GBS.

■ Prognosis

The course of GBS is usually progressive for the first 2 weeks of illness, followed by 2 to 4 weeks of a plateau phase, and then a recovery phase. Disease progression for more than 8 weeks is consistent with the diagnosis of chronic inflammatory demyelinating polyneuropathy (CIDP). Poor prognostic factors include older age, rapid onset, preceding diarrheal illness, respiratory failure, and distal CMAP amplitudes <20% of normal. Overall, 85% of GBS patients achieve a full functional recovery within 6 to 12 months. The mortality rate is generally <5%, but up to 15% of patients may have neurologic sequelae. Of those who become ventilator dependent, the mortality rate is 20%. Outcome depends on the GBS variant. Patients with AIDP typically do better than axonal variants, with remyelination occurring over several weeks to months. In a small fraction of AIDP patients there is superimposed axonal degeneration leading to incomplete or delayed recovery. Relapses occur in up to 10% of GBS patients, and 2% of patients develop CIDP.[10,11]

Pearls and Pitfalls

- Ascending weakness and areflexia are the cornerstones of clinical diagnosis.
- CSF and EMG/NCS are the major elements of the diagnostic evaluation.
- GBS patients can deteriorate very rapidly and should be closely observed.
- Elective intubation is recommended for a VC <10 to 15 mL/kg and/or NIF worse than −20 cm H_2O or steadily declining NIF and/or VC.
- GBS is treated with plasma exchange or IVIG. There is no role for corticosteroids.

References

1. Seneviratne U. Guillain-Barré syndrome. Postgrad Med J 2000;76(902):774–782
2. Ropper AH. The Guillain-Barré syndrome. N Engl J Med 1992;326(17):1130–1136
3. Zochodne DW. Autonomic involvement in Guillain-Barré syndrome: a review. Muscle Nerve 1994;17(10):1145–1155
4. Felz MW, Smith CD, Swift TR. A six-year-old girl with tick paralysis. N Engl J Med 2000;342(2):90–94
5. Criteria for diagnosis of Guillain-Barré syndrome. Ann Neurol 1978;3(6):565–566
6. Raphael JC, Chevret S, Hughes RA, Annane D. Plasma exchange for Guillain-Barré syndrome. Cochrane Database Syst Rev 2002; (2):CD001798
7. Hughes RA, Raphaël JC, Swan AV, et al. Intravenous immunoglobulin for Guillain-Barré syndrome. Cochrane Database Syst Rev 2006; (1):CD002063
8. Hughes RA, Wijdicks EF, Barohn R, et al. Quality Standards Subcommittee of the American Academy of Neurology. Practice parameter: immunotherapy for Guillain-Barré syndrome: report of the Quality Standards Subcommittee of the American Academy of Neurology. Neurology 2003;61(6):736–740
9. Hughes RA, Swan AV, van Koningsveld R, van Doorn PA. Corticosteroids for Guillain-Barré syndrome. Cochrane Database Syst Rev 2006; (2):CD001446
10. Asbury AK. New concepts of Guillain-Barré syndrome. J Child Neurol 2000;15(3):183–191
11. Odaka M, Yuki N, Hirata K. Patients with chronic inflammatory demyelinating polyneuropathy initially diagnosed as Guillain-Barré syndrome. J Neurol 2003;250(8):913–916

13 Critical Illness Polyneuropathy and Myopathy

Valerie Dechant, Eduardo Adonias de Sousa, and Kiwon Lee

Critically ill patients are at risk for developing severe weakness secondary to critical illness polyneuropathy (CIP) and/or critical illness myopathy (CIM). Weakness may progress to severe quadriparesis and muscle wasting.[1] The incidence of CIP/CIM in critically ill patients has been reported as 33 to 44% of patients with prolonged admission to critical care settings. The incidence increases to nearly 70% when considering only patients with sepsis.[1-5] Risk factors that have been suggested for CIP and CIM include:

- Sepsis/systemic inflammatory response syndrome (SIRS):[2,3,5,6] Sepsis/SIRS are proinflammatory states that result in the release of cytokines as well as microcirculatory changes. These inflammatory changes can result in CIP by direct injury to the nerve as well as increased permeability of the endoneurium to neurotoxins. The activation of proteosomes in the proinflammatory state can lead directly to muscle protein breakdown, leading to CIM. Elevations in proteosomes have been detected as early as 1 week into intensive care unit (ICU) treatment.[7] Nerve conductions studies done as early as 3 days post-sepsis onset have shown findings consistent with CIP.[2,4,6,8]

- Neuromuscular blocking agents (NMBAs): The role of NMBAs as a risk factor for CIM has been debated. Some authors suggest that the use of NMBAs, particularly aminosteroidal (vecuronium, pancuronium, rocuronium) NMBAs or NMBAs used in conjunction with corticosteroids or aminoglycosides increase the risk of CIM.[9] These agents have been found to cause pharmacological muscle denervation, resulting in upregulation of acetylcholine receptors and glucocorticoid receptors in muscle.[5,6]

- Corticosteroids: The risk of developing CIM/CIP from steroid use is dose dependent with higher doses and longer uses. High-dose steroids contribute to muscle wasting by decreasing myosin synthesis and increasing muscle turnover, as well as triggering skeletal muscle apoptosis. Patients with sepsis may be at a higher risk of steroid-induced CIM, as glucocorticoid receptors of muscle may be unregulated in the septic state.[6,7]

- Hyperglycemia: Elevated blood sugars lead to insulin resistance that can prevent glucose uptake in skeletal muscle, leading to a depletion of energy stores. Tight control of blood sugars has been shown to reduce the risk of CIP.[10]

Case Example

A 57-year-old woman was initially admitted to the ICU with a chronic obstructive pulmonary disease (COPD) exacerbation. Despite treatment with prednisone and β agonist nebulizers, she subsequently developed respiratory failure and became ventilator dependent. Her hospital course was complicated by sepsis. It became difficult to wean the patient from the ventilator. On morning rounds she was noted to have decreased motor function in withdrawing from painful stimuli in all four extremities.

Questions

- What was the dose and duration of steroid use?
- Has the patient been persistently hyperglycemic?
- Did the patient receive neuromuscular blockers, and if so, for how long?
- What antibiotics did the patient receive?
- Does the patient have any known neurologic history that may account for the weakness (i.e., underlying peripheral neuropathy)?

Urgent Orders

- Discontinue neuromuscular blockade, steroids, and aminoglycosides if possible.

■ History and Examination

History

- CIM: Failure to wean from the ventilator, generalized weakness of subacute onset (reports of acute onset do exist)

- CIP: Failure to wean from the ventilator, generalized weakness onset over first 1 to 2 weeks in ICU
- Assess for history of sepsis, steroid use, neuromuscular blockade, antibiotic use, and hyperglycemia.

Physical Examination

Assess for symmetry in the exam: gross asymmetry (hemiparesis, paraparesis, hemisensory loss or crossed signs) suggests an etiology other than CIP/CIM. Prominent mental status changes, cranial nerve involvement, pain, bowel or bladder involvement, cerebellar signs or a sensory level should prompt further work-up.

Neurologic Examination

- A full neurologic examination, including assessment of mental status, cranial nerves, motor skills, and reflexes, as well as a sensory and cerebellar exam, should be performed on all patients.
- CIM: Mental status not affected; flaccid quadriparesis proximal > distal; muscle atrophy; facial weakness is common, but extraocular muscle weakness is uncommon; reflexes normal; sensation intact
- CIP: Mental status not affected, preservation of cranial nerve function, limb weakness, atrophy, fasciculations possible, reduced or absent reflexes, length dependent loss of sensation (test with painful stimuli in less responsive/nonverbal patients)

■ Differential Diagnosis

1. *CIP/CIM*
2. *Guillain-Barré syndrome (GBS)*: GBS is an acute demyelinating polyneuropathy that typically begins as an ascending paralysis accompanied by areflexia and sometimes follows a diarrheal illness. Coincidental occurrence of GBS in a critically ill patient is relatively rare. However, if the history is suspicious, a lumbar puncture can be done (best yield is 1 to 2 weeks from symptom onset). Elevated protein without elevation in leukocytes would be suspicious for GBS. Cerebrospinal fluid (CSF) studies should be normal in CIP/CIM. Nerve conduction studies in GBS should be consistent

with a demyelinating neuropathy in the AIDP (acute inflammatory demyelinating polyneuropathy) subtype (i.e., severely prolonged distal motor latencies, severe motor conduction velocity slowing, severely prolonged F waves), often with an acquired demyelinating component (i.e., partial conduction blocks and abnormal temporal dispersion). The axonal variant of GBS seems to be less frequent in the Western world and more frequent in China and Japan.

3. *Cachetic myopathy*: Critically ill patients can develop a subacute myopathy due to protein catabolism and disuse. Patients develop weakness and muscle atrophy. Type II muscle atrophy is seen histologically.

4. *Spinal cord lesions*: A lesion to the cervical spinal cord can result in tetraparesis and should be considered if the clinical setting is appropriate. Lesions in the cord can initially cause flaccid paresis with decreased reflexes, followed subacutely by hyperreflexia and increased tone. A sensory level may be evident in a patient who is able to participate in a sensory examination. If the history or examination is suspicious, a magnetic resonance imaging (MRI) scan of the cervical cord with and without contrast may be appropriate.

5. *Underlying neuropathy—Toxins and medication effects*: Often medications used in the ICU (i.e., neuromuscular blocking agents) can result in prolonged weakness and sedation. A nerve conduction study may help in this case. For patients who have been treated with neuromuscular blocking agents, "a train of four" (slow repetitive stimulation at 2 to 3 Hz at the median or ulnar nerve) may be used to determine if the medication's effect is persisting.

Life-Threatening Diagnoses Not to Miss

- *Spinal cord lesion*

■ Diagnostic Evaluation

- Electromyography/nerve conduction study (EMG/NCS) findings:
  - CIP: CIP is an acute axonal sensorimotor polyneuropathy. Nerve conduction studies show amplitude reduction of both motor and sensory action potentials and normal or mildly slowed conduction velocities.

○ CIM: CIM is an acute primary myopathy (i.e., it is not due to muscle denervation). Routine electrodiagnostic studies often reveal nonspecific findings, including normal sensory nerve action potentials with small compound muscle action potentials and early recruitment, fibrillation potentials, and positive sharp waves on EMG.

Studies that have employed both biopsy and advanced electrodiagnostic studies suggest that CIM is as common as CIP and that the two often coexist. Differentiation between the two based on physical exam or even basic electrodiagnostic testing can be extremely difficult.[5,6]

Direct muscle stimulation (DMS) has been suggested as a technique to differentiate CIP and CIM. Compound muscle action potential (CMAP) amplitudes derived from direct muscle stimulation (DMS) may be inexcitable (absent) or decreased (<2 mV) in CIM, while they remain normal in CIP. However, nerve-evoked CMAPs are reduced in both CIP and CIM. Thus, a ratio of nerve-evoked CMAP to DMS CMAP would be >0.5 in patients with CIM and <0.5 in patients with CIP (**Table 13.1**).

- Muscle biopsy: Although biopsy is the gold standard for diagnosis of CIM, it is not commonly necessary. Both fiber types I and II are generally affected, but type II myofibers are sometimes more affected. Atrophic myofibers (predominantly type II) with basophilic cytoplasm on hemolytic and eosin (H&E) stain are seen under light microscopy. Electron microscopy shows loss of myosin filaments with relative sparing of actin filaments (patchy thick filament loss). The presence of necrosis is variable, ranging from absent to diffuse lesions described in acute necrotizing myopathy. Inflammatory changes are usually absent, and angulated fibers, rimmed vacuoles, and fatty degeneration may be seen. In patients with CIP, neuropathic features are seen on biopsy, including grouped atrophy, fiber-type grouping, and target fibers.

- Imaging studies: Computed tomography (CT) or MRI of the brain or spinal cord may be appropriate to rule out other etiologies when physical examination and electrodiagnostic studies are not conclusive or if electrodiagnostic studies are not available urgently. These studies may help to eliminate other emergent illnesses.

- Laboratory studies: Serum creatine phosphokinase (CPK) is usually normal or only mildly elevated in CIP/CIM. A lumbar puncture

Table 13.1 Comparison of Critical Illness Polyneuropathy (CIP) and Critical Illness Myopathy (CIM) on Electrodiagnostic Studies

	Motor Nerve Conduction Studies (NCS)	Sensory NCS	Needle Electromyography	Direct Muscle Stimulation
CIP	Low amplitude CMAPs, minimal or no conduction velocity slowing	Low amplitude SNAPs. Absence of conduction block or prolongation of F waves	Fibrillation potentials and PSW; reduced recruitment patterns. Long duration, high amplitude polyphasic motor unit potential after weeks. Absence of decremental response on repetitive stimulation	neCMAP amplitude is reduced; dmCMAP amplitude is proportionally higher than neCMAP.
CIM	Low amplitude CMAPs, normal conduction velocities	Usually normal SNAPs	Fibrillation potentials and PSW; complex repetitive discharges may be present; myopathic units (short duration and polyphasic motor unit action potentials); early, normal, or reduced recruitment patterns. Absence of decremental response on repetitive stimulation	Muscle membrane may be inexcitable—some muscles may be inexcitable to both nerve-evoked and direct muscle needle stimulation. Both neCMAP and dmCMAP are reduced.

Abbreviations: CMAPs, compound muscle action potentials; dmCMAP, direct muscle CMAP; neCMAP, nerve-evoked CMAP; SNAPs, sensory nerve action potentials; PSW, positive sharp waves.

for cerebrospinal fluid (CSF) analysis may be appropriate only if the clinical picture is unclear. This may be especially helpful to differentiate CIP/CIM from Guillain-Barré syndrome. CSF studies should be normal in CIP/CIM.

■ Treatment and Prognosis

Patients with CIP/CIM may be more difficult to wean from mechanical ventilation and require prolonged rehabilitation. The mortality rate of patients with CIP has been reported as ranging from 26 to 71% and may be significantly higher than for patients with similar underlying illness without evidence of CIP.[4,5] Patients who survive their underlying illness may recover some strength within weeks to months; however, many may have residual functional deficits. In one review, 68.4% of patients discharged from the ICU with CIP/CIM regained the ability to breathe and walk independently, while 28.1% had persistent severe disability.[5] There is no specific therapy available for CIP/CIM. If possible, avoid the use of neuromuscular blocking agents and prolonged use of corticosteroids. Physical therapy is recommended to potentially speed recovery.

Pearls and Pitfalls

- Have a high suspicion for CIP/CIM in patients with sepsis or systemic inflammatory response syndrome (SIRS).
- Early nerve conduction studies after 1 week may help in diagnosis.
- Failure to think of CIP/CIM may lead to errors in prognostication, as many patients with CIM/CIP may recover substantially over weeks to months.

References

1. Garnacho-Montero J, Amaya-Villar R, Garcia-Garmendia JL, Madrazo-Osuna J, Ortiz-Leyba C. Effect of critical illness polyneuropathy on the withdrawal from mechanical ventilation and the length of stay in septic patients. Crit Care Med 2005;33(2):349–354
2. de Letter MA, Schmitz PI, Visser LH, et al. Risk factors for the development of polyneuropathy and myopathy in critically ill patients. Crit Care Med 2001;29(12):2281–2286
3. Hund E. Myopathy in critically ill patients. Crit Care Med 1999;27(11):2544–2547
4. Kane SL, Dasta JF. Clinical outcomes of critical illness polyneuropathy. Pharmacotherapy 2002;22(3):373–379
5. Latronico N, Fenzi F, Recupero D, et al. Critical illness myopathy and neuropathy. Lancet 1996;347(9015):1579–1582

6. Bird SJ. Diagnosis and management of critical illness polyneuropathy and critical illness myopathy. Curr Treat Options Neurol 2007;9(2):85–92

7. Friedrich O. Critical illness myopathy: what is happening? Curr Opin Clin Nutr Metab Care 2006;9(4):403–409

8. Tennila A, Salmi T, Pettila V, Roine RO, Varpula T, Takkunen O. Early signs of critical illness polyneuropathy in ICU patients with systemic inflammatory response syndrome or sepsis. Intensive Care Med 2000;26(9):1360–1363

9. Murray MJ, Brull SJ, Bolton CF. Brief review: nondepolarizing neuromuscular blocking drugs and critical illness myopathy. Can J Anaesth 2006;53(11):1148–1156

10. Van den Berghe G, Schoonheydt K, Becx P, Bruyninckx F, Wouters PJ. Insulin therapy protects the central and peripheral nervous system of intensive care patients. Neurology 2005;64(8):1348–1353

14 Brain Death and Organ Donation

Jennifer A. Frontera

Brain death, which is equivalent to legal death, is defined as the irreversible loss of brain and brainstem function. There is no universal policy governing the declaration of brain death, and protocols vary from hospital to hospital, although many states have issued guidelines. The declaration of pediatric brain death follows different parameters, and adult brain death will be the focus of this chapter. In the United States, top etiologies for brain death include subarachnoid hemorrhage, traumatic brain injury, intracerebral hemorrhage, and hypoxic ischemic injury.

According to the United Network for Organ Sharing (UNOS), there were over 98,000 patients awaiting transplant in 2007, yet only 14,000 donors. In 2005, 18 patients died each day awaiting transplant.[1] Although historically most organ donations have come after neurologic death, donation after cardiac death (DCD) and tissue donation (cornea, skin, bone, and musculoskeletal tissue) are also possible. Patients with terminal injuries and intent to withdraw life support are potential donors if cardiac death is expected within 60 minutes of withdrawal of support (DCD). For DCD, withdrawal of life-sustaining measures is performed in the operating room. Typically, morphine and benzodiazepines are administered for comfort after withdrawal of support.

Final decisions over suitability of a donor should be arbitrated by the regional organ donor center, not the physician (**Table 14.1**). Because the progression from brain death to somatic death results in the loss of 10 to 20% of potential donors, intensive monitoring and care are needed to preserve organs for donation.[2]

Table 14.1 Contraindications to Organ Donation

Contraindication	Notes
Multisystem organ failure due to sepsis	
History of cancer	EXCEPT: Skin cancer other than melanoma, certain primary brain tumors, remote prostate cancer
Viral infections	HIV, HTLV-1 and 2, rabies, reactive HbsAg, measles, West Nile virus, SARS, adenovirus, enterovirus, parvovirus, active HSV, VZV, EBV, viral encephalitis/meningitis Hepatitis B or C organs can be transplanted into recipients with the same virus CMV+ organs can be transplanted—better success if recipient is prophylaxed
Bacterial infections	Tuberculosis, gangrenous bowel, bowel perforation, intra-abdominal sepsis
Fungal infections	Active *Cryptococcus, Aspergillus, Histoplasma, Coccidioides, Candidemia*, invasive yeast infections
Parasitic infections	*Leishmania, Trypanosoma, Strongyloides*, malaria
Prion disease	CJD, vCJD, fatal familial insomnia, Gerstmann-Sträussler-Scheinker syndrome

Abbreviations: CJD, Creutzfeldt-Jakob disease; CMV, cytomegalovirus; EBV, Epstein-Barr virus; HbsAg, hepatitis B surface antigen; HIV, human immunodeficiency virus; HSV, herpes simplex virus; HTLV-1, human T-lymphotropic virus 1; SARS, severe acute respiratory syndrome; vCJD, variant CJD; VZV, varicella zoster virus.

Case Example

You are called to the medical intensive care unit (ICU) to evaluate a 53-year-old man who suffered a cardiac arrest 3 days ago. The medical team has noticed that the patient has no brainstem reflexes and no response to painful stimuli.

Questions

- Has the patient received any sedation recently, and if so, what?
- What are the patient's temperature and vital signs?

- Does the patient have any severe electrolyte or acid–base abnormalities?
- Is the patient overbreathing the ventilator?

Urgent Orders

- Discontinue any sedation the patient may be receiving.
- If the patient is hypothermic, place a rewarming blanket.

■ History and Examination

History

Certain clinical criteria are necessary prior to the diagnosis of brain death:

- A diagnosis compatible with brain death (e.g., intracranial hemorrhage [ICH], subarachnoid hemorrhage [SAH])
- Exclusion of confounding factors: no severe electrolyte, endocrine, or acid–base abnormalities
- Exclusion of intoxicating drugs, poisoning, or neuromuscular blockade
  - Midazolam has active metabolites, and propofol can accumulate. Effects can be seen for prolonged periods after discontinuation of medications. Check urine toxicology for opiates or benzodiazepines and illicit drugs. Benzodiazepines can be reversed with flumazenil and opiates with naloxone. There is no urine or blood test for propofol.
  - Reverse neuromuscular blockade with neostigmine/glycopyrrolate; check a train-of-four stimulus to confirm reversal. On the maximal stimulus over the median nerve four sharp twitches of the thumb and fingers should be seen if neuromuscular blockade is reversed.
  - If a known drug cannot be quantified, the patient should be observed for 4x the half-life of the drug prior to proceeding with the brain death examination, or a confirmatory test can be performed (see below).
- Patient must not be hypothermic (core temperature <32°C) or hypotensive (systolic blood pressure [SBP] <90 mm Hg).

Physical Examination

Brain death is a clinical diagnosis based on the physical examination. In most hospitals the brain death exam can be performed by a neurologist, neurosurgeon, or other specially designated physicians. Typically, two neurologic exams performed 6 hours apart and an apnea test are required to confirm brain death.

- Vitals: Assess for hypothermia, urine output (assess for diabetes insipidus, urinary output [UOP] $\geq$5 cc/kg/h $\times$ 2 hours, or urine-specific gravity <1.005), and hypotension.

Neurologic Examination

- Mental status: Patient should have no response to verbal, tactile, or painful stimuli.
- Cranial nerves (**Table 14.2**)
- Motor: No response to deep nail bed pressure in any extremity
- Sensory: No motor or hemodynamic (tachycardia) response to pain.
- Reflexes: Brisk reflexes do not exclude brain death. A variety of exam findings, including C-spine reflexes (seen in 44–75% of patients)[3,4] can be compatible with brain death (**Table 14.3**).

Table 14.2 Neurologic Examination of Cranial Nerves in a Brain-Dead Patient

Brainstem Reflex	Cranial Nerves Tested	Response
Pupillary reflex	Afferent: II, Efferent: III	Midposition fixed (4 mm) or fixed and dilated (9 mm)
Corneal reflex	Afferent: V, Efferent: VII	No blink bilaterally to limbus stimuli
Oculocephalic/ doll's eye	Afferent: VIII, Efferent: III, IV, VI	Eyes move with head as head is turned (no doll's eye effect)
Oculovestibular/ cold calorics	Afferent: V, VIII, Efferent: III, VI	No eye movement bilaterally when 60 cc of cold water instilled on intact tympanic membrane bilaterally (5 minutes apart)
Cough/gag	Afferent: IX, X, Efferent: X	Absent cough/gag

Table 14.3 Reflexes that Can Be Seen in Brain-Dead Patients

• Triple flexion	• Undulating toe (flexion/extension)	• Sweating, flushing, tachycardia, blood pressure swings
• Babinski	• Finger flexor movement	• Opisthotonus
• Lazarus (looks like Moro reflex)	• Semirhythmic facial spasm (due to denervated seventh nerve)	• Tonic neck flexion (passive neck movement induces fencer posturing or stereotyped trunk or extremity movement)

■ Differential Diagnosis

1. *Brain death*
2. *Locked-in syndrome* (pontine ischemia or hemorrhage): Evaluate for command following with vertical eye movement or blinking.
3. *Drug intoxication, neuromuscular blockade*

Life-Threatening Diagnoses Not to Miss

- *Hypothermia*: Temperature must be $\geq 32°C$ to proceed with brain death testing.
- *Metabolic disarray (i.e., acidosis)*
- *Endocrine abnormalities: Hypothyroidism/myxedema coma*

■ Diagnostic Evaluation

Apnea Test

Complications occur in 25% of patients undergoing an apnea test, most often in patients with inadequate preoxygenation, acid–base or electrolyte abnormalities, or preexisting arrhythmia.[5] To avoid such complications, normalize pH, preoxygenate to PO_2 >200 mm Hg, and ensure that core temperature >36.5°C. CO_2 rises roughly 3 mm Hg per minute. Follow steps shown in **Table 14.4**.

Table 14.4 Performing the Apnea Test

1.	Check baseline ABG. A baseline $pCO_2 \geq 40$ mm Hg makes it more likely that the apnea test will reach target pCO_2 levels.
2.	While the patient is connected to an O_2 sat monitor and BP monitor, disconnect the ventilator and use 100% 6 L/min flow-by.
3.	A physician designated to declare brain death monitors for chest excursion or respiratory effort after ventilator disconnect.
4.	Check an ABG after 8 min.
5.	If $pCO_2 \geq 60$ mm Hg or increased by 20 mm Hg over baseline pCO_2 and no respiratory movement observed: the apnea test supports brain death.
6.	Abort the test and reconnect the ventilator if the SBP < 90 mm Hg, the patient has a significant desaturation, or an arrhythmia develops. Draw an immediate ABG.
7.	If the patient cannot tolerate an apnea test, a confirmatory test must be performed.

Abbreviations: ABG, arterial blood gas; BP, blood pressure; sat, saturation; SBP, systolic blood pressure.

Confirmatory Tests

Confirmatory tests are necessary when there is severe facial or C-spine trauma (do not perform doll's eye maneuver on patients with C-spine injury), surgical pupils or preexisting pupillary abnormality, sleep apnea or chronic obstructive pulmonary disease (COPD) with chronic CO_2 retention or toxic levels of sedatives, aminoglycosides, tricyclic antidepressants, anticholinergics, chemotherapeutics, or neuromuscular blockade. Examples of confirmatory tests include:

- Digital subtraction angiography (DSA): Gold standard—absence of intracranial blood flow at the level of carotid bifurcation or circle of Willis. The external carotid artery typically fills. Bilateral anterior circulation and posterior circulation injections are required.
- Computed tomography angiography (CTA) or magnetic resonance angiography (MRA): similar to above.
- Transcranial Doppler ultrasound: Isolated systolic flow (no diastolic flow) or reverberating flow are compatible with brain death. Both

bilateral anterior circulation and posterior circulation must be insonated and reveal isolated systolic or reverberating flow. The sensitivity of TCD for brain death is 91 to 99%, and the specificity is 100%. Absent temporal windows occur in 10% of the population.[6]

- Electroencephalography (EEG)–electrical-cerebral silence: Criteria include >2 microvolt sensitivity, 1 to 30 Hz, minimum of eight electrodes 10 cm apart, impedance 100 to 10,000 Ω, and 30 minutes of recording. Due to frequent ICU artifact, it is difficult to use EEG to confirm brain death.

- Radionucleotide study (technetium single-photon emission computed tomography [SPECT]): Empty lightbulb sign. No radionucleotide uptake intracranially.

- Somatosensory evoked potential (SSEP): Absent N20–P22 bilaterally; less useful in patients with neuropathy or primary brainstem pathology.

Notification of Next of Kin

The physician is responsible for informing the next of kin of the patient's prognosis, though consent is not needed to perform a brain death examination. Once a patient is declared brain dead, the patient is legally dead and can be extubated unless the patients next of kin has consented to organ donation. Reasonable accommodations should be made for the family's religious and moral beliefs, and life support should be continued for a reasonable amount of time based on family wishes. Brain-dead patients can survive typically for only 1 to 2 weeks after brain death is declared (97% suffer cardiac death within 7 days).[7]

Notification of Organ Donor Services

Regional organ donor networks should be informed when:
- Impending brain death is suspected
- Withdrawal of care is planned
- After all deaths for potential cornea or tissue donation

Organ donor representatives, rather than the primary physician team, should reach out to the family for potential donation to avoid a conflict of interests. This is typically done after the second brain death examination and apnea test have been performed.

■ Treatment and Care for the Potential Organ Donor

Sympathetic Surge

The final stage of brain death is typically medullary-level death, at which point a sympathetic surge occurs with subsequent hypertension, and potentially, cardiac stunning with myocyte necrosis and troponin leak. Intracranial pressure (ICP) is typically elevated, and a Cushing's triad (elevated ICP, bradycardia, and abnormal respiratory pattern) may be seen. Spinal cord ischemia coincides with herniation, resulting in deactivation of the sympathetic nervous system and hypotension.

Pan-Hypopituitary State

With brain death comes a pan-hypopituitary state with concomitant diabetes insipidus and hypotension. Hormonal therapy addresses this pan-hypopituitary state and has been shown to reduce cardiovascular lability, electrocardiogram (ECG) abnormalities, and acid–base disturbances. Hormonal therapy has been shown to improve transplant rates and graft function. Patients refractory to volume and vasopressors have been shown to have a significant response to hormonal therapy such that >50% can be weaned off other vasopressors.[8] In a study of 10,292 brain-dead donors, hormonal therapy with thyroxine, insulin, and pitressin yielded 22.5% more organs with significant increases in kidney, heart, liver, lung, and pancreas donation.[9] Graft loss and graft dysfunction posttransplantation are significantly lower in organs that were managed preoperatively with hormonal therapy.[10] Means of employing hormonal therapy are outlined below.

Flowsheet of Organ-Sparing Therapy

Organ-sparing therapy should be initiated as soon as brain death is evident or impending brain death is suspected (**Fig. 14.1**).

1. *Assess hemodynamics.*
   - Is the patient hemodynically unstable (SBP <90 mm Hg, mean arterial pressure (MAP) <60 mm Hg)?
     ◦ Make sure central line and A-line are in place; order transthoracic echocardiography (TTE)
   - Is the patient hypovolemic (central venous pressure [CVP] <5 mm Hg, pulmonary capillary wedge pressure [PCWP] <8 mm Hg, UOP < 0.5 mL/kg/h, or fluid deficit > 2 L in 24 hours)?

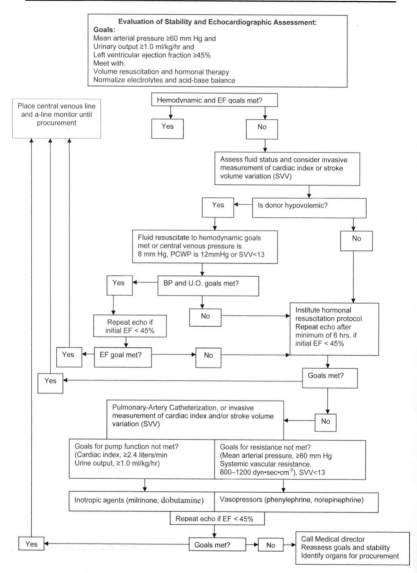

Fig. 14.1 Evaluation of stability and echocardiographic assessment. U.O., urine output; EF, ejection fraction.

- Bolus 10 mL/kg normal saline (NS); continue to infuse 2 to 3 mL/kg/h until goal SBP ≥90 mm Hg, MAP ≥60 mm Hg, CVP ≥5 mm Hg, or PCWP ≥8 mm Hg.

- Use NS if Na$^+$ ≤155 mg/dL, 1/2 NS if Na$^+$ 156 to 164, and 1/4 NS or 5% dextrose in water (D5W) if Na$^+$ >165 mg/dL.
- Maintain fluids at 1.5 to 2 mL/kg/h (use above saline strategy depending on Na$^+$ level).
- Is the patient actively bleeding?
  ∘ Use colloids (packed red blood cells [pRBC], fresh frozen plasma [FFP], etc.) if patient is actively bleeding.
- Does the patient have diabetes insipidus (UOP ≥5 cc/kg/h for ≥2 hours, urine-specific gravity <1.005, serum Na >145 mEq/dL, *or* serum osmolality >305 mg/dL)? Of note, hyponatremia can also occur as part of triphasic diabetes insipidus (initial hypernatremia followed by hyponatremia and then hypernatremia again), which occurs more commonly after pituitary surgery.
  ∘ Bolus vasopressin 0.5 U intravenously (IV), then begin infusion (25 U in 250 mL NS or D5W) at 0.5 U/h; titrate to UOP 1 to 2 mL/kg/h, max dose 6 U per hour.
  ∘ Avoid D5W, as glucose load can lead to osmotic diuresis and worsen hypotension.

2. *Treat hypopituitary state with hormonal resuscitation.*
   - This regimen should be initiated in all brain-dead patients. Thyroxine (synthroid) and vasopressin act as pressors and should be titrated to maintain SBP ≥90 mm Hg or MAP ≥60 mm Hg. Thyroxine has inotropic properties as well. (**Table 14.5**).

3. *Meet hemodynamic goals.*
   - SBP ≥90 mm Hg, MAP ≥60 mm Hg, UOP ≥1.0 mL/kg/h, Ejection fraction (EF) ≥45%
     ∘ If the above goals are not met, place a pulmonary artery catheter or a continuous cardiac index monitor (PiCCO [Pulsion Medical Systems, Munich, Germany], Flotrac [Edwards Lifesciences, Irvine CA], LiDCO [LiDCO Ltd., Cambridge, UK], etc.).
     ∘ If cardiac index ≤2.4 L/min and UOP ≤1.0 mL/kg/h, initiate inotrope (milrinone or dobutamine).
     ∘ If MAP ≤60 mm Hg or systemic vascular resistance (SVR) ≤800 dyn · sec/cm^5, use vasopressor (phenylephrine, norepinephrine).

Table 14.5 Organ-Sparing Therapy

Drug	Dosage	Comments
Thyroxine T4	Administer 10 U regular insulin with 1 ampule of 50% dextrose (unless glucose >300 mg/dL); then 20 µg T4 IV bolus (mixed 200 µg in 500 mL NS) followed by 10 µg/h of T4 IV Maximum dose 20 µg/h	Inotropic effect, can be used as a pressor Causes hyperkalemia with bolus; must administer insulin and D50 prior to initiation T4 shown to be more beneficial than T3.
Vasopressin	0.5 U/h IV (25 U in 250 mL NS or D5W) Maximum dose 6 U/h	Check for DI: UOP ≥5 cc/kg/h for ≥2 h, urine-specific gravity <1.005, serum Na >145 mEq/dL, or serum osmolality >305 mg/dL Titration should be based on BP, UOP, Na$^+$ levels, and urine-specific gravity.
Insulin	1 U/h IV (25 U in 250 mL NS)	Adjust to maintain glucose 80–110 mg/dL.
Methylprednisolone	15 mg/kg IV bolus; repeat daily	Leads to better yield for lung donation

Abbreviations: BP, blood pressure; D5W, 5% dextrose in water; DI, diabetes insipidus; IV, intravenous; NS, normal saline; UOP, urinary output.

4. *Organ-specific management:*

- *Lung:* The rate of lung recovery is lower than that of other organs. Empiric Zosyn (Wyeth Pharmaceuticals, Philadelphia, PA) or Unasyn (Pfizer U.S. Pharmaceuticals, New York, NY) is recommended by most organ donor foundations, and methylprednisolone 15 mg/kg IV leads to better lung procurement rates. Bronchoscopy is necessary to assess the lungs for transplant and can be therapeutic for mucous plugging (washings should not be performed).

  ○ Ventilator settings: Start with tidal volume (TV) 8 to 10 mL/kg; use 6 mL/kg in cases of acute lung injury or acute respiratory distress syndrome (ALI/ARDS); avoid atelectasis with positive end expiratory pressure (PEEP) $\geq$5 mm Hg, goal PaO_2/FIO_2 >300, plateau pressure $\leq$30 mm Hg.

- ◦ Recruitment maneuvers: If decreased PO_2 or chest x-ray (CXR) with atelectasis, increase PEEP to 30 mm Hg × 30 seconds (dial up over 5 to 10 seconds). Increase baseline PEEP and repeat in 5 minutes. Beware of hypotension during increased PEEP. Such recruitment maneuvers have not been shown useful in ALI/ARDS patients,[11] but they still appear in some regional management protocols. Bilevel and APRV (airway pressure release ventilation) are used by some centers to improve recruitment.

- *Heart*: Some patients will experience neurogenic stunned myocardium after brain death, which is reversible. Initial low EF may not preclude cardiac donation. TTE should be repeated after hemodynamic goals are optimized. Cardiac catheterization is typically performed prior to donation. This procedure is considered emergent because longer medical care prior to donation has been shown to lead to lower cardiac allograft yield.

5. *Other laboratories and studies*:
   - Organ donor representative sends: human immunodeficiency virus (HIV) 1/2; (HTLV-) 1, 2; rapid plasma reagin (RPR), toxoplasmosis immunogammaglobulin (IgG); cytomegalovirus (CMV) IgG; Epstein-Barr virus (EBV) IgG; varicella zoster virus (VZV) IgG; herpes simplex virus (HSV-) 1, 2; hepatitis A, B, C.
   - Physician sends: chemistry panel, liver function tests (LFTs), complete blood count (CBC), coagulation profile, amylase, lipase, and troponin every 6 hours, daily CXR, and electrocardiogram (ECG).

■ Prognosis

Aggressive management with hormonal therapy and hemodynamic monitoring have been shown to improve organ procurement rates.[12]

Pearls and Pitfalls

- Brain death is a clinical diagnosis comprised of two neurologic examinations 6 hours apart.
- Organ-sparing therapy, including hemodynamic management, and hormonal resuscitation should be initiated as soon as brain death becomes evident to preserve the choice for donation for families and increase organ procurement rates.
- Rapid referral to the local organ donor network can help improve donation rates.

References

1. www.unos.org Accessed 7/08.
2. Kutsogiannis DJ, et al. Medical management to optimize donor organ potential: review of the literature. Can J Anaesth 2006;53(8):820–830
3. Saposnik G, et al. Spontaneous and reflex movements in 107 patients with brain death. Am J Med 2005;118(3):311–314
4. Ivan LP. Spinal reflexes in cerebral death. Neurology 1973;23(6):650–652
5. Goudreau JL, Wijdicks EF, Emery SF. Complications during apnea testing in the determination of brain death: predisposing factors. Neurology 2000;55(7):1045–1048
6. Wijdicks EF, et al. Practice parameter: prediction of outcome in comatose survivors after cardiopulmonary resuscitation (an evidence-based review): report of the Quality Standards Subcommittee of the American Academy of Neurology. Neurology 2006;67(2):203–210
7. Hung TP, Chen ST. Prognosis of deeply comatose patients on ventilators. J Neurol Neurosurg Psychiatry 1995;58(1):75–80
8. Salim A, Vassiliu P, Velmahos GC, et al. The role of thyroid hormone administration in potential organ donors. Arch Surg 2001;136(12):1377–1380
9. Rosendale JD, Kauffman HM, McBride MA, et al. Hormonal resuscitation yields more transplanted hearts, with improved early function. Transplantation 2003;75(8):1336–1341
10. Rosendale JD, Chabalewski FL, McBride MA, et al. Increased transplanted organs from the use of a standardized donor management protocol. Am J Transplant 2002;2(8):761–768
11. Meade MO, Cook DJ, Guyatt GH, et al. Ventilation strategy using low tidal volumes, recruitment maneuvers, and high positive end-expiratory pressure for acute lung injury and acute respiratory distress syndrome: a randomized controlled trial. JAMA 2008;299(6):637–645
12. Wood KE, Becker BN, McCartney JG, D'Alessandro AM, Coursin DB. Care of the potential organ donor. N Engl J Med 2004;351(26):2730–2739

15 Management of Elevated Intracranial Pressure

David Seder, Stephan A. Mayer,
and Jennifer A. Frontera

The cranial vault has a fixed volume comprised of the brain parenchyma (80% or ~1200 mL), blood (10% or ~150 mL), and cerebrospinal fluid (CSF; 10% or ~150 mL produced at a rate of 20 mL/h or 500 mL/day). Because the volume of the intracranial vault is fixed, intracranial pressure (ICP) increases when additional volume overwhelms the modest buffering capacity afforded by an extracranial shift of CSF and venous blood (**Fig. 15.1** and **Fig. 15.2**). Pressure and volume are related by compliance (Δvolume/Δpressure). In non-

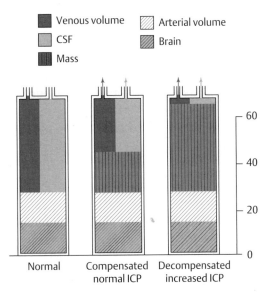

Fig. 15.1 Intracranial pressure (ICP) compensation. Under normal conditions the cranial vault contents include the brain, arterial and venous blood, and cerebrospinal fluid (CSF). When a mass is present, extrusion of venous blood and CSF allows for a compensated ICP. If a mass becomes large enough, ICP increases.

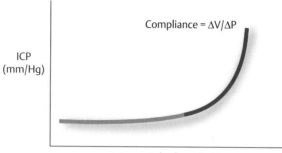

Fig. 15.2 Monroe-Kellie doctrine. Over a range of intracranial vault volumes, the intracranial pressure (ICP) remains relatively constant due to compensation, such as increased outflow of venous blood and cerebrospinal fluid. At an inflection point ICP increases exponentially when compensation measures are exhausted or in noncompliant systems.

compliant systems, small changes in volume will result in exponential pressure changes. Neuronal injury results from reductions in cerebral blood flow (CBF) and resulting ischemia as cerebral perfusion pressure (CPP) is compromised or from direct tissue compression when the brain moves along pressure gradients and herniates between fixed compartments (**Fig. 15.3**). Etiologies of elevated ICP are outlined in **Table 15.1**. Elevated intracranial pressure is a medical and surgical emergency, in which irreversible brain injury or death may be averted by timely intervention.

Case Example

A previously healthy 35-year-old woman at 34 weeks' gestation with preeclampsia and hemolysis, elevated liver enzyme levels, and a low platelet count (HELLP syndrome) is admitted and emergently delivered. She complains of extreme headache and vomiting. A computed tomography (CT) scan of the brain shows diffuse cerebral edema, and an ICP monitor is inserted. The initial ICP is 38 mm Hg, and the CPP is 55 mm Hg.

Questions

- Are the hemodynamic data believable? Make sure the ICP monitor and arterial catheter are properly leveled and zeroed. The

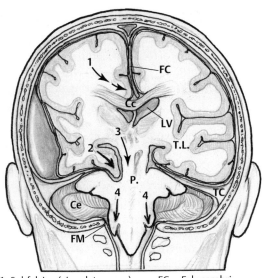

1. Subfalcine (cingulate gyrus) herniation
2. Uncal herniation into tentorial hiatus
3. Caudal displacement of brainstem
4. Cerebellar (tonsillar) herniation through foramen magnum

FC - Falx cerebri
LV - Lateral ventricle
TC - Tentorium cerebelli
FM - Foramen magnum
P. - Pons
Ce - Cerebellum
Cc - Corpus callosum
T.L. - Temporal lobe

Fig. 15.3 Coronal diagram demonstrating different patterns of brain herniation.

Table 15.1 Etiologies of Raised Intracranial Pressure

Primary Pathology	Examples
Mass lesions	Tumor, hematoma, air, abscess, foreign body
CSF accumulation	Hydrocephalus: obstructive or communicative (tumor, intraventricular hemorrhage, ventriculitis/meningitis, direct compression of ventricular drainage), overproduction (papilloma)
Vascular	Input failure (increased CBF or CBV due to exhausted autoregulation) or output failure (venous congestion or sinus thrombosis)
Cerebral edema	
Vasogenic	Vessel damage due to tumor, infection/abscess, contusion
Cytotoxic	Cell membrane/pump failure, ischemia
Hydrostatic	Transmural pressure due to hydrocephalus
Hypo-osmolar	For example, due to hyponatremia

Abbreviations: CBF, cerebral blood flow; CBV, cerebral blood volume; CSF, cerebrospinal fluid.

ICP reading should display a physiologic waveform, and the CPP should be calculated from an arterial catheter placed at the level of the foramen of Monroe (tragus of ear) with a reliable pressure tracing. ICP rises with cough or lowering of the head of the bed.

- What is the patient's neurologic status?
- What mechanism caused the acute increase in ICP?

Urgent Orders

- Address airway, breathing, circulation (ABCs): Assess the patient's need for intubation. If the patient has a decreased mental status and cannot protect her airway, proceed to intubation immediately. When intubating a patient with elevated ICP, measures should be taken to avoid coughing and bucking during intubation. Lidocaine 1% 1 mL/kg intravenously (IV) suppresses the cough reflex, may lower cerebral oxygen demand, reduces bronchospasm, and should be used as premedication for intubation in addition to standard intubation medications (see Chapter 16).

- Elevate head of bed to 30 to 45 degrees, and keep head midline to promote venous drainage.

- Treat agitation and pain.

- Prescribe mannitol 20% 1.0 to 1.5 g/kg rapid intravenous (IV) infusion or 23% hypertonic saline, 30 mL over 10 to 20 minutes via a central line.

- Hyperventilate to pCO_2 ~30 mm Hg (short term and only if the patient is herniating). If the patient is acutely herniating, disconnect the patient from the ventilator and manually bag into endotracheal tube (ETT) for hyperventilation.

- Order a noncontrast CT scan of the head.

- Pursue a neurosurgical consultation for ICP monitoring and/or possible decompressive surgery.

■ History and Examination

History

Note acuity of onset: rapid onset suggests hemorrhage, acute hydrocephalus, or trauma; gradual onset suggests tumor, long-standing hydrocephalus, or abscess, for example. Previous history of cancer, weight loss, smoking, drug use, coagulopathy, trauma, or ischemic disease may point toward an etiology. Headache is caused by pressure exerted on the dural pain fibers of cranial nerve V. Nausea and vomiting are common accompaniments of elevated ICP.

Physical Examination

- Breathing patterns can help localize the level of injury (**Fig. 15.4**).
- Vital signs: Cushing's triad (hypertension, bradycardia, respiratory irregularity) implies elevated ICP.

Neurologic Examination

- A full neurologic examination, including assessment of mental status, cranial nerves, motor skills, and reflexes, as well as a sensory and cerebellar exam, should be performed on all patients.
- Mental status changes range from inattention to coma.
- Cranial nerve examination: Pupillary findings can be localizing (**Fig. 15.5**). Third nerve palsy (clue to uncal herniation, posterior communicating artery [PCOMM] aneurysm rupture), sixth nerve palsy (nonlocalizing), and papilledema (unreliable finding; the presence of venous pulsations is reassuring for normal ICP, but they are sometimes not seen in normal patients).
- Motor examinaton: Posturing—decorticate or flexor posturing is classically due to lesions anywhere from the cortex to the red nucleus. Decerebrate or extensor posturing is classically due to lesions below the level of the red nucleus. These fixed anatomic localizations of posturing do not always apply. Note that mixed posturing can be seen in one limb, or different types of posturing can be seen on opposite sides of the body.

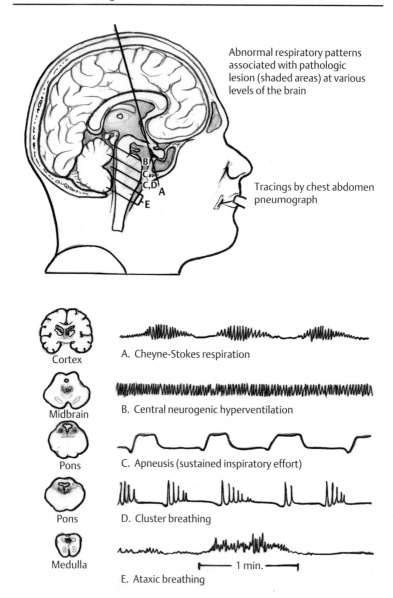

Abnormal respiratory patterns associated with pathologic lesion (shaded areas) at various levels of the brain

Tracings by chest abdomen pneumograph

Cortex

A. Cheyne-Stokes respiration

Midbrain

B. Central neurogenic hyperventilation

Pons

C. Apneusis (sustained inspiratory effort)

Pons

D. Cluster breathing

Medulla

⊢——— 1 min. ———⊣

E. Ataxic breathing

Fig. 15.4 Abnormal respirator patterns associated with pathologic lesions at various levels of the brain. Tracings represent chest and abdomen pneumographs.

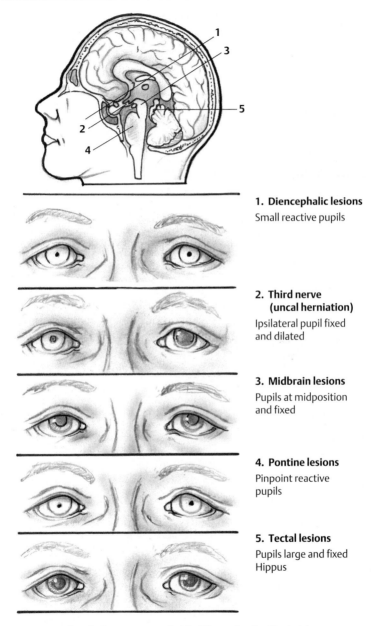

1. Diencephalic lesions
Small reactive pupils

**2. Third nerve
   (uncal herniation)**
Ipsilateral pupil fixed
and dilated

3. Midbrain lesions
Pupils at midposition
and fixed

4. Pontine lesions
Pinpoint reactive
pupils

5. Tectal lesions
Pupils large and fixed
Hippus

Fig. 15.5 Pupillary findings associated with different levels of brain injury.

- Kernohan's notch phenomenon (long track signs/weakness ipsilateral to the lesion due to herniation and compression of the contralateral cerebral peduncle) is an ominous sign.

■ Differential Diagnosis

1. *Elevated ICP*
2. *Seizures* (tonic-clonic activity can occasionally be mistaken for posturing, and coma due to nonconvulsive seizures could be mistaken for possible ICP elevation)
3. *Metabolic coma can cause mental status changes.* Pupillary reactivity should be spared. Diabetic third nerve palsies are pupil sparing (because the pupil fibers laminate the outside of the nerve, and diabetes causes microvascular infarcts affecting the central nerve fibers).
4. A blown pupil in the context of a normal mental status almost never is consistent with herniation. Be on the lookout for *medications that cause fixed pupillary dilation* (any local β agonist or anticholinergic medication: nebulizers—both ipratropium and albuterol are notorious culprits). *Physiologic anisocoria* occurs in 10% of the population and is characterized by asymmetric though reactive pupils. New-onset anisocoria requires determination of which pupil is affected. This can be differentiated by examining anisocoria in the light and dark. More prominent anisocoria in the dark suggests a sympathetic lesion (with failure to dilate), whereas more pronounced anisocoria in bright light suggests a parasympathetic lesion (with failure to constrict).
5. *Meningeal irritation* (infectious or sterile) can cause headache, photophobia, nausea, and vomiting and mental status changes (if there is associated encephalitis).
6. *Migraine* can present with acute headache, nausea, vomiting, photophobia, and focal deficits (complicated migraine). Because mass lesions can present with migrainous-type headache, all patients with new-onset migraines should have brain imaging.

Life-Threatening Diagnoses Not to Miss

- *Herniation*
- *Acute hydrocephalus*
- *Surgical mass lesions*

■ Diagnostic Evaluation

ICP Monitoring

Although there is no level 1 evidence demonstrating the benefit of ICP monitoring, ICP monitoring has been shown in small traumatic brain injury (TBI) series to reduce mortality. A large, randomized study demonstrating improved outcomes with ICP monitoring would require 700 patients at an estimated cost of $5 million to detect a 10% mortality difference.[1] The only way to reliably diagnose elevated ICP is to measure it directly. This can be accomplished by performing a lumbar puncture, but this does not allow for continuous ICP monitoring. Additionally, lumbar puncture should not be performed in patients with significant posterior fossa mass lesions, patients with significant midline shift, or patients with third or fourth ventricular hemorrhage. Different ICP monitors are shown in **Fig. 15.6** and described below. For all monitors, transducers should be placed at the level of the foramen of Monroe (tragus of the ear) (**Table 15.2**).

Patients with symptomatic hydrocephalus or a noncommand-following neurologic examination and suspected elevated ICP should undergo ICP monitoring. According to the Brain Trauma Foundation,[1] indications for placing an ICP monitor in TBI patients include:

- Glasgow Coma Scale (GCS) ≤8 with abnormal CT
- GCS ≤8 with normal CT if two thirds of the following risk factors are present:
  - Age >40 years
  - Posturing
  - Systolic blood pressure (SBP) < 90 mm Hg

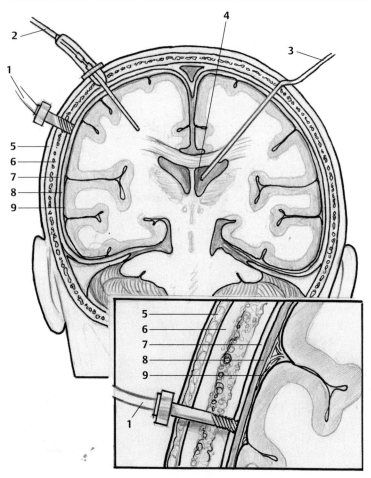

1. Subdural bolt
2. Intraparenchymal monitor
3. External ventricular drain
4. Lateral ventricle
5. Skin
6. Skull
7. Dura
8. Subdural space
   (this is a potential spac
9. Arachnoid layer

Fig. 15.6 Types of intracranial pressure monitors.

Table 15.2 Intracranial Pressure Monitors

Type of Monitor	Pro	Con
Intraventricular	Gold standard, more global ICP measurement, allows for diagnosis and treatment	Highest infection rate (5–20%), risk of hemorrhage (2%)
Intraparenchymal	Infection and hemorrhage rate low (1%), easy to place	Measures regional ICP, cannot recalibrate after placement, drift (readings may vary by 3 mm Hg)
Subarachnoid/ subdural	Infection and hemorrhage rate low	Unreliable measurements, not often used
Epidural	Low risk of hemorrhage compared with intraventricular and intraparenchymal monitors, occasional use with coagulopathic liver patients	Unreliable measurements

Abbreviation: ICP, intracranial pressure.

Normal ICP is defined as 20 mm Hg or 25 cm H_2O (there is a 3:4 ratio for mm Hg to cm H_2O). Aside from absolute ICP values, ICP waveforms can provide information about compliance. The ICP waveform is characterized by P1, P2, and P3 components, with each element of the wave smaller than the prior (**Fig. 15.7**). The P1 wave represents an arterial wave, P2 represents rebound, and P3 represents venous outflow. An elevated P2 wave is a sign of poor compliance. Compliance can be measured by draining a set volume of CSF and examining the change in pressure that this creates (compliance = Δvolume/Δpressure). Critically low intracranial compliance, coupled with inadequate tissue perfusion, may result in Lundberg waves (**Fig. 15.8**).

Lundberg A waves (plateau waves) are sudden increases in ICP of 20 to 100 mm Hg that last for minutes to hours, causing reduced CBF/CPP

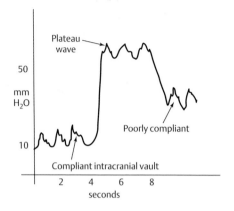

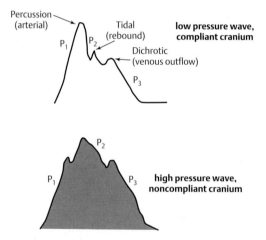

Fig. 15.7 Intracranial pressure waveform. Components of ICP waveform in compliant and noncompliant cranial systems.

and brain ischemia. Lundberg B waves are smaller increases, usually of 5 to 20 mm Hg, that last 1 to 5 minutes, may be related to respiratory variation, and are characterized by a sharpened waveform. Lundberg waves are a marker for critically low intracranial compliance and probably result from a spiral of tissue hypoperfusion, progressive arteriolar dilation, and increased cerebral blood volume, which worsens ICP and feeds back to exacerbate the initial problem of hypoperfusion. The cycle

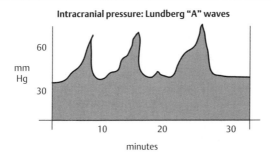

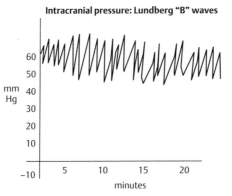

Fig. 15.8 Pathologic (plateau) intracranial pressure waveforms. Lundberg waves A (top) and B (bottom).

is ultimately broken by a sympathetic-mediated blood pressure surge known as the "termination spike," which serves to restore brain perfusion and break the cycle of cerebral vasodilation. Lundberg A waves should be treated aggressively by increasing CPP with vasopressors, and decreasing ICP with osmotic therapy and hyperventilation.

It is important to note that patients can herniate with normal ICP values. Patients sitting on the asymptote of their compliance curve may have precipitous rises in ICP (such as with turning or coughing). Pressure gradients between brain compartments can cause shift and herniation, even though the absolute ICP in any given compartment is <20 mm Hg. Significant ICP gradients are present when there is >3 mm of shift seen radiographically. When basal cisterns are effaced, ICP gradients can rise quickly.

Imaging

Head CT scan without contrast may show mass effect with midline shift or effacement of the basal cisterns and sulci, global, or focal edema, acute and/or subacute hemorrhage or contusion, and/or infarction. Head CT alone is not a reliable marker for elevated ICP. Fifty to 60% of TBI patients who are comatose and have an abnormal CT will have an elevated ICP, whereas an additional 10 to 15% of comatose TBI patients with a normal CT will have an elevated ICP. Thirty-three percent of comatose TBI patients with a normal head CT and two of the following: age >40 years, posturing, or SBP <90 mm Hg, will have an elevated ICP.

Noninvasive Measurements

Elevated pulsatility index (systolic–diastolic pressure/average pressure) as measured by transcranial Doppler can be a marker for elevated ICP, though the sensitivity and specificity of pulsatility index are suboptimal. In cases of extremely elevated ICP, as occurs with brain death, isolated systolic flow with no diastolic flow is seen.

Advanced Monitoring

Microdialysis technology, placed intracranially in an at-risk area, employs high-performance liquid chromatography to measure tissue levels of lactate, pyruvate, and glucose. Brain tissue oxygen monitoring provides an averaged measure of capillary and interstitial brain oxygen pressure. It is important to understand the limitations of brain with monitoring. PbO_2 is not equivalent to oxygen extraction fraction or the oxygen delivered to the brain tissue but rather, represents the partial pressure of brain oxygen, or the dissolved oxygen content in the brain. Thus, PbO_2 values are more representative of oxygen diffusion than oxygen delivery or metabolism.[2] The combination of microdialysis technology with a brain tissue oxygen sensor, ICP and, CBF monitoring, sometimes in combination with continuous electroencephalogram (EEG), is known as multimodality monitoring. Multimodality monitoring offers a sophisticated biochemical profile of the regional brain environment around the probes. Although the ideal parameters of multimodality monitoring data are yet to be determined, below are listed accepted thresholds for normal and abnormal values. Where multimodality monitoring is available, the trends of these numbers, in conjunction with CPP and the clinical examination, can be useful in guiding medical and surgical management (**Table 15.3**).

Table 15.3 Accepted Thresholds for Normal and Abnormal Values of Multimodality Monitoring

Microdialysis	
Normal	Glucose >2 mmol/L
	Glutamate <15 mmol/L
	Lactate/pyruvate 15–25 mmol/L
Abnormal	Glucose <2 mmol/L
	Glutamate >15 mmol/L
	Lactate/pyruvate >25–40 mmol/L
Brain tissue O_2	
Normal	PbO_2 20–40 mm Hg
Abnormal	PbO_2 <10–15 mm Hg ischemic/inadequate O_2 delivery or excessive demand
	PbO_2 >50 mm Hg hyperemia, elevated FIO_2 or inability to extract O_2
PET	
Normal	$CMRO_2$ 3.0 mL/100 g/min
	CMRglucose 25 µmol/100 g/min
	CBF 50 mL/100 g/min
	CBV 4 mL/100 mL
	OEF 30–40%
Abnormal	$CMRO_2$ <1.25 mL/100 g/min
	CMRglucose < 25 µmol/100 g/min
	CBF
	<20 mL/100 g/min ischemia,
	<10 mL/100 g/min infarction
	CBV < 3 mL/100 mL
	OEF
	>40% inadequate O_2 delivery or excessive demand,
	<20% metabolic downregulation
$SjvO_2$	
Normal	60–80%
Abnormal	<60% inadequate O_2 delivery or excessive demand,
	>80% hyperemia, or inability to extract O_2

Abbreviations: CBF, cerebral blood flow; CBV, cerebral blood volume; OEF, oxygen extraction fraction; PET, positron emission tomography; $CMRO_2$, cerebral metabolic rate of O_2; CMRglucose, cerebral metabolic rate of glucose.

■ Treatment

Prevention of Elevated ICP in Brain-Injured Patients at Risk

- Elevate the head of the bed to 30 to 45 degrees. Keep the head midline to promote venous drainage.

- Avoid all free water and maintain normal or elevated serum osmolarity.

- Place a central venous catheter to infuse vasoactive or hyperosmolar medications as needed. Hypotension will exacerbate elevated ICP, and mean arterial pressure (MAP) <65 mm Hg should be immediately corrected.

- Avoid fever and treat shivering, which increases cerebral metabolic rate ($CMRO_2$), increases ICP, activates intracellular apoptotic mechanisms, and worsens brain injury.

- Prevent seizures that may cause a catastrophic increase in ICP.

- Control pain (fentanyl) and agitation (Versed, propofol).

- Consider lidocaine 1% 10 cc into ETT before suctioning.

- Maintain normocarbia ($PaCO_2$ 35 to 40 mm Hg).

- Maintain euvolemia with normal saline or albumin (please note that CVP is an unreliable measurement of volume status in intensive care unit [ICU] patients).

■ Treatment of Elevated ICP (Fig. 15.9)

1. *Consider urgent neurosurgical referral for evacuation or ventricular drainage.* Lesions causing mass effect and elevated ICP, such as subdural or epidural hematomas, tumors, abscesses, and, in some cases, ischemic lesions or intracerebral hemorrhages, may require evacuation. Decompressive craniectomy with durotomy can be performed for ICP that is refractory to medical therapy and has been shown to lower ICP by up to 70%. Options include hemicraniectomy and bifrontal craniectomy. Although decompressive craniectomy is a highly effective means of decreasing ICP, patients

can suffer from focally or globally elevated ICP and herniation even after surgical decompression.

2. *Optimize CPP by adding vasopressors and/or isotonic fluids if CPP < 60 mm Hg, or by reducing blood pressure if the CPP >110 mm Hg.* CPP, the driving force for brain perfusion, is mathematically derived by the equation $CPP = MAP - ICP$. The relationship of CBF, CPP, and ICP must be understood in the context of autoregulation. Autoregulation is the ability to maintain constant CBF over a wide range of arterial blood pressures and is primarily maintained by the changing caliber of arterioles, as demonstrated in **Fig. 15.10**. In the autoregulation breakthrough zone, arterioles passively dilate under extremes of elevated systemic blood pressure. Because cerebral blood volume (CBV) increases, ICP will also increase. In the vasodilatory cascade zone, arterioles are also maximally dilated to maintain CBF in the face of falling systemic blood pressure. Again, because CBV is elevated, ICP will increase. This is the rationale for maintaining a CPP between 60 and 110 mm Hg. In certain disease states, autoregulation is lost, and a direct relationship between systemic blood pressure and CBF exists. CBF is further related to metabolic demand such that more active tissue preferentially receives more blood flow.

In most cases, the ICP should be kept below 20 mm Hg, while maintaining CPP between 60 to 100 mm Hg. Unfortunately, achieving these hemodynamic parameters does not guarantee adequate local tissue perfusion. Pathological dysregulation of local vasomotor tone, variable pressure between brain compartments, and metabolic factors create a situation in which brain tissue may be hypoperfused or hyperemic despite a seemingly appropriate CPP. In these circumstances, clinicians should change CPP goals (closely monitoring for changes in clinical and neurologic status) and consider the insertion of an adjunct monitoring device (microdialysis or brain oxygen monitoring), allowing for the titration of diuretics, fluids, vasopressors, FiO_2, or pCO_2 in response to biochemical markers of ischemia.

3. *Osmotic therapy.* Osmotic therapy draws water into the intravascular space along an osmotic gradient. Both mannitol and hypertonic saline have the additional rheologic benefits of lowering blood viscosity and decreasing the rigidity and volume of red blood cells.

Flowsheet for Management of Elevated ICP

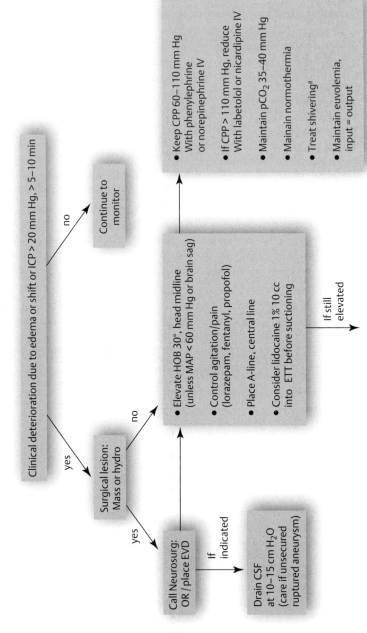

Clinical deterioration due to edema or shift or ICP > 20 mm Hg, > 5–10 min

no → Continue to monitor

yes ↓

Surgical lesion: Mass or hydro

yes → Call Neurosurg: OR / place EVD

If indicated → Drain CSF at 10–15 cm H_2O (care if unsecured ruptured aneurysm)

no →
- Elevate HOB 30°, head midline (unless MAP < 60 mm Hg or brain sag)
- Control agitation/pain (lorazepam, fentanyl, propofol)
- Place A-line, central line
- Consider lidocaine 1% 10 cc into ETT before suctioning

→
- Keep CPP 60–110 mm Hg With phenylephrine or norepinephrine IV
- If CPP > 110 mm Hg, reduce With labetolol or nicardipine IV
- Maintain pCO_2 35–40 mm Hg
- Mainain normothermia
- Treat shivering[a]
- Maintain euvolemia, input = output

If still elevated →

212

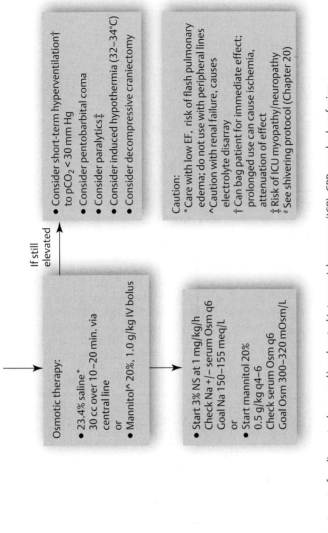

Osmotic therapy:

- 23.4% saline*
  30 cc over 10–20 min. via
  central line
  or
- Mannitol^ 20%, 1.0 g/kg IV bolus

↓

- Start 3% NS at 1 mg/kg/h
  Check Na +/− serum Osm q6
  Goal Na 150–155 meq/L
  or
- Start mannitol 20%
  0.5 g/kg q4–6
  Check serum Osm q6
  Goal Osm 300–320 mOsm/L

If still elevated →

- Consider short-term hyperventilation†
  to $pCO_2 < 30$ mm Hg
- Consider pentobarbital coma
- Consider paralytics‡
- Consider induced hypothermia (32–34°C)
- Consider decompressive craniectomy

Caution:

* Care with low EF, risk of flash pulmonary
  edema; do not use with peripheral lines
^ Caution with renal failure, causes
  electrolyte disarray
† Can bag patient for immediate effect;
  prolonged use can cause ischemia,
  attenuation of effect
‡ Risk of ICU myopathy/neuropathy
⁑ See shivering protocol (Chapter 20)

Fig. 15.9 Treatment of malignant edema and/or elevated intracranial pressure (ICP). CPP, cerebral perfusion pressure; CSF, cerebrospinal fluid; CVP, central venous pressure; EF, ejection fraction; ETT, endotracheal tube; EVD, external ventricular drain; HOB, head of bed; ICU, intensive care unit; IV, intravenous; MAP, mean arterial pressure; NS, normal saline; OR, operating room; q6, every 6 hours; OSM, osmolality; Na, serum sodium.

213

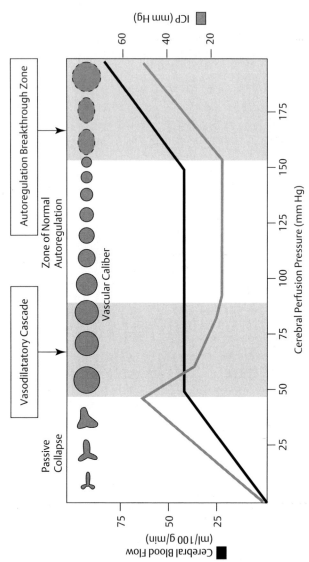

Fig. 15.10 Autoregulation curve. Cerebral blood flow, (dark line), is maintained relatively constant over a wide range of cerebral perfusion pressures. At extremely high cerebral perfusion pressure (CPP), cerebral blood flow (CBF) increases as arterioles passively dilate (autoregulation breakthrough zone), and at extremely low CPP, CBF decreases as arterioles collapse (vasodilatory collapse). Intracranial pressure (ICP), (light grey line) increases both in the autoregulation breakthrough zone and in the vasodilatory cascade zone because CBF increases when arterioles are maximally dilated.

Hypertonic saline improves CPP, and both are free radical scavengers.

- Hypertonic saline: Loading dose 30 mL of 23% saline pushed over 10 to 20 minutes via a central line, maintenance dose of 3% saline 1 mg/kg/h titrated to a serum Na of 150 to 155 mEq/h. Na should be checked every 6 hours. Administration of hypertonic saline is associated with pulmonary edema and can cause hypotension if pushed too rapidly.

- Mannitol 20%: Loading dose of 1 g/kg (or 100 g if weight unknown), followed by a maintenance dose of 0.5 g/kg every 4 to 6 hours titrated to a serum osmolarity of 300 to 320 mOsm or an osmolal gap (measured Osm − calculated Osm) of 50 mOsm/kg. Serum osmolarity should be checked every 6 hours. The half-life of mannitol is 0.16 hour. Efficacy is seen in 15 to 30 minutes, and the duration of effect is 90 minutes to 6 hours. Mannitol has an osmotic reflection coefficient of 0.9, while hypertonic saline has a reflection coefficient of 1.0. Thus, mannitol is slightly more likely to cross the blood–brain barrier and undergo a degradation of gradient.

- Hypertonic saline bolusing has been shown to reduce ICP faster than mannitol and is effective even in patients who are refractory to mannitol.

- Both mannitol and hypertonic saline can cause rebound cerebral edema during tapering. Both drugs should be slowly and cautiously tapered to avoid this devastating consequence. Three percent saline can be weaned to 2% and then normal saline. Use extra caution in patients with cerebral salt wasting as Na values can drop precipitously during tapering (**Table 15.4**).

4. *Other options:*

- Short-term hyperventilation to $PaCO_2$ 25 to 30 mm Hg. Reduction in $PaCO_2$ by 1 mm Hg will reduce CBF by 3%. The effect of hyperventilation lasts 1 to 24 hours and is short-lived because the CSF buffers the effect. Hyperventilation causes vasoconstriction and increases the risk of tissue ischemia. Use only for short periods, for example, in actively herniating patients.

- Barbiturates: Pentobarbital 5 to 20 mg/kg bolus followed by 1 to 4 mg/kg/h titrated to burst suppression on EEG can be used in patients refractory to other ICP treatments. Barbiturates reduce metabolic demand and consequently CBF, CBV, and ICP if

Table 15.4 Osmotic Therapy

	Pros	Cons	Use if	Avoid if
Hypertonic saline	Can be given as continuous infusion, ease of titration, improves CPP, volume expands, effective in lowering ICP in patients refractory to mannitol	Volume overload, flash pulmonary edema, extreme hypernatremia, rebound cerebral edema upon tapering, renal insufficiency (less common than with mannitol), single case report of CPM when used in chronic hyponatremia	Want to volume expand or improve CPP	Decompensated CHF, care if baseline hyponatremia >24 hours (risk of CPM)
Mannitol	Can use through a peripheral line, bolus dosing	Volume depletion, MUST REPLETE UOP ML/ML WITH SALINE, ESPECIALLY IN TBI AND SAH, hypotension, rebound cerebral edema upon tapering, hypernatremia, renal insufficiency (reversible, seen if >200 g used daily or osmolal gap > 60–75 mOsm/kg)	Want to diurese, no central line access	Renal failure, hypotension

Abbreviations: CHF, congestive heart failure; CPM, central pontine myelinolysis; CPP, cerebral perfusion pressure; ICP, intracranial pressure; SAH, subarachnoid hemorrhage; TBI, traumatic brain injury; UOP, urine output.

metabolic coupling is intact. Major risks include hypotension, inability to examine the patient due to sedative effects of barbiturates, cardiosuppression, and immunosuppression. According to the Brain Trauma Foundation,[1] there is no role for prophylactic barbiturates after TBI.

- Induced hypothermia to 32 to 34°C can reduce CBF and ICP by reducing metabolic demand if metabolic coupling is intact. Every 1°C reduction in temperature reduces cerebral oxygen metabolism ($CMRO_2$) by 7%. Hypothermia also reduces inflammation. Side effects of hypothermia include systemic infection, and bacteremia, coagulopathy, pneumonia, hypokalemia, and arrhythmias. Side effects of rewarming include pulmonary edema, systemic inflammatory response syndrome (SIRS) and rebound cerebral edema. (See Chapter 20).

- Steroids have been shown to increase mortality after TBI[3] and have been shown to be ineffective after ischemic stroke and ICH.[4–7] Steroids are useful for edema related to tumors and certain infections.

- Paralytics can be used to lower refractory ICP, but they carry a risk of ICU myopathy/neuropathy and can mask seizures. Paralytics must be used in conjunction with an amnesic sedative.

■ Prognosis

The prognosis in patients with elevated ICP is directly related to the severity of the underlying pathophysiology, efficacy of management, and the age and medical comorbidities of the patient. In general, disease-specific prognostic scores should be consulted. *The appearance of a herniation syndrome (i.e., blown pupil or motor posturing) does not always imply an irreversible and hopeless outcome.*

Pearls and Pitfalls

- Comatose patients suspected of having elevated ICP should always be managed in an ICU environment with invasive ICP monitoring and established CPP goals.

- Adequate CPP does not guarantee adequate tissue perfusion, but it is essential and is the cornerstone of therapy for elevated ICP.

- Elevated ICP can usually be controlled by observing basic "ICP housekeeping" measures, with sedation, maintenance of volume status and CPP, and osmotherapy. A stepwise treatment algorithm is the most effective way to guide treatment.

References

1. Brain Trauma Foundation. Brain Trauma Foundation Guidelines 2007. Available at: www.braintrauma.org. Accessed 10/20/2008.
2. Rosenthal G, Hemphill JC, 3rd, Sorani M, Martin C, Morabito D, Obrist WD, Manley GT. Brain tissue oxygen tension is more indicative of oxygen diffusion than oxygen delivery and metabolism in patients with traumatic brain injury. Crit Care Med 2008;36:1917–1924
3. Edwards P, Arango M, Balica L, et al. Final results of MRC CRASH, a randomised placebo-controlled trial of intravenous corticosteroid in adults with head injury-outcomes at 6 months. Lancet 2005;365(9475):1957–1959
4. Donley RF, Sundt TM Jr. The effect of dexamethasone on the edema of focal cerebral ischemia. Stroke 1973;4(2):148–155
5. Poungvarin N, Bhoopat W, Viriyavejakul A, et al. Effects of dexamethasone in primary supratentorial intracerebral hemorrhage. N Engl J Med 1987;316(20): 1229–1233
6. Qizilbash N, Lewington SL, Lopez-Arrieta JM. Corticosteroids for acute ischaemic stroke. Cochrane Database of Systematic Reviews (Online) 2002(2):CD000064
7. Tellez H, Bauer RB. Dexamethasone as treatment in cerebrovascular disease: 1. A controlled study in intracerebral hemorrhage. Stroke 1973;4(4):541–546

16 Airway Management and Sedation

*David C. Kramer, Irene Osborn, and
Meagen Gaddis*

When evaluating a neurocritical care patient for intubation, the following considerations must be assessed: (1) urgency of airway management, (2) assessment of ability to secure the airway, (3) issues related to "full stomach" and aspiration risk, (4) intracranial pressure, (5) hemodynamics, and (6) immobilization and restraints as impediments to securing the airway. The basic pharmacokinetics and clinical application of commonly used drugs to facilitate induction, intubation, and sedation will be reviewed.

Case Example

A 64-year-old male presents with confusion, lethargy, and new left hemiparesis. His blood pressure is 180/105 mm Hg, and his heart rate is 43. His head computed tomography (CT) scan shows a large right-sided intracerebral hemorrhage with edema and a midline shift. The patient had previously undergone a tracheostomy at age 33 after a motor vehicle accident.

Questions

- Is the patient protecting his airway?
- What is the O_2 saturation and arterial blood gas (ABG)?
- Has the patient received any sedation?
- Has the patient received any treatment for elevated intracranial pressure (ICP)?

Urgent Orders

- If the patient is not oxygenating (O_2 saturation <90% or PaO_2 <60 mm Hg), is retaining CO_2, is showing signs of respiratory distress (dyspnea, retracting, nasal flaring, paradoxical abdominal breathing, cyanosis), or is not protecting his airway due to neurologic injury, a member of the medical team should begin manual bag ventilation with 100% O_2 at a rate of 12 breaths per minute. Brief hyperventilation can be a strategy for ICP reduction in patients who are herniating, but prolonged and excessive hyperventilation (to a $PaCO_2$ <25 mm Hg) is not recommended, as this can precipitate regional cerebral ischemia (see Chapter 15). Patients with craniofacial trauma are at risk for pneumocephalus with bag mask ventilation. This risk should be assessed prior to bagging such patients, and preemptive controlled intubation should be undertaken when necessary.

- Suction and airway equipment must be available. The location of the difficult airway cart should be ascertained prior to attempts at intubation of the neurocritical care patient.
- In any airway that is deemed truly difficult, a second experienced anesthesiologist should be present.
- If the airway presents more than the usual degree of challenge, an otolaryngologist should be present at the bedside, along with a tracheostomy tray, to aid in securing the airway or providing an emergency surgical airway.
- Obtain free-flowing intravenous access.
- Order medications to the bedside that might be needed for intubation (propofol, etomidate, neuromuscular blocking agents, phenylephrine, and/or ephedrine).

■ History and Examination

History

Determine the mechanism of injury and whether there is any associated trauma (craniofacial, thoracic, or pulmonary) or spinal cord injury. If there is a plan for surgery, the patient may need to be intubated for general anesthesia. Assess for previous history of a difficult airway, including a history of prolonged intubation, head or neck radiation or surgery, history of rheumatoid arthritis (associated with atlantoaxial subluxation), Down's syndrome (associated with abnormal airway anatomy and atlantoaxial subluxation), ankylosing spondylitis (which may limit neck movement), or a history of tracheostomy. A cardiac and pulmonary history should be assessed as well as a history of smoking. A history of last ingestion should be undertaken to ascertain aspiration risk.

Physical Examination

It is critical to assess for difficulty in securing an airway, which can occur in roughly 10% of intensive care unit (ICU) patients (see H-LEMOON below). Neuro-ICU (NICU) patients have additional risks related to elevated ICP, craniofacial trauma, or cervical spine immobilization.

Neurologic Examination

- A full neurologic examination, including assessment of mental status, cranial nerves, motor skills, and reflexes, as well as a sensory and cerebellar exam, should be performed on all patients, once the patient is stabilized.
- Particular attention should be given to mental status and the ability of the patient to protect his or her airway. Patients with neuromuscular weakness or fatigable weakness should be assessed according to parameters described in Chapters 11 and 12.

■ Differential Diagnosis

- Indications for intubation include failure to protect the airway, failure to maintain the airway, failure of oxygenation, failure of ventilation, anticipated clinical deterioration (neurologic worsening, expanding neck mass, etc.), and the need for general anesthesia (planned surgery, status epilepticus management, etc.).
- Contraindications to intubation include total loss of facial landmarks, total airway obstruction, and an anticipated difficult airway (relative contraindication).

Life-Threatening Diagnoses Not to Miss

- *Airway obstruction requiring emergency tracheostomy*
- *Unstable C-spine requiring precautions during intubation*
- *Craniofacial trauma or surgery that places patients at risk for pneumocephalus with bag mask ventilation*

■ Diagnostic Evaluation

1. *Assess difficulty of airway.* The pneumonic H-LEMOON can be applied (**Table 16.1**). In patients in whom the difficult airway may be anticipated, alternative airway devices such as the Rusch FlexiSlip (Teleflex Medical, Research Triangle Park, NC) stylet, the gum elastic

Table 16.1 The H-LEMOON Pneumonic

	Less Difficult Airway	More Difficult
History	No history of difficult intubation	History of difficult intubation or tracheostomy
Look externally	Normal face and neck No facial or cervical pathology	Abnormal facial shape Facial hair Overhanging incisors Narrow mouth Inability to protrude mandible Micrognathia Poor temporomandibular joint mobility Long, high-arched palate Facial or cervical pathology Short, thick neck Tracheal deviation Presence of vomitus or blood in oropharynx
Evaluate the 3-3-2 rule	Mouth opening >3 finger breadths (4 cm) Hyoid–chin distance >3 finger breadths (4 cm) Thyroid cartilage–mouth of floor > 2 finger breadths	Mouth opening <3 finger breadths (4 cm) Hyoid–chin distance <3 finger breadths (4 cm) Thyroid cartilage–mouth of floor <2 finger breadths
Mallampati classification (best performed with the patient sitting, tongue protruding, and not phonating)	Class I: Fully visible tonsils, uvula, and soft palate Class II: Visibility of hard and soft palate and upper portion of the tonsils and uvula	Class III: Soft and hard palate and base of uvula are visible Class IV: Only hard palate visible
Obstruction and Obesity	No airway obstruction BMI <30 kg/m^2 and/or neck circumference <60 cm	Pathology in or surrounding the upper airway, difficulty swallowing secretions, stridor (ominous and occurs when <10% of airway patent), muffled (hot-potato) voice BMI >30 kg/m^2 and/or neck circumference >60 cm
Neck mobility	Complete flexion and extension of neck	Limited ROM of neck Presence of halo or neck immobilization devices History of cervical instrumentation

Abbreviations: BMI, body mass index; ROM, range of motion.

bougie, the fiberoptic scope, video laryngoscopes, or an intubating laryngeal mask airway (ILMA) may prove helpful. A laryngeal mask airway (LMA) of the appropriate size should be readily available for the patient in whom intubation is anticipated to be difficult.

2. *Assess aspiration risk.* Pneumonia secondary to aspiration and microaspiration is a common source of infection following intubation. Neurocritically ill patients have potential for aspiration secondary to decreased or altered level of consciousness, decreased gastric motility, increased sympathetic tone, and intermittent feeds. The goal of aspiration preventive measures is to decrease gastric stomach content volume, raise the pH of stomach content to greater than 7.25, and decrease the time of induction of unconsciousness to intubation.

   The American Society of Anesthesiology has suggested a period of 2 hours after the ingestion of clear liquids, 6 hours after a "light meal," and 8 hours after a meal of fried or fatty food be utilized as a guideline for surgical patients undergoing elective surgical procedures.[1] The administration of 100% oxygen to preoxygenate the patient, avoidance of positive-pressure ventilation during induction, the use of rapid sequence induction (RSI), and the institution of cricoid pressure have been advocated to decrease the risk of aspiration.

3. *Assess ICP.* It is essential for the laryngoscopist to take maneuvers to minimize elevations of ICP, such as to minimize laryngeal stimulation and to use maneuvers to avoid bucking, movement, and vomiting. Lidocaine 1% 1.0 mg/kg IV suppresses the cough reflex, may lower cerebral oxygen demand, reduces bronchospasm, and should be used in patients with suspected elevated ICP.

4. *Assess hemodynamics.* Intubation in the intensive care unit is often complicated by hemodynamic compromise and cardiovascular collapse. As many as a quarter of ICU patients may experience hemodynamic collapse, 10% experience cardiac arrhythmias, and 2% have cardiac arrest coincident with endotracheal intubation. Should multiple attempts at intubation be required, the incidence of cardiac arrest increases 1600%.[1]

   In the hypovolemic patient who is hypotensive, a bolus of intravenous (IV) fluid is indicated. The judicious use of vasopressor agents may be indicated should hypotension persist. The use of etomidate as an induction agent should be considered in patients who are elderly, critically ill, or have tenuous hemodynamics.

Etomidate (even a single dose) can suppress steroidogenesis and cause delayed hypotension after intubation related to relative adrenal insufficiency.

5. *Assess immobilizations and restraints.* Neurocritical care patients may sometimes be immobilized to prevent movement, which could be detrimental or dangerous to their condition. Devices such as hard cervical collars and halo frames restrict neck mobility. In patients with C-spine precautions who require emergent intubation, a two-person intubation can be undertaken, with one person providing in-line mobilization once the anterior portion of the cervical collar is removed. In the nonemergent setting, fiberoptic bronchoscopy should be strongly considered.

The halo device provides the most rigid form of external cervical immobilization and prevents proper positioning for laryngoscopy by restricting atlanto-occipital extension. Oral intubation is often possible, but it is a function of other variables, such as mouth opening, tongue size, upper dentition, and ability to prognath the lower jaw forward. Techniques include awake or sedated fiberoptic intubation and the ILMA performed awake or asleep. Video laryngoscopy may be successful, but it requires expertise, and mask ventilation is often possible with the addition of oral airways. It is imperative that clinicians involved have: (1) skills and equipment for alternative intubation techniques, (2) a neurosurgeon or professional who can safely remove the halo if necessary, and (3) a rescue plan in case of failed ventilation in these challenging patients.

■ Treatment

Intubation

1. *Equipment and preparation.* The most commonly used laryngoscope is a Mac #3 curved blade, and in circumstances of larger patients, a Mac #4. A Miller #3 or #4 (straight blade) can also be used. A Mac blade is placed in the vallecula, while a Miller blade is placed over the epiglottis and lifted. Video-assisted laryngoscopes are gaining popularity and allow for group visualization of the airway. Such devices include the Glidescope (Saturn Biomedical System Inc., Burnaby, BC, Canada), the McGrath

(Aircraft Medical, Edinburgh, Scotland), Airtraq (Prodol, Meditec S.A., Vizcaya, Spain), and the AWS (Pentax Corp., Montvale, NJ) (**Table 16.2**).

As part of the preparation for intubation, the cuff of the endotracheal tube (ETT) should be checked and lubricated, the light source on the laryngoscope should be confirmed, contraindications to medications should be reviewed, free-flowing IV access should be present, and blood pressure (BP), O_2, and heart rate (HR) continuous monitoring should be applied. In case of hypotension related to induction, the laryngoscopist should have available phenylephrine (mix 10 mg in 250 mL of normal saline (NS), 40 µg/mL; *never inject phenylephrine directly from vial without dilution*). In patients who are bradycardic and hypotensive, ephedrine is preferred (50 mg in 10 mL; 5 mg/mL).

2. *Positioning.* Place the patient in sniffing position (neck flexion and head extension) or neck extension to obtain adequate visualization of the glottic opening. Avoid this in patients with known or suspected C-spine injury.

3. *Pretreatment.* Preoxygenate with 100% O_2 for at least 1 minute prior to attempted intubation, and ensure that the O_2 saturation is at least 95% prior to an attempt. Lidocaine 1% 1.0 mg/kg IV suppresses the cough reflex, may lower cerebral oxygen demand, and reduces bronchospasm. Lidocaine spray can rarely cause

Table 16.2 Equipment Checklist

Endotracheal tube with a stylet (usually 8.0 in men and 7.0 in women)
Ambu bag with PEEP device attached to 100% O_2
Suction
10 mL syringe
Intubating laryngeal mask airway
Capnometer/CO_2 detector
Oral and nasal airway
Tape and tincture of benzoin

Abbreviation: PEEP, positive end expiratory pressure.

methemoglobinemia, but it can be used to blunt coughing and gagging. IV lidocaine should be used in any patient with intracranial pathology, as it may blunt increases in ICP.

4. *Induction* (**Table 16.3**)[2]

Paralysis is not always necessary. Many practitioners avoid paralysis of neurologic patients so as not to confound the examination. How-

Table 16.3 Induction medications

Induction Agents	Induction Dosage	Sedation Dosage	Comments
Propofol	1.5–2.5 mg/kg	0.5–1 mg/kg	Induction dose unchanged by renal or liver disease. Associated with hypotension and bradycardia (particularly in volume-depleted patients). Causes cardiosuppression, immunosuppression. Infusion may be associated with propofol infusion syndrome (PRIS).*
Etomidate	0.2–0.5 mg/kg		Induction dose unchanged by renal or liver disease. Does not cause hypotension or cardiosuppression. Inhibits adrenal steroidogenesis via inhibition of mitochondrial hydroxylase, even after a single induction dose. Can cause delayed hypotension due to adrenal insufficiency, particularly in patients previously medicated with steroids. Caution in patients with sepsis.
Ketamine	1–2 mg/kg IV 5–10 mg/kg IM	0.25–0.5 mg/kg IV	Induction dose unchanged by renal or liver disease. Bronchodilator. May cause increased ICP, hypertension, tachycardia, arrhythmia, dissociative psychological effects, and delirium.

*Typically in doses over 5 mg/kg/h and associated with refractory lactic acidosis, rhabdomyolysis, renal failure, hyperkalemia, cardiovascular collapse, and death. This is more common in children, but it has been described in adults as well. The concommitant use of steroids or sympathomimetic agents can increase the risk of PRIS.

Abbreviations: ICP, intracranial pressure; IM, intramuscularly; PO, by mouth.

Data from: Walz JM, Zayaruzny M, Heard SO. Airway management in critical illness. Chest 2007;131(2):608–620.

ever, the laryngoscopist should have paralytics available should they be necessary to perform a safe intubation. Prolonged neuromuscular blockade has been described with both aminosteroids and benzylisoquiniliniums. Risk factors for prolonged blockade include organ dysfunction, sepsis, magnesium therapy, acidosis, steroid therapy, and prolonged infusion. Use a train of four to check for prolonged blockade (anything less than four strong twitches suggests blockade). Infusions of neuromuscular blocking agents are discouraged because they increase the risk of ICU myopathy/neuropathy. There are many contraindications to succinylcholine in NICU patients that should carefully be considered before its use (**Table 16.4**).

Table 16.4 Paralysis

Muscle Relaxants	Mechanism	Induction Dosage	Comments
Succinylcholine	Depolarizing	0.6 mg/kg IV 3–4 mg/kg IM	Induction dosage unchanged by renal disease. Prolonged effect in liver disease. Prolonged paralysis in those with pseudocholinesterase deficiency. Can cause malignant hyperkalemia in patients immobilized >24 h (due to upregulation of extrajunctional embryonic nicotinic receptors), patients with neurologic injury, crush injuries, burns, or preexisting hyperkalemia. Malignant hyperthermia is related to a defect in ryanodine receptor. Can cause elevated ICP and intraocular pressure. We do no recommend use of succinylcholine in most NICU patients.
Vecuronium	Nondepolarizing aminosteroid	0.1 mg/kg IV	Induction dose unchanged by renal disease. Prolonged effect in liver disease. Active metabolite may accumulate in renal insufficiency.

(Continued on next page)

Table 16.4 Paralysis (continued)

Muscle Relaxants	Mechanism	Induction Dosage	Comments
Pancuronium	Nondepolarizing aminosteroid	0.1–0.2 mg/kg IV	Causes sympathetic effect (strong vagolytic effect) with bolus dosing (vecuronium does not). Active metabolite.
Cisatracurium	Nondepolarizing benzyliso-quinolinium	0.2 mg/kg IV	Hoffman elimination (not renally or hepatically cleared): can be used in either renal or liver failure. Preferred to atracurium, which causes histamine release. No active metabolite.
Rocuronium	Nondepolarizing aminosteroid	0.6 mg/kg IV	Induction dose unchanged by renal disease. Prolonged action in hepatic disease. No hemodynamic effects. No active metabolite. Alternative to succinylcholine for rapid sequence intubation.

Abbreviations: ICP, intracranial pressure; IM, intramuscularly; IV, intravenously; NICU, neuro-intensive care unit.

5. *Placement*
   - Once the patient is adequately sedated, scissor open the mouth with the thumb and index fingers of the right hand and insert the laryngoscope with the left hand.
   - Place the blade on the right side of the patient's mouth and sweep the tongue to the left.
   - Advance the laryngoscope slightly until the tip of the epiglottis can be seen posterior to the back of the tongue (**Fig. 16.1**).
   - If using a Mac blade, place the tip in the vallecula and lift the handle up and away (taking care not to rock the blade and injure the dentition) to reveal the vocal cords.
   - With the right hand, insert the ETT through the vocal cords and advance until the cuff passes through the cords.

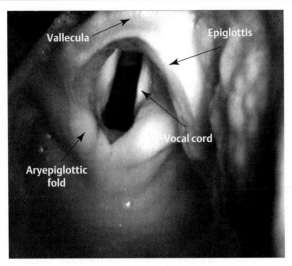

Fig. 16.1 View of the airway during laryngoscopy.

- Remove the laryngoscope and the stylet and inflate the cuff with 10 mL of air.

6. *Confirmation*
   - Visualize the ETT passing through the vocal cords.
   - Look for condensation in the tubing.
   - Look for a symmetrical rise in the chest wall with bagging.
   - Auscultate over the stomach and over each lateral lung field. In the event of right mainstem bronchus intubation, deflate the cuff and pull the ETT back 2 to 3 cm.
   - Apply a newly opened capnometer (most change color from purple to yellow to detect CO_2). Typically, capnometers detect a CO_2 concentration of 0.5 to 2%. This is an essential step even if you feel confident of placement. In the event of an esophageal intubation, there may be an initial yellow color change, but this is not sustained with subsequent bagging. In the event of intubation of a patient with low cardiac output, the capnometer may show a low but persistent level of end-tidal CO_2.

7. *Postintubation management.* Tie or tape the ETT securely at 22 to 24 cm at the teeth. Initiate mechanical ventilation and confirm appropriate depth of the ETT with a chest x-ray (CXR).

8. *Rapid sequence intubation.* Patients who are not NPO (nothing by mouth), obese, and gravid pose an aspiration risk, and rapid sequence intubation with preoxygenation but no bag mask ventilation is preferred. Cricoid pressure using Sellick's maneuver can be applied to compress the esophagus and limit aspiration.

9. *Alternatives to intubation.* Alternatives include tracheostomy and cricothyroidotomy. Patients who have undergone nasal intubation should be changed over to oral-tracheal intubation when possible, to limit the risk of sinusitis.

Sedation

The choice of sedation should be made based on whether analgesia (opioids), amnesia (benzodiazepines), anxiolysis (benzodiazepine or dexmedetomidine), or sedation/hypnosis (propofol, benzodiazepines) is desired. A combination of agents can be used to meet different needs (**Table 16.5**). In neurologic patients, the minimum

Table 16.5 Common Sedative Medications

Medication	Mechanism	Bolus Dose	Infusion Dose	Comments
Fentanyl	Opioid analgesic	0.35–1.5 μg/kg IV	0.7–10 μg/kg/h IV	Induction dose is minimally changed in hepatic disease. Causes respiratory suppression, constipation. No active metabolite.
Morphine	Opioid analgesic	0.01–0.15 mg/kg IV	0.07–0.5 mg/kg/h IV	Prolonged half-life in liver disease. Renal failure leads to accumulation. Causes respiratory suppression, constipation. Histamine release causes itching.
Hydro-morphone	Opioid analgesic	10–30 μg/kg IV	7–15 μg/kg/h IV	No active metabolite. Can be used in renal failure (whereas fentanyl and morphine accumulate).

(Continued)

Table 16.5 Common Sedative Medications (continued)

Medication	Mechanism	Bolus Dose	Infusion Dose	Comments
Propofol	Sedative, hypnotic, anticonvulsive, antiemetic, no analgesia	1.5–2.5 mg/kg	0.3–4.0 mg/kg/h	See Table 16.3. Additionally, large lipid load can cause pancreatitis. No active metabolite.
Midazolam	Benzodiazepine, anxiolysis, amnesia, anticonvulsive, no analgesia	0.02–0.04 mg/kg	0.02–0.2 mg/kg/h IV	Active metabolite; can lead to prolonged sedation in liver and renal failure. Binds to GABA receptor. Benzodiazepines are highly lipid soluble with rapid diffusion into CNS and redistribution to inactive tissue. Benzodiazepines are extensively albumin bound. Duration of action is limited by metabolism and elimination.
Lorazepam	Benzodiazepine, anxiolysis, amnesia, anticonvulsive, no analgesia	0.02–0.06 mg/kg IV	0.01–0.1 mg/kg/h IV	Solvent related (propylene glycol) acidosis/renal failure in high doses. Longer half-life than midazolam but similar pharmacokinetics as above. No active metabolite. Binds to GABA receptor.
Dexmedetomidine	Central α2 agonist, analgesic, antishivering, sedative, hypnotic, and anxiolytic effects	0.5 µg/kg IV	0.2–0.7 µg/kg/h IV	Minimal respiratory or neurologic depression. Hypotension and bradycardia with bolus dosing. Can reduce CBF. Contraindicated in heart block. No active metabolite. Synergistic with other sedatives/analgesics, particularly opiates. With long duration of use can produce withdrawal symptoms similar to clonidine. Inhibits cortisol synthesis at high doses.

Abbreviations: CBF, cerebral blood flow; CNS, central nervous system; GABA, gamma-aminobutyric acid; ICP, intracranial pressure; IV, intravenously

Table 16.6 Ramsay Scale

Score	Patient Description
1	Awake, anxious, agitated, restless
2	Cooperative, oriented, tranquil
3	Responds to commands only
4	Eyes closed, awakens to glabellar tap or loud auditory stimulus
5	Sluggish response to glabellar tap or loud auditory stimulus
6	No response to glabellar tap or loud auditory stimulus

Data from: Ramsay MA, Savege TM, Simpson BR, et al. Controlled sedation with alphaxalone-alphadolone. BMJ 1974;2(5920):656–659.

amount of sedation to provide comfort should be applied so that the neurologic examination can be followed. Daily sedation interruption is important for shortening the duration of mechanical ventilation.[3] More frequent sedation interruption is typically needed in the NICU to perform exam checks. Benzodiazepines can be reversed with flumazenil (not recommended because flumazenil can precipitate seizures), and opiates can be reversed with naloxone. Sedation scales are sometimes employed (**Table 16.6**).[4]

■ Prognosis

The patient's prognosis depends largely on the underlying mechanism leading to intubation. Serious complications are estimated to occur in roughly 25% of intubations. These include: dental trauma, esophageal intubation, perforation of the larynx, pharynx, trachea, or esophagus (with potential pneumothorax or pneumopericardium [rare]), vocal cord avulsion, dislocation of arytenoid cartilage, mainstem bronchus intubation, aspiration/pneumonia, hypotension, arrhythmias, laryngeal spasm, bronchospasm, increased ICP, and hypoxia.

Pearls and Pitfalls

- Intubation should be performed in a controlled and well-planned manner.

- ICP and C-spine instability are special concerns during intubation of neurologic patients.

- The choice of sedation in neurologic patients should be guided by the need for analgesia, anxiolysis, or hypnosis. Frequent sedation interruption should be preformed for neuro-checks and to facilitate ventilator weaning.

- Paralysis should be used cautiously due to risks of ICU myopathy/neuropathy.

References

1. Practice guidelines for preoperative fasting and the use of pharmacologic agents to reduce the risk of pulmonary aspiration: application to healthy patients undergoing elective procedures: a report by the American Society of Anesthesiologist Task Force on Preoperative Fasting. Anesthesiology 1999;90(3):896–905

2. Walz JM, Zayaruzny M, Heard SO. Airway management in critical illness. Chest 2007;131(2):608–620

3. Kress JP, Pohlman AS, O'Connor MF, Hall JB. Daily interruption of sedative infusions in critically ill patients undergoing mechanical ventilation. N Engl J Med 2000;342(20):1471–1477

4. Ramsay MA, Savege TM, Simpson BR, et al. Controlled sedation with alphaxalone-alphadolone. BMJ 1974;2(5920):656–659

17 Ventilator Management

Mariana Nunez, Roopa Kohli-Seth, Zinobia Khan, Moses Bachan, and Jennifer A. Frontera

Mechanical ventilation (also known as respiratory failure) is common in critically ill patients. Neurologic patients often require mechanical ventilation for failure to protect the airway due to poor mental status or neuromuscular disease, rather than for pulmonary insufficiency. Noninvasive positive pressure ventilation (NPPV) which is commonly used in COPD exacerbation, can be used in amyotrophic lateral sclerosis (ALS), Guillain-Barré, or myasthenia gravis patients when there is a minimal aspiration risk. Decreased mental status is a contraindication to NPPV. This chapter will focus on positive pressure ventilation in intubated patients. For details on intubation, see Chapter 16.

Case Example

You are called to the neuro-intensive care unit (NICU) to see a ventilated patient who recently underwent a laparotomy and who has a peak airway pressure of 55 cm H_2O on assist control/volume control (AC/VC) at a rate of 12 breathes per minute, fraction inspired oxygen (FIO_2) 40%, and positive end-expiratory pressure (PEEP) 5 cm H_2O.

Questions

- What are the most recent arterial blood gas (ABG) and O_2 saturation?
- Does the patient have a history of bronchospasm or mucous plugging?
- What is the pulmonary history?
- When was the patient intubated?
- Is the patient biting the ETT? Is there any kinking of the ETT?

Urgent Orders

- Remove the patient from the ventilator and manually bag on 100% O_2 to assess resistance. High resistance might be due to mucous plugging or to the patient biting the endotracheal tube (ETT).
- Check the ventilator circuit for kinking or fluid pooling.
- Check the ventilator settings: Excessively high tidal volume or flow rate could contribute to elevated peak airway pressure.
- Auscultate the lungs: Wheezing indicates bronchospasm; decreased breath sounds may indicate intrinsic lung disease or the ETT in the right mainstem bronchus.
- Check an inspiratory pause: If both peak and plateau pressures are high, there is an issue of poor compliance; if only peak airway pressures are high, the problem is high airway resistance.
- Abdominal compartment syndrome can also lead to elevated peak inspiratory and mean airway pressures, hypotension, and oliguria. Abdominal compartment syndrome should be suspected in patients with recent abdominal surgery and can be assessed by checking a bladder pressure (a pressure >15 mm Hg is abnormal, and >25 to 35 mm Hg often requires surgical treatment).

■ History and Examination

History

Assess pulmonary and cardiac history (history of pneumonia, COPD, reactive airway disease, pulmonary emboli, congestive heart failure, myocardial infarction (MI), smoking history), details of intubation (including if it was a difficult, complicated intubation), duration of mechanical ventilation, and modes used. Look for a recent history of secretions (noting their color and character), mucous plugging, or atelectasis.

Physical Examination

Assess vital signs, oxygenation, and end-tidal CO_2; check ETT position (should be ~22 to 24 cm at the lips, depending on the patient's size), assess for ETT air leak (listen at mouth for gurgling with inspiration), assess for signs of respiratory distress (tachypnea, diaphoresis, retraction, paradoxic abdominal breathing, cyanosis), and auscultate the lungs and heart. Assess for excessive secretions and sputum production.

Neurologic Examination

- A full neurologic examination, including assessment of mental status, cranial nerves, motor skills, and reflexes, as well as a sensory and cerebellar exam, should be performed on all patients.
- Particular attention should be given to mental status and the potential for ventilator liberation.

■ Differential Diagnosis

Indications for mechanical ventilation include

1. *Airway protection*
   - Bulbar dysfunction, decreased consciousness, for example, head injury with Glasgow Coma Score (GCS) <8 (to prevent massive aspiration)
   - Airway obstruction (e.g., acute laryngeal edema)
   - Loss of airway (e.g., neck trauma)

2. *Ventilation failure*
   - Neurologic disease
     ◦ Loss of ventilatory drive due to sedation, narcosis, or brain injury
     ◦ Spinal cord injury or lesions (e.g., high cord lesions)
     ◦ Peripheral nerve injury (e.g., phrenic nerve in surgery), Guillain-Barré syndrome, poliomyelitis, motor neuron disease
   - Muscular disease (e.g., myasthenia crises)
   - Chest wall trauma (e.g., flail chest, pneumothorax)

3. *Oxygenation failure*
   - Ventilation perfusion mismatch (e.g., pulmonary embolus)
   - Diffusion abnormalities (e.g., pulmonary edema, pneumonia)

4. *Need for moderate-profound sedation,* for example, for surgery, status epilepticus treatment, or elevated intracranial pressure (ICP) management

■ Diagnostic Evaluation

The following suggest the need for mechanical ventilation:

- Vital capacity (VC): <10–15 mL/kg
- Negative inspiratory force (NIF): Weaker than -20 cm H_2O
- Tidal volume (TV): <5 mL/kg
- Respiratory rate (RR): >35 breaths/minute
- Minute ventilation (TV × RR): <10 L/minute
- Rise in pCO_2: >10 mm Hg
- Alveolar-arterial gradient ($FiO_2 = 1.0$): >450
- PaO_2 with supplemental O_2: <55 mm Hg
- PaO_2/FiO_2 (P/F): <150
- Physical appearance: Labored breathing, retracting, nasal flaring, paradoxic abdominal breathing
- Mental status: Comatose or not protecting the airway

Life-Threatening Diagnoses Not to Miss

- *Respiratory failure due to massive pulmonary embolism or pneumothorax* (both require emergent treatment)
- *Respiratory failure due to insecure airway* (accidental extubation, esophageal intubation, or obstructed airway)

■ Treatment

Basic Ventilator Settings

- *Tidal volume (TV):* A typical initial TV is 8 to 10 mL/kg. Higher TV (10 to 15 mL/kg) is associated with barotrauma. In patients with acute lung injury (ALI) or acute respiratory distress syndrome (ARDS), lung protective ventilation with 6 mL/kg of predicted body weight is recommended. There are some data that TV of 6 mL/kg might be protective in other disease processes as well. $\uparrow TV = \downarrow PaCO_2$ and $\uparrow pH$.

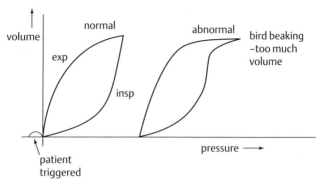

Fig. 17.1 Tidal volume: Pressure volume curves demonstrating both patient triggered breaths and if patient is receiving too much tidal volume.

The pressure volume curves in **Fig. 17.1** demonstrate both patient triggered breaths and if the patient is receiving too much tidal volume.

- *Respiratory rate (RR):* Initial RR is often set at 12 breaths per minute. In patients with ALI/ARDS, low-volume, high-frequency respiration is sometimes used. ↑RR = ↓$PaCO_2$ and ↑pH.

- *Fraction of inspired oxygen (FiO2):* Oxygenation goals are to maintain an O_2 saturation ≥90% and a PaO_2 >60 mm Hg utilizing the lowest FiO_2 possible to avoid oxygen toxicity and free radical injury. Typical initial setting is FiO_2 of 40%. A PaO_2 slightly <60 mm Hg can be accepted in the setting of ARDS if the tradeoff is higher plateau pressures and greater volutrauma. Causes of hypoxia include endobronchial intubation, accidental extubation, ventilator dysfunction, pneumothorax, pulmonary embolus, and primary pulmonary pathology (pneumonia, reactive airway disease, ARDS, pulmonary contusion, etc.). In patients with methemoglobinemia, ABGs will reveal normal PaO_2 in the context of cyanosis. The oxygen saturation on the ABG will be abnormally low. Pulse oximetry is unreliable in methemoglobinemia and tends to 85% regardless of the true oxygenation status or changes in FiO_2. In carbon monoxide poisoning, the pulse oximetry reveals a summation of oxyhemoglobin and carboxyhemoglobin and may give a falsely reassuring value in the face of arterial oxygen desaturation. Screening for either carboxyhemoglobin or methemoglobin can be done with co-oximetry. To troubleshoot hypoxia, increase the FiO_2 to 100%, auscultate the chest, check the ETT position, suction the patient and manually bag with 100% O_2, check the ventilator circuitry, check a chest x-ray (CXR), adjust FiO_2 and PEEP as needed, and treat the underlying pathology.

- *Positive end-expiratory pressure (PEEP):* PEEP prevents alveoli from collapsing on expiration and facilitates alveoli expansion with subsequent breaths. Increases in PEEP (which affects mean alveolar pressure) and mean airway pressure can improve oxygenation and lung recruitment. PEEP may improve secretion drainage from otherwise closed alveoli and can reduce right ventricular venous return and also lower left ventricular afterload. The disadvantages of PEEP include risk of barotrauma and worsening hypoxemia in patients with localized lung disease such as pneumonia (lung heterogeneity). Because increasing PEEP will increase mean intrathoracic pressure as well, elevated PEEP can lead to decreased preload and hypotension. PEEP that exceeds central venous pressure can theoretically lead to elevations in ICP, though studies with PEEP up to 15 cm H_2O do not show a significant effect on ICP or cerebral perfusion pressure (CPP).[1] Other disadvantages include the risk of increased cardiac shunt, especially in patent foramen ovale, hepatic congestion, and decreased renal perfusion. PEEP over 20 cm H_2O is rarely beneficial and results in additional pressure-induced lung injury.

Extrinsic PEEP is the PEEP set on the ventilator (typically beginning at 5 cm H_2O). Intrinsic PEEP is also known as stacking or auto-PEEP and occurs when there is insufficient time for complete expiration of a tidal volume. On ventilator flow curves (see below), the expiratory phase fails to return to baseline when the inspiratory phase starts. An expiratory pause maneuver allows quantification of auto-PEEP (normal auto-PEEP should be zero). With auto-PEEP there is increase work of breathing because the patient must generate enough pressure to overcome this intrinsic PEEP and trigger the ventilator. The easiest way to treat auto-PEEP is to slow the RR and allow for additional expiratory time (this may require sedation). Other options include increasing flow rates to allow for a longer expiratory phase and applying extrinsic PEEP ($\leq$80% of auto-PEEP) to ease the work of breathing. Lower TV can limit the risk of hyperinflation as well. COPD patients are particularly susceptible to auto-PEEP. Excessive auto-PEEP, just like extrinsic

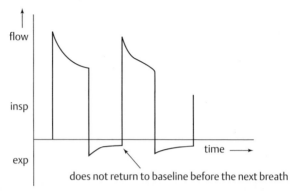

flow

insp

exp

time →

does not return to baseline before the next breath

Fig. 17.2 Intrinsic positive end-expiratory pressure (PEEP): On ventilator flow curves the expiratory phase fails to return to baseline when the inspiratory phase starts.

PEEP, can lead to hypotension due to elevated intrathoracic pressures and decreased venous return (**Fig. 17.2**).

- *Flow rate and inspiratory:expiratory (I:E):* The peak flow rate determines the maximal inspiratory flow. A normal flow rate is 60 L/minute. Increasing the flow rate will shorten the inspiratory time and prolong the expiratory time. This may be useful in patients with reactive airway disease. Conversely, slowing the flow rate will inverse the normal I:E (1:2) and can be employed to improve oxygenation in cases of ALI/ARDS, but at the expense of potential auto-PEEP.

Ventilator Modes

Volume Cycled Ventilation

In this mode, inspiration is terminated after a present TV is delivered a set number of times per minute. The pressure delivered depends on the lung mechanics (resistance and compliance). Advantages of this mode are that TV and minute ventilation are guaranteed, but disadvantages are that the airway pressure is not controlled, and this mode is somewhat less comfortable than other modes. Troubleshoot peak and plateau airway pressures. Examples of volume cycled ventilation include:

- *Controlled mechanical ventilation (CMV):* The ventilator is preset to give only a certain number of breaths per minute of a set volume. The patient is not able to trigger any additional breaths. This mode

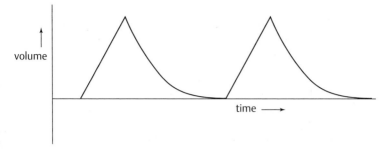

Fig. 17.3 Controlled mechanical ventilation (CMV): The ventilator is preset to give only a certain number of breaths per minute of a set volume.

is uncomfortable and requires sedation or paralysis and is infrequently used. CMV can lead to diaphragm dysfunction (**Fig. 17.3**).

- *Assist control/volume control (AC/VC):* In this mode, the ventilator provides full tidal volume at a minimum preset rate with additional full tidal volumes given if the patient initiates extra breaths. The pressure varies with each breath. It provides near complete resting of ventilatory muscles and can be effectively used in awake, sedated, or paralyzed patients. However, patients can hyperventilate and become alkalotic or can "stack" breaths and develop barotrauma, making this a less appealing mode in patients with obstructive lung disease. This is one of the most widely used basic modes of ventilation. Note in **Fig. 17.4** that the dip before the assisted breath indicates patient initiation.

- *Synchronized intermittent mandatory ventilation (SIMV):* The ventilator provides set TV at a preset rate. When a ventilator breath is programmed to occur, the ventilator waits a predetermined trigger period. The patient can take additional breaths,

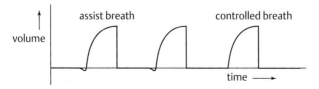

Fig. 17.4 Assist control/volume control (AC/VC): The dip before the assisted breath indicates patient initiation.

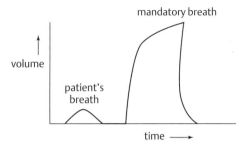

Fig. 17.5 Synchronized intermittent mandatory ventilation (SIMV): Ventilator provides set tidal volume (TV) at a preset rate. The patient can take additional breaths, but the TV of these extra breaths is dependent on the patient's inspiratory effort.

but the TV of these extra breaths is dependent on the patient's inspiratory effort. SIMV can be combined with pressure support to augment spontaneous breaths with a prespecified pressure (pressure support). SIMV can cause chronic respiratory fatigue if the set ventilatory rate is too low, resulting in high respiratory rate, rising pCO_2, increased work of breathing, greater oxygen consumption, and elevated blood pressure. SIMV is not a favored mode of ventilation because of increased work of breathing (**Fig. 17.5**).

Pressure Cycled Ventilation

Inspiration is terminated when a preset pressure is delivered a set number of times per minute. The volume delivered depends on the lung mechanics (resistance and compliance). Advantages of pressure cycled ventilation are that airway pressures are controlled, and this mode is frequently more comfortable than volume cycled modes. Disadvantages are that TV and minute ventilation are not guaranteed. Troubleshoot TV and minute ventilation. Examples of this mode include:

- *Assist control/pressure control (AC/PC) ventilation:* In this mode the ventilator delivers a set pressure (15 cm H_2O typically) at a set rate (12 breaths per minute). If the patient initiates a breath, the same preset pressure is delivered. The maximum airway pressure is the preset pressure plus the PEEP. There is no guaranteed tidal volume, and thus there is no guaranteed minute ventilation in this mode. Unstable reactive airways disease can dramatically affect minute ventilation. Air trapping and CO_2 retention can occur, al-

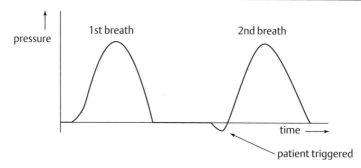

Fig. 17.6 Assist control/pressure control (AC/PC) ventilation: Ventilator delivers a set pressure (15 cm H_2O typically) at a set rate (12 breaths per minute). If patient initiates a breath, the same preset pressure is delivered. Maximum airway pressure is equal to the preset pressure plus the positive end-expiratory pressure (PEEP).

though this may be acceptable in "permissive hypercapnia" strategies for ventilation of some patients with acute respiratory failure (**Fig. 17.6**).

- *Pressure control–inverse ratio ventilation (PC-IRV):* This mode is a version of AC/PC with high initial flow rates, rapid inflation, and therefore an inversed I:E. This leads to prolonged inspiration and improved alveolar recruitment and compliance. This mode can lead to higher mean airway pressures, is uncomfortable (often requiring sedation for patient tolerance), and can lead to auto-PEEP.

- *Airway pressure release ventilation (APRV):* The ventilator cycles between high continuous and low continuous airway pressure. Spontaneous breathing primarily occurs during high airway pressure. A very brief pressure release expiratory phase provides an inverse I:E and aids in alveolar recruitment and oxygenation. When patients do not overbreathe the ventilator, this is the same as PC-IRV. Compared with PC-IRV, this mode is more comfortable, is associated with less barotrauma and circulatory compromise, and improves V/Q (ventilation/perfusion) matching.

- *Bilevel:* In this mode there are pressure-controlled mandatory breaths at a set rate and pressure-supported patient-initiated breaths. Like APRV, the ventilator cycles between high and low continuous pressure. This mode is more comfortable than PC-IRV, helpful for recruitment, causes less ventilator dyssynchrony than APRV, and is sometimes used in patients with ARDS.

- *Pressure regulated volume controlled (PRVC):* The ventilator adjusts pressure from breath to breath to deliver the set tidal volume with the lowest possible peak pressure by varying flow. The maximum pressure delivered is up to 5 cm H_2O above the set pressure limit (typically 35 to 40 cm H_2O). Barotrauma is rare in this ventilation mode.

Flow Cycled Ventilation

Inspiration is terminated after a set flow rate is reached. Examples include:

- *Pressure support ventilation (PSV):* Pressure support is a method of assisting spontaneous breathing in a ventilated patient. When a patient triggers a demand valve, a preset pressure is delivered until the flow rate tapers (usually to ~25% of its maximal value). Tidal volume and minute ventilation are dependent on the patient effort, and neither is guaranteed. Pressure support overcomes the resistance in the ventilator circuit. Higher pressure support settings allow patients to inspire larger TV. In patients with small ETT (<7.0), a higher PS may be necessary to overcome the resistance of the ETT. PS can be used as a partial or full support mode (i.e., patients can be rested on PS when they are spontaneously breathing). It is advantageous because it avoids patient–ventilator asynchrony, and patients are often more comfortable because they have full control over their ventilatory pattern and minute ventilation. This mode often avoids breath stacking and auto-PEEP, especially in patients with COPD. It has the ability to permit self-determination of respiratory rate and permit forced exhalation, which offers substantial advantages in status asthmaticus. Pressure support is used to assist spontaneous breaths in SIMV ventilation and bilevel ventilation. It cannot be used in heavily sedated, paralyzed, or comatose patients, and respiratory muscle fatigue can develop if the pressure support is set too low (**Fig. 17.7**).

- *Volume support ventilation (VSV):* In VSV, a target TV is set, and the ventilator adjusts the pressure support applied to reach this TV. This mode is patient triggered. It can be used as a liberation mode. It is similar to PSV, but the tidal volume is set, and the pressure varies.

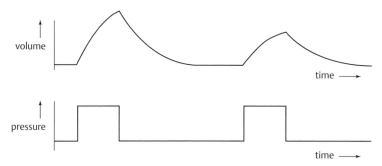

Fig. 17.7 Pressure support ventilation (PSV): When the patient triggers the demand valve, a preset pressure is delivered until flow rate tapers (usually to ~25% of its maximal value). Tidal volume (TV) and minute ventilation are dependent on the patient effort.

Time Cycled Ventilation

Inspiration is terminated after a set time, and both volume and airway pressures vary as a function of lung mechanics (resistance and compliance). Examples of time cycled ventilation include CMV (which is both time and volume cycled) and APRV (which is both time and pressure cycled).

Ventilator Weaning

Adverse effects of invasive mechanical ventilation include hemodynamic compromise due to elevated intrathoracic pressure, pneumonia, oxygen toxicity, alveolar edema, epithelial sheering, ICU myopathy/ neuropathy (in patients that require neuromuscular blockade for ventilation), and barotrauma (e.g., tension pneumothorax, particularly in patients with COPD receiving high TV or PEEP). Be alert to decreased breath sounds and hypotension. This emergency can be treated with a 16-gauge angiocatheter in the second intercostal space at the midclavicular line). To avoid complications, it is important to frequently assess patients for liberation from the ventilator. The two most important factors in shortening the duration of mechanical ventilation (MV) are daily weaning trials[2] and sedation vacation.[3] In a randomized controlled trial of sedated mechanically ventilated patients, those who underwent daily sedation vacation had significantly shorter MV duration (4.9 vs 7.3 days, $p = .004$) and shorter mean ICU length of stay (6.4 vs 9.9 days, $p = .02$) compared with those who did not undergo daily sedation vacation.

Sedation vacation led to an increased discovery of neurologic complications but did not increase accidental extubation rates.[3] Daily interruption of sedation is now a standard of care and is supported by the Joint Commission for the American Hospital Organization.

- Readiness to wean criteria are listed in **Table 17.1**.[4]

- *Weaning and extubating comatose patients:* Whether or not comatose patients can be extubated has been a matter of some controversy. In a prospective study of 242 patients with neurologic injury, 81% of those with a Glasgow Coma Score (GCS) ≤8 and 89% of those with absent or weak gag were successfully extubated. The presence of a cough and infrequent need for suctioning predicted successful extubation. In this study, those who were extubated regardless of mental status had significantly less pneumonia, shorter ICU and hospital length of stay, lower hospital costs, and lower mortality.[5] In a randomized controlled trial of 100 neurosurgical

Table 17.1 Criteria for Readiness to Wean

Oxygenation	PaO_2 >60 mm Hg on FiO_2 40% or O_2 saturation ≥90%, PEEP ≤5 cm H_2O, P/F >200[†], alveolar-arterial gradient <350 mm Hg
Ventilation	RR/TV <105 breaths/min/L, * NIF better than −30 cm H_2O, VC >10–15 mL/kg, minute ventilation <10–12 L/min, requires suctioning <2 times/h
Hemodynamic status	SBP >90 mm Hg, HR <140 beats per minute
Neurologic status	ICP <20 mm Hg, alert or command following (unless aphasic),[‡] cough present

Abbreviations: HR, heart rate; ICP, intracranial pressure; NIF, negative inspiratory force; PEEP, positive end-expiratory pressure; P/F, ratio of PaO_2 to FiO_2; RR, respiratory rate; TV, tidal volume; VC, vital capacity.

[†] P/F <300 = ALI and <200= ARDS in the context of normal left atrial pressure and bilateral opacities on CXR.

*Rapid shallow breathing index[§]: It does not need to be <105 to initiate a weaning trial, but it does predict successful extubation.

[‡] Mental status necessary for extubation is a matter of controversy.

[§] Index data from: Yang KL, Tobin MJ. A prospective study of indexes predicting the outcome of trials of weaning from mechanical ventilation. N Engl J Med 1991;324(21): 1445–1450.

patients, the odds of a successful extubation increased by 39% with each incremental increase in GCS. Those with a GCS ≥8 had a 75% successful extubation rate versus 33% in those with a GCS <8 ($p <$ .0001).[6] Though extubation of comatose patients with minimal secretions and good cough may be safe, most practitioners opt for early tracheostomy and wean to trach collar in such patients. Comatose patients should undergo daily weaning trials and sedation vacation even if a tracheostomy is planned because this may expedite weaning to trach collar and liberation from the ventilator.

- *Weaning modes:* In a pivotal randomized controlled trial of 120 mechanically ventilated patients randomized to T-piece trial once a day versus twice a day versus IMV versus PS, patients who received once or twice daily T-piece trials had significantly higher rates of successful weaning and shorter duration of mechanical ventilation.[2] In a subsequent randomized trial of 526 mechanically ventilated patients, those who received 30 versus 120 minutes of a spontaneous breathing trial (SBT) had similar reintubation rates, indicating that a 30-minute SBT is sufficient.[7] Others have shown a shorter duration of mechanical ventilation with PS weaning compared with T-piece or IMV weaning (5.7 days with PS versus 8.5 days with T-piece and 9.9 days with IMV).[8] In a meta-analysis of 16 randomized controlled trials, different methodologies for readiness to wean and different extubation criteria seemed to overwhelm the effect of alternative weaning mode choices. Nonetheless, multiple daily T-piece trials or PS trials are superior to SIMV weaning.[9,10] SIMV has been shown to increase the work of breathing by up to 2 times that of resting modes. The difficulty of brain respiratory centers in adjusting to intermittent support may account for part of this effect. SIMV, therefore, is not recommended as a weaning mode. PS has been a preferred mode of weaning because most ventilators provide backup assist control ventilation in patients who are failing in this mode or are apneic, increasing the safety of PS over T-piece. Many ventilators have tube compensation modes that mimic T-piece by providing continuous airway support to overcome the resistance in the circuit, while still allowing for backup ventilation in the case of apnea.

A typical weaning protocol might entail PS 5 or 10 mm Hg, tube compensation, or T-piece trial for 30 minutes followed by extubation. In patients with small ETT, a higher PS may be required to overcome the resistance in the ETT. An ABG prior to extubation is needed only if there is concern regarding CO_2 retention; otherwise O_2 saturation can be followed to monitor oxygenation. Always check for an air leak before extubation (to ensure that serious laryngeal edema is not present) by deflating the ETT cuff (removing 10 mL of air) and listening for gurgling at the mouth or observing lower tidal volumes on an assist control mode. If an air leak is not present, the patient *should not be extubated*. Steroids (e.g., dexamethasone 4 mg every 6 hours) can be administered to control edema until an air leak is noted.

Patients with COPD or neuromuscular disease often have successful PS trials only to fatigue after extubation. It is recommended that these patients undergo a T-piece or tube compensation trial for at least 30 minutes prior to extubation. Patients with neuromuscular disease should have a VC >10–15 mL/kg and an NIF better than −30 cm H_2O prior to extubation.

A pressure support trial is considered unsuccessful if RR >35 breaths/minute, O_2 saturation <90%, heart rate (HR) >140 beats per minute, or there are signs of fatigue such as retraction, diaphoresis, nasal flaring, or paradoxical abdominal breathing. If a weaning trial is unsuccessful, the patient should be rested on an assist control mode or a higher level of pressure support, and a weaning trial should be attempted again the next day. Even patients who are likely to require tracheostomy should undergo daily weaning trials, as this may expedite time to trach collar and ventilator liberation.

Early Tracheostomy

Tracheostomy not only provides a secure airway, but makes pulmonary and oral hygiene easier, decreases dead space and airway resistance, thus making ventilation more efficient, decreases the need for sedation, decreases the work of breathing and attenuates complications of prolonged intubation, including ulceration, granulation tissue formation, subglottic edema, and tracheal and laryngeal stenosis. Once the patient is weaned off the ventilator, by using a speaking valve the patient can talk and eat, thus providing comfort and allowing communication with the medical staff and family. This is a reversible procedure, and the tracheostomy site closes on it own once the tube is removed.

In a randomized controlled trial of mechanically ventilated patients projected to require >14 days of MV (with an APACHE-2 score >25), those randomized to early percutaneous tracheostomy within 48 hours versus delayed tracheostomy at 14 to 16 days had a lower mortality (32% vs 62%, p = .005), less pneumonia (5% vs 25%, p = .005), shorter ICU length of stay (5 vs 16 days, p = .001), and shorter duration of MV (8 vs 17 days, p = .001).[11] Similarly, early tracheostomy in neurologic patients has been shown to reduce MV time, length of stay, and pneumonia. Early tracheostomy should be considered in patients who have profound neurologic injury and who are not likely to protect their airway or tolerate weaning. Tracheostomy should not be performed in patients with elevated and unstable ICP. Open tracheostomy and percutaneous tracheostomy are both options. Contraindications to percutaneous tracheostomy include high FiO_2 or PEEP requirement (as is the case in open tracheostomy), unstable cervical spine, goiter, and mediastinal irradiation.

Acute Lung Injury and Acute Respiratory Distress Syndrome

According to the ARDSnet study,[12] the following steps can be followed for patients with ALI/ARDS (ALI/ARDS is defined by bilateral opacities on chest x-ray (CXR), P/F <300 = ALI, and <200 = ARDS in the context of normal left atrial pressure):

1. *Initial mode AC/VC with TV 8 mL/kg predicted body weight (PBW) and RR <35 breaths per minute to match baseline minute ventilation.* Reduce TV to 7 mL/kg and then 6 mL/kg PBW over 1 to 3 hours.

2. *Plateau pressure goal ≤30 cm H_2O.* Check inspiratory pause at least every 4 hours and after each change in TV or PEEP. If the plateau pressure is >30 cm H_2O, reduce TV by 1 mL/kg PBW (to minimum of 4 mL/kg PBW). If the plateau pressure is <25 cm H_2O and the TV is <6 mL/kg, increase TV by 1 mL/kg until plateau pressure >25 cm H_2O or TV = 6 mL/kg. If auto-PEEP or dyspnea occurs, the TV may be increased to 8 mL/kg PBW if the plateau pressure remains ≤30 cm H_2O.

3. *Oxygenation goal 55 to 80 mm Hg or O_2 saturation 88 to 90%.* Use the FiO_2/PEEP sliding scale (**Table 17.2**).

4. Using high or low PEEP in addition to these guidelines has not been shown to affect outcome.[13]

Table 17.2 FiO_2/PEEP Sliding Scale

FiO_2	0.3	0.4	0.5	0.6	0.7	0.8	0.9	1.0
PEEP	5	5–8	8–10	10	10–14	14	14–18	18–22

Abbreviation: PEEP, positive end-expiratory pressure.

■ Prognosis

The patient's prognosis depends largely on the underlying mechanism leading to intubation. Shorter duration of MV and early tracheostomy may lead to better outcomes in neurologic patients.

Pearls and Pitfalls

- AC/VC is the most commonly used ventilation mode.
- Daily sedation vacation and weaning trials are essential to limiting the duration of MV.
- PS or T-piece trials are reasonable modes for weaning.
- Early tracheostomy should be considered in patients who are unlikely to be successfully extubated.
- Lung protective ventilation using TV of 6 mL/kg PBW and maintaining a plateau pressure ≤30 cm H_2O is recommended in ALI/ARDS.

References
1. McGuire G, Crossley D, Richards J, Wong D. Effects of varying levels of positive end-expiratory pressure on intracranial pressure and cerebral perfusion pressure. Crit Care Med 1997;25(6):1059–1062
2. Esteban A, Frutos F, Tobin MJ, et al. A comparison of four methods of weaning patients from mechanical ventilation. Spanish Lung Failure Collaborative Group. N Engl J Med 1995;332(6):345–350
3. Kress JP, Pohlman AS, O'Connor MF, Hall JB. Daily interruption of sedative infusions in critically ill patients undergoing mechanical ventilation. N Engl J Med 2000;342(20):1471–1477
4. Yang KL, Tobin MJ. A prospective study of indexes predicting the outcome of trials of weaning from mechanical ventilation. N Engl J Med 1991;324(21):1445–1450

5. Coplin WM, Pierson DJ, Cooley KD, Newell DW, Rubenfeld GD. Implications of extubation delay in brain-injured patients meeting standard weaning criteria. Am J Respir Crit Care Med 2000;161(5):1530–1536

6. Namen AM, Ely EW, Tatter SB, et al. Predictors of successful extubation in neurosurgical patients. Am J Respir Crit Care Med 2001;163(3 Pt 1):658–664

7. Esteban A, Alía I, Tobin MJ, et al. Effect of spontaneous breathing trial duration on outcome of attempts to discontinue mechanical ventilation. Spanish Lung Failure Collaborative Group. Am J Respir Crit Care Med 1999;159(2):512–518

8. Brochard L, Rauss A, Benito S, et al. Comparison of three methods of gradual withdrawal from ventilatory support during weaning from mechanical ventilation. Am J Respir Crit Care Med 1994;150(4):896–903

9. Meade M, Guyatt G, Cook D, et al. Predicting success in weaning from mechanical ventilation. Chest 2001; 120(6, Suppl):400S–424S

10. Meade M, Guyatt G, Sinuff T, et al. Trials comparing alternative weaning modes and discontinuation assessments. Chest 2001; 120(6, Suppl):425S–437S

11. Rumbak MJ, Newton M, Truncale T, Schwartz SW, Adams JW, Hazard PB. A prospective, randomized, study comparing early percutaneous dilational tracheotomy to prolonged translaryngeal intubation (delayed tracheotomy) in critically ill medical patients. Crit Care Med 2004;32(8):1689–1694

12. Ventilation with lower tidal volumes as compared with traditional tidal volumes for acute lung injury and the acute respiratory distress syndrome. The Acute Respiratory Distress Syndrome Network. N Engl J Med 2000;342(18):1301–1308

13. Brower RG, Lanken PN, MacIntyre N, et al; National Heart, Lung, and Blood Institute ARDS Clinical Trials Network. Higher versus lower positive end-expiratory pressures in patients with the acute respiratory distress syndrome. N Engl J Med 2004;351(4):327–336

18 Prophylaxis

Sherry Hsiang-Yi Chou

Critically ill neurologic patients are at high risk for venous thromboembolism (VTE), nosocomial infection, gastric ulcer, and anemia. Prophylaxis can minimize the risk of these hospital complications.

- *Venous thromboembolism (VTE)*: The prevalence of deep vein thrombosis (DVT) among various neurologic populations is listed in **Table 18.1**.[1]

  Pulmonary emboli (PE) account for 10% of hospital deaths and carry an in-hospital case fatality rate of 10% and a 1-year fatality rate of 30%. PE is the most preventable cause of in-hospital death. The risk for VTE depends on the patient's age, history of hypercoagulability, prior VTE, history of cancer, and type of surgery (if any) **Table 18.2**.[1]

- *Nosocomial infections* are common among neurologic patients, given the increased incidence of abnormal mental status, coma, aspiration, and concomitant trauma that occurs in this patient group. Additionally, such patients may be susceptible to different infections, such as ventriculitis or meningitis, as compared with other

Table 18.1 The Prevalence of Deep Vein Thrombosis among Various Neurologic Populations

Neurosurgery	15–40%
Stroke	20–50%
Spinal cord injury	60–80%
Critically ill	10–80%

Data from: Geerts WH, Bergqvist D, Pineo GF, et al; American College of Chest Physicians. Prevention of venous thromboembolism: American College of Chest Physicians Evidence-Based Clinical Practice Guidelines (8th ed.). Chest 2008; 133(6, Suppl):381S–453S

Table 18.2 Preventive Measures for Deep Vein Thrombosis (DVT) and Pulmonary Embolism (PE) Based on Level of Risk

Risk of VTE	DVT % without Prophylaxis	PE % without Prophylaxis	Prevention
Low risk Minor surgery in mobile patients, medical patients who are fully mobile	<10	0.2	Early mobilization
Moderate risk Most general, open gynecologic or urologic surgery patients, medical patients (bed rest or sick)	10–40	1–2	LMWH (at recommended doses), low-dose unfractionated heparin q 12 h, fondaparinux
Moderate risk plus bleeding risk			Mechanical thromboprophylaxis, including GCS, IPC; consider switch to anticoagulant thromboprophylaxis when high bleeding risk decreases
High-risk hip or knee arthroplasty, hip fracture surgery, major trauma, spinal cord injury	40–80	4–10	LMWH (at recommended doses), fondaparinux, warfarin (INR 2–3)
Highest risk plus high bleeding risk			Mechanical thromboprophylaxis, including GCS, IPC; consider switch to anticoagulant thromboprophylaxis when high bleeding risk decreases

Abbreviations: LMWH, low molecular weight heparin; GCS, graded compression stockings; INR, international normalized ratio; IPC, intermittent pneumatic compression; q, every; VTE, venous thromboembolism.

Data from: Geerts WH, Bergqvist D, Pineo GF, et al; American College of Chest Physicians. Prevention of venous thromboembolism: American College of Chest Physicians Evidence-Based Clinical Practice Guidelines (8th ed.). Chest 2008; 133(6, Suppl):381S–453S

critically ill patients. The most commonly documented infections are pneumonia (3 to 12 per 100 patients), urinary tract infection (UTI; 3 to 9 per 100 patients), bloodstream infection (1 to 2 per 100 patients), meningitis or ventriculitis (1 to 9 per 100 patients), and surgical wound infections.[2–5] There are many preventive measures that should be undertaken to limit the incidence of nosocomial infections. Antibiotic prophylaxis must be cautiously administered to balance against the risks of antimicrobial resistance and *Clostridium difficile* infection.

• *Anemia* occurs frequently in neurologically critically ill patients and can be due to blood loss during surgery, active bleeding, disseminated intravascular coagulopathy (DIC)/hemolysis, chronic anemia, or frequent phlebotomy. Theoretical benefits of red cell transfusion include increased O_2 delivery and tissue perfusion. Downsides of transfusion include:
  ◦ acute and delayed hemolytic reaction
  ◦ volume overload
  ◦ pulmonary edema (FFP worst offender)
  ◦ transfusion related acute lung injury (TRALI: noncardiogenic pulmonary edema; must occur within 6 hours of transfusion; is immune mediated; more common with FFP occurs also with packed red blood cells (RBCs); must distinguish from volume overload)
  ◦ acute respiratory distress syndrome (ARDS)
  ◦ disseminated intravascular coagulation (DIC)
  ◦ posttransfusion purpura (7 to 10 days after transfusion)
  ◦ nosocomial infection
  ◦ hypothermia
  ◦ alkalosis/citrate toxicity
  ◦ hypocalcaemia.

• Fresh blood releases 23% of carried O_2; however, stored blood releases only 6% (due to depletion of 2,3-diphosphoglycerate (DPG) and a left shift in the oxyhemoglobin curve), leading to diminishing returns from transfusion.

• *Gastric ulcer*: Severe physiologic stress such as critical illness, burns, surgery, and neurologic injury can increase the risk of peptic ulcers. Risk factors for stress ulcer development and gastrointestinal (GI) bleeding in critically ill patients include coagulopathy (most potent risk factor), mechanical ventilation, renal failure, burn injury, and neurologic injuries.[6]

Case Example

You are called to assess a patient with a C3-level cord compression who underwent anterior surgical decompression and fusion 24 hours ago. His hemoglobin is 8.4 mg/dL. You are asked to recommend DVT, antibiotic, and gastric ulcer prophylaxis. The neurosurgeon asks you if the patient should receive a red blood cell transfusion.

Questions

- Does the patient have any evidence of active bleeding?
- Is the patient mechanically ventilated?
- Is the patient receiving steroids?
- Is there any evidence of active infection?

Urgent Orders

- Check complete blood count (CBC), iron studies, vitamin B12, folate, coagulation studies, and guaiac stool; consider DIC panel.

■ History and Examination

History

Assess for history of cancer, hypercoagulability, previous VTE, coagulopathy, past GI bleed, anemia, steroid or nonsteroidal antiinflammatory drug (NSAID) use, and immunosuppressed state. Assess timing and type of surgery performed (if any).

Physical Examination

Venous Thromboembolism

- Asymmetric swelling, redness, and warmth of extremities are suggestive of DVT. Absence of clinical signs and symptoms does not rule out VTE. The majority of VTEs are clinically asymptomatic.
- Oxygen desaturation, A-a gradient, refractory hypoxia, sinus tachycardia, and hypotension may all be signs of clinically significant PE. Sinus tachycardia is the most common abnormality on ECG with PE. An S wave in lead I, Q wave in lead III and T wave in lead III ($S_1Q_3T_3$) is considered a classic finding with PE.

- Obesity, venous stasis ulcers in the lower extremities, indwelling central catheters, and hemiparesis are factors that increase the patient's risk for VTE.

Nosocomial Infection

- Fever, elevated white blood cell (WBC) count, respiratory distress, crackles, rhonchi, pleuritic rubs on chest auscultation, and excessive purulent sputum production are suggestive of pneumonia. Absence of fever or elevated WBC does not rule out pneumonia, particularly in immune-suppressed patients. UTIs are typically asymptomatic in the ICU. Meningitis/ventriculitis is characterized by cerebrospinal fluid (CSF) pleocytosis (typically polymorphonuclear cells), elevated protein, and low glucose. Patients who have had recent neurosurgery or intracranial hemorrhage can develop aseptic chemical meningitis, which can have a similar CSF profile. CSF cultures can help distinguish between the two, though if the patient has been receiving antibiotics at the time of CSF sampling, CSF cultures are unreliable. Wound infections are characterized by erythema, induration, and purulent drainage.

- Patients who are edentulous or have poor dentition, who have - pharyngeal or laryngeal weakness, or who consume alcohol in excess may be at increased risk of nosocomial pneumonia.

Gastric Ulcer/Anemia

- Anemia, melanotic stool, and coffee-ground aspirates from a nasogastric tube suggest the presence of an upper GI bleed. Absence of these signs does not rule out stress ulcers.

- Examine wounds from trauma and/or surgical site for evidence of ongoing hemorrhage. Ongoing hemorrhage in the pleural, peritoneal, and retroperitoneal cavities may not be visible on general physical examination. Remember to examine the pelvis and groin for signs of deep expanding hematoma.

Neurologic Examination

- A full neurologic examination, including assessment of mental status, cranial nerves, motor skills, and reflexes, as well as a sensory and cerebellar exam, should be performed on all patients.

■ Prophylaxis and Preventive Strategies

Evidence-based guidelines for preventing hospital complications are often "bundled" to allow for most effective implementation. Many government (Joint Commission on the Accreditation of Healthcare Organizations [JCAHO]) and state organizations support such bundles.

Venous Thromboembolism

General Principles

- In most neurologically critically ill patients, use compression boots plus heparin 5000 units twice daily (b.i.d.) or three times daily (t.i.d.) (if >60 years old, cancer, hypercoagulable state, or history of VTE) or Enoxaparin 40 mg subcutaneously every day.

- Enoxaparin is superior to unfractionated heparin for VTE prophylaxis in patients with ischemic stroke or acute spinal cord injury.[7,8]

- Low molecular weight heparin (LMWH) causes less heparin-induced thrombocytopenia (HIT) and less osteopenia than unfractionated heparin. It can be administered once a day instead of b.i.d. or t.i.d., but only 60–75% reversal can be achieved with protamine for enoxaparin and even less reversibility is possible with other types of LMWH. Unfractionated heparin is preferred in patients with renal insufficiency.

- Fondaparinux is a synthetic heparin analogue that binds antithrombin. It does not prolong activated partial prothrombin time (aPTT), prothrombin time (PT), or bleeding time, or alter platelet function or fibrinolysis. Fondaparinux has a long half-life and no antidote.

- There are no recommendations to support the use of prophylactic inferior vena cava (IVC) filters.

- Timing of initiation of VTE prophylaxis:
  - Craniotomy: Postop 24 to 48 h if hemostasis[9]
  - Acute spinal cord injury (SCI): As soon as hemostasis is achieved[1]
  - Intracerebral hemorrhage (ICH): post 3 to 4 days[10]

Table 18.3 Specific Recommendations

Disease Category	Recommendation	Level of Recommendation
General	Mechanical methods alone have not been shown to reduce PE or death in any group.	
	Use mechanical methods alone in patients at high risk of bleeding, or as an adjunct to anticoagulant based prophylaxis.	Grade 1A (ACCP) Grade 2A (ACCP)
	Aspirin is not recommended as prophylaxis for any group.	Grade 1A (ACCP)
	Routine screening Doppler in asymptomatic patients is not cost effective and not recommended.	Grade 1A (ACCP)
Craniotomy	Compression boots for all patients	Grade 1A (ACCP)
	Heparin SQ or LMWH are options.	Grade 2B, 2A (ACCP)
	A randomized controlled trial of enoxaparin plus compression stockings started 24 h postop compared with compression stockings alone in elective neurosurgery patients showed significantly fewer DVT/PE in the enoxaparin group, with no significant increase in bleeding.	
	Heparin SQ or LMWH plus compression boots are recommended for high-risk patients.	Grade 2B (ACCP)
Elective spine surgery	Early mobilization and no prophylaxis if no risk factors	Grade 2C (ACCP)
	Use some form of prophylaxis in older patients, history of cancer, previous VTE, neurologic deficit, or anterior approach. Options:	Grade 1B (ACCP)
	Heparin SQ	Grade 1C (ACCP)
	LMWH SQ	Grade 1B (ACCP)
	Compression boots alone	Grade 1B (ACCP)
	GCS alone	Grade 2B (ACCP)
	If multiple risk factors: SQ heparin or LWMH plus GCS and/or compression boots	Grade 2C (ACCP)
Acute spinal cord injury (SCI)	LMWH commenced as soon as hemostasis present	Grade 1B (ACCP)
	Alternatives: compression boots + unfractionated heparin or LMWH	Grade 1B (ACCP) Grade 1C (ACCP)

(Continued)

Table 18.3 Specific Recommendations *(continued)*

Disease Category	Recommendation	Level of Recommendation
	If anticoagulant thromboprophylaxis is contraindicated because of high bleeding risk, compression boots or GCS is recommended.	Grade 1A (ACCP)
	When bleeding risk decreases, pharmacologic prophylaxis should be substituted or added.	Grade 1C (ACCP)
	For patients with an incomplete SCI associated with spinal hematoma on CT or MRI, use mechanical thromboprophylaxis at least for the first few days after injury.	Grade 1C (ACCP)
	Recommend against unfractionated heparin alone	Grade 1A (ACCP)
	A randomized controlled trial in SCI patients of heparin t.i.d. + compression boots vs LMWH found VTE in 16% of heparin group and 12% in LMWH group, major bleeding in 5% of heparin group, and 3% of LMWH group.	
	Recommend against IVC filter as primary prophylaxis	Grade 1C (ACCP)
	IVC filters do NOT prevent DVTs. Complications of IVC filter placement include erosion/perforation of IVC wall, filter migration, improper initial placement, distal thrombi formation, arterial-venous fistula at insertion site, infection, IVC occlusion, and 0.12% incidence of death.	
Intracerebral hemorrhage	All patients should have compression stockings.	Class I, level B (AHA/ASA)
	After documentation of cessation of bleeding, SQ heparin or LMWH may be started in patients with hemiplegia after 3–4 days.	Class IIb, level B (AHA/ASA)
	In a randomized trial, 68 patients with ICH were treated with SQ heparin at days 2, 4, and 10 postbleed. Rates of PE were 0, 4, and 13% at each time epoch with no increase in bleeding in the early time group.	
Traumatic brain injury	Compression boots recommended in patients who do not have lower extremity injury	Level III (Brain Trauma Foundation)

(Continued on next page)

Table 18.3 Specific Recommendations *(continued)*

Disease Category	Recommendation	Level of Recommendation
	SQ heparin or LMWH + mechanical prophylaxis may be used.	Level III (Brain Trauma Foundation)
Ischemic stroke	Early mobilization is recommended.	Class I, level C (AHA/ASA)
	SQ administration of anticoagulants to prevent DVT in immobilized patients is recommended. The timing for starting these medications is not known. In a randomized trial of 1,335 ischemic stroke patients to enoxaparin vs. SQ heparin b.i.d., those who received enoxaparin had significantly fewer VTE, DVT, and PE without any significant increase in intracranial or clinically significant bleeding.	Class I, level A (AHA/ASA)
	Aspirin is a potential intervention to prevent DVT, but it is not as effective as SQ anticoagulants.	Class IIa, level A (AHA/ASA)
	Compression stockings are recommended for patients who cannot receive SQ anticoagulants.	Class IIa, level B (AHA/ASA)

Abbreviations: ACCP, American College of Chest Physicians; AHA/ASA, American Heart Association/American Stroke Association; b.i.d., twice a day; CT, computed tomography; DVT, deep vein thrombosis; GCS, Graded Compression Stocking; GBM, glioblastoma multiforme; ICH, intracerebral hemorrhage; IVC, inferior vena cava; LMWH, low molecular weight heparin; MRI, magnetic resonance imaging; PE, pulmonary embolism; SCI, spinal cord injury; SQ, subcutaneus; t.i.d., three times a day; VTE, venous thromboembolism.

Data from: Geerts WH, Bergqvist D, Pineo GF, et al; American College of Chest Physicians. Prevention of venous thromboembolism: American College of Chest Physicians Evidence-Based Clinical Practice Guidelines (8th ed.). Chest 2008; 133(6, Suppl):381S–453S. Agnelli G, Piovella F, Buoncristiani P, et al. Enoxaparin plus compression stockings compared with compression stockings alone in the prevention of venous thromboembolism after elective neurosurgery. N Engl J Med 1998;339(2):80–85. Broderick J, Connolly S, Feldmann E, et al; American Heart Association. American Stroke Association Stroke Council; High Blood Pressure Research Council; Quality of Care and Outcomes in Research Interdisciplinary Working Group. Guidelines for the management of spontaneous intracerebral hemorrhage in adults: 2007 update: a guideline from the American Heart Association/American Stroke Association Stroke Council, High Blood Pressure Research Council, and the Quality of Care and Outcomes in Research Interdisciplinary Working Group. Stroke 2007;38(6):2001–2023. *(Continued)*

Table 18.3 Specific Recommendations *(continued)*

Disease Category	Recommendation	Level of Recommendation
Brain tumor	All cancer patients are high risk for VTE SQ heparin or LMWH + compression boots No evidence for IVC filter Prophylactic IVC filter carries high complication rates in cancer patients and risks often outweigh benefits Incidence of VTE: meningioma (72%), GBM (60%), metastasis (20%)	No society guidelines

Data from (continued): Spinal Cord Injury Thromboprophylaxis Investigators. Prevention of venous thromboembolism in the acute treatment phase after spinal cord injury: a randomized, multicenter trial comparing low-dose heparin plus intermittent pneumatic compression with enoxaparin. J Trauma 2003;54(6):1116–1124.

Boeer A, Voth E, Henze T, Prange HW. Early heparin therapy in patients with spontaneous intracerebral haemorrhage. J Neurol Neurosurg Psychiatry 1991;54(5):466–467.

Guidelines for the management of severe traumatic brain injury. J Neurotrauma 2007;24(Suppl 1):S1–S106.

Adams HP Jr, del Zoppo G, Alberts MJ, et al; American Heart Association. American Stroke Association Stroke Council; Clinical Cardiology Council; Cardiovascular Radiology and Intervention Council; Atherosclerotic Peripheral Vascular Disease and Quality of Care Outcomes in Research Interdisciplinary Working Groups. Guidelines for the early management of adults with ischemic stroke: a guideline from the American Heart Association/American Stroke Association Stroke Council, Clinical Cardiology Council, Cardiovascular Radiology and Intervention Council, and the Atherosclerotic Peripheral Vascular Disease and Quality of Care Outcomes in Research Interdisciplinary Working Groups: the American Academy of Neurology affirms the value of this guideline as an educational tool for neurologists. Stroke 2007;38(5):1655–1711.

Sherman DG, Albers GW, Bladin C, et al. PREVAIL Investigators. The efficacy and safety of enoxaparin versus unfractionated heparin for the prevention of venous thromboembolism after acute ischaemic stroke (PREVAIL Study): an open-label randomised comparison. Lancet 2007;369(9570):1347–1355.

Sawaya R, Zuccarello M, Elkalliny M, Nishiyama H. Postoperative venous thromboembolism and brain tumors: Part i. Clinical profile. J Neurooncol. 1992;14:119–125.

Sawaya R, Glas-Greenwalt P. Postoperative venous thromboembolism and brain tumors: Part ii. Hemostatic profile. J Neurooncol. 1992;14:127–134.

Sawaya R, Highsmith RF. Postoperative venous thromboembolism and brain tumors: Part iii. Biochemical profile. J Neurooncol. 1992;14:113–118.

- Patients with type II HIT, (heparin induced thrombocytopenia) whether or not complicated by thrombosis, should be treated with a nonheparin anticoagulant such as a direct thrombin inhibitor (lepirudin—American College of Chest Physicians [ACCP] grade 1C, argatroban—ACCP grade 1C, bivalirudin—ACCP grade 2C), danaparoid (ACCP grade 1B), or fondaparinux (ACCP grade 1C). Patients with HIT should be screened for DVT (ACCP grade 1C). Warfarin can be started once the platelet count recovers (to at least $150 \times 10^9/L$) and should be overlapped with the nonheparin anticoagulant for at least 2 days with the international normalized ratio (INR) in therapeutic range (ACCP grade 1B). Anticoagulation should be continued for 6 months.[9]

- PE is typically diagnosed by chest computed tomography angiogram (CTA), and in patients without any contraindications, anticoagulation should be started immediately.

Table 18.4 Nosocomial Infection

Infection Type	Preventive Strategy
Ventilator-associated pneumonia	Aggressive weaning Daily sedation vacation Early tracheostomy Consider noninvasive ventilation Oral ETT (rather than nasal intubation) ETT cuff pressure >20 cm H_2O Semirecumbent position 30–45 degrees unless contraindicated Oral hygiene (every 4 h and prn) Enteral feedings rather than total parenteral nutrition Pneumococcal vaccine for patients >65 years
Catheter-related bloodstream infection	Maximal sterile barrier Preferential use of subclavian line site (greater infection risk: femoral > internal jugular > subclavian) 2% chlorhexidine skin preparation Use of preassembled insertion kits Use catheters with least number of ports needed Replace transparent dressings when loose, damp, or otherwise every 7 days Replace gauze when loose, damp, or otherwise every 2 days

(Continued)

Table 18.4 Nosocomial Infection *(continued)*

Infection Type	Preventive Strategy
	No routine line replacement
	No guide wire exchanges
	Selective use of antimicrobial/antiseptic impregnated catheters
	Remove lines when no longer needed
	Glycemic control
Surgical site infection (SSI)	Most SSIs occur between days 5–10 postop.
	Smoking cessation
	Shower preop with antimicrobial soap.
	Patient should not shave operative field.
	Intraop skin prep with chlorhexidine
	Surgeon hand and forearm surgical scrub × 5 minutes preop
	Use closed suction drains and insert through a separate incision.
	Keep operative incision covered for 48 h postop,
	then keep primarily closed incision open after 48 h.
	Change dressing with sterile technique.
	Maintain normoglycemia.
	Minimize periop transfusions.
	<u>Perioperative antibiotics.</u>
	First dose to start within 60 minutes before incision.
	A single preoperative dose is the recommended standard, but antibiotics can be continued for a maximum of 24 h, except in cardiothoracic surgery (48–72 hours) and in solid organ transplant (48 h).
	For craniotomy, spine surgery, transsphenoidal surgery, and CSF shunting procedures, use:
	Cefuroxime 1.5 g IV q 6 h *or* cefazolin 1 g IV q 4 h intraoperatively (to be D/C'd after 24 hours)
	For neurosurgery with entry into the sinuses:
	Cefuroxime 1.5 g IV q 6 h *and* ampicillin 1 g IV q 6 h
	<u>For immediate-type penicillin (PCN) allergy:</u>
	Vancomycin 1000 mg IV q 12 h *and*
	gentamicin 1.5 mg/kg (ideal body weight) q 8 h (to be D/C'd after 24 h)
	For trauma: first- or third-generation cephalosporin, given for no longer than 24 h, even in colon injuries, as long as trauma is >4 h old.
	Routine vancomycin and third-generation cephalosporin prophylaxis should not be given.

(Continued on next page)

Table 18.4 Nosocomial Infection *(continued)*

Infection Type	Preventive Strategy
Clostridium difficile diarrhea	Judicious use of antibiotics Place infected patients on contact precautions. Meticulous hand washing with antiseptic soap and water before and after each contact Alcohol/Purell does not kill C. *difficile* spores. Dedicated single-use patient care items for those infected Terminally clean (with bleach) rooms of those infected. Treat clinically infected (not carriers) patients who have active diarrhea with PO or IV metronidazole or PO vancomycin (if refractory to metronidazole).
Meningitis/ ventriculitis	A randomized trial did not show any benefit to routine EVD change (risk of infection rises over the first 4 d, but then plateaus). A retrospective study of 308 patients showed the same meningitis/ventriculitis rate (4%) for those who received only periprocedural antibiotics compared with those who had antibiotics for the duration the drain was in place. Using only periplacement antibiotics would save $80,000 a year. A prospective study of 228 patients showed that those who got periprocedure Unasyn had an 11% CSF infection rate and a 42% extracranial infection rate, compared with those who had Unasyn and aztreonam for the duration of catheter placement (3% CSF infection, 20% extracranial infection). Those who received antibiotics for the duration grew more MRSA and *Candida*. Both chemical and infectious meningitis can produce CSF leukocytosis and low glucose. Using prophylactic antibiotics for the duration of drain placement makes cultures unreliable and selects for resistance. Tunneling and surveillance protocols can limit infection. Minimize shunt manipulation and tapping. Use sterile technique with shunt tapping. Antibiotic-coated catheters are associated with fewer positive CSF cultures.

Abbreviations: CSF, cerebrospinal fluid; D/C, discontinue; ETT, endotracheal tube; EVD, external ventricular drain; IV, intravenously; MRSA, methicillin-resistant *Staphylococcus aureus*; prn, as needed; PO, by mouth; q, every.

(Continued)

Table 18.4 Nosocomial Infection *(continued)*

Infection Type	Preventive Strategy
Indwelling catheter-related infection	Prophylactic antibiotics have not been shown to be useful for central lines, Foley catheters, lumbar drains, JP drains, or a Hemovac, and can breed resistance. We do not recommend prophylactic antibiotics for drains of any kind.

Data from: Hemovac autotransfusion system; Zimmer Orthopaedic Surgical Products, Dover, OH. Gojo, Akron, OH. Pfizer Pharmaceuticals, New York, NY. Niederman MS. The clinical diagnosis of ventilator-associated pneumonia. Respir Care 2005;50(6):788–796, discussion 807–812.

Szalados, JE, ed. Adult Multiprofessional Critical Care Review. Mount Prospect, IL: Society of Critical Care Medicine; 2007.

O'Grady NP, Alexander M, Dellinger EP, et al. Guidelines for the prevention of intravascular catheter-related infections. Centers for Disease Control and Prevention. MMWR Recomm Rep 2002;51(RR-10):1–29.

Pronovost P, Needham D, Berenholtz S, et al. An intervention to decrease catheter-related bloodstream infections in the ICU. N Engl J Med 2006;355(26): 2725–2732.

Bratzler DW, Houck PM. Antimicrobial prophylaxis for surgery: an advisory statement from the National Surgical Infection Prevention Project. Am J Surg 2005;189(4):395–404.

Surgical Care Improvement Project. Available at: www.medqic.org. Accessed August 10, 2008.

Wong GK, Poon WS, Wai S, Yu LM, Lyon D, Lam JM. Failure of regular external ventricular drain exchange to reduce cerebrospinal fluid infection: result of a randomised controlled trial. J Neurol Neurosurg Psychiatry 2002;73(6):759–761.

Alleyne CH Jr, Hassan M, Zabramski JM. The efficacy and cost of prophylactic and perioprocedural antibiotics in patients with external ventricular drains. Neurosurgery 2000;47(5):1124–1127, discussion 1127–1129.

Poon WS, Ng S, Wai S. CSF antibiotic prophylaxis for neurosurgical patients with ventriculostomy: a randomised study. Acta Neurochir Suppl (Wien) 1998;71:146–148.

Zabramski JM, Whiting D, Darouiche RO, et al. Efficacy of antimicrobial-impregnated external ventricular drain catheters: a prospective, randomized, controlled trial. J Neurosurg 2003;98(4):725–730.

Table 18.5 Anemia

Product	Transfusion/Administration Indication
Packed red blood cells	Transfuse for active bleeding Transfuse for a hematocrit <30% for acute ischemia (MI, consider for acute cerebral ischemia, SAH with vasospasm). For all other critically ill patients, restrict transfusion for those with Hgb <7 g/dL. TRICC trial randomized 838 critically ill patients to restricted transfusion for a Hgb <7.0 g/dL vs. liberal transfusion for a Hgb <10 g/dL, 26% of patients had a history of CAD, and 5% had a neurologic diagnosis. Overall, there was no difference in survival between the restrictive and liberal transfusion groups. Subgroups with APACHE score <20 or age <55 years had significantly better survival with restricted transfusion. The restrictive group had significantly fewer cardiac complications, MI, pulmonary edema, and multisystem organ dysfunction. In a retrospective study of 78,974 patients >65 years old with acute MI, transfusion for a hematocrit <30% was associated with a lower 30-day mortality.
Erythropoietin	Restrict use of erythropoietin to those with anemia receiving renal replacement therapy (target Hgb 7–9 mg/dL). In a randomized controlled trial of 1460 critically ill medical, surgical, and trauma patients, weekly erythropoietin did not decrease the number of patients who required an RBC transfusion or the number of units transfused (Hgb target 7–9 g/dL). Treatment with erythropoietin was associated with a significantly higher risk of thrombotic events.
Fresh frozen plasma	Transfuse for patients with vitamin K deficiency or warfarin therapy and active bleeding (if significantly increased PT, INR, or PTT). Transfuse for patients with vitamin K deficiency or warfarin therapy who require surgery or an invasive procedure (if significantly increased PT, INR, or PTT). Transfuse for patients with liver disease and active bleeding (if significantly increased PT, INR, or PTT). Transfuse for patients with liver disease before surgical or invasive procedures (except percutaneous liver biopsy, paracentesis, or thoracentesis) (if significantly increased PT, INR, or PTT). Transfuse for acute DIC with treatable triggering condition and active bleeding (if significantly increased PT, INR, or PTT).

(Continued)

Table 18.5 Anemia *(continued)*

Product	Transfusion/Administration Indication
	Transfuse for TTP/HUS and initial plasmapheresis. Transfuse acquired deficiencies of a single coagulation factor when DDAVP or appropriate factor concentrates are ineffective/unavailable and there is serious bleeding or before emergency surgical or invasive procedure. Give FFP along with massive transfusion of RBCs (>1 blood volume and significantly increased or unknown PT, INR, or PTT).
Platelets	Risk of severe bleeding rises when platelets <5–10,000/UL Risk of spontaneous intracranial hemorrhage when platelets <1000/UL (0.76% per day) Platelets are not indicated for stable thrombocytopenic patients with counts >10,000/UL. Consider maintaining platelets >50,000/UL in patients with recent intracranial or spinal hemorrhage. Consider maintaining platelets >50,000/UL in patients who require invasive procedures. Transfuse platelets for patients with defective platelets (due to antiplatelet medication, EtOH, renal failure, etc.), who are actively bleeding, had a recent intracranial or spinal hemorrhage, or are having an invasive procedure. Platelet transfusion (in addition to cryoprecipitate) is recommended for patients with bleeding after tPA. Platelet transfusion can worsen TTP and HIT.

Abbreviations: CAD, coronary artery disease; DDAVP, 1,desamino-8-D-arginine vasopressin; DIC, disseminated intravascular coagulation; EtOH, ethyl alcohol; ETT, endotracheal tube; FFP, fresh frozen plasma; Hgb, hemoglobin; HIT, heparin-induced thrombocytopenia; HUS, hemolytic uremic syndrome; INR, international normalized ratio; MI, myocardial ischemia; PT, prothrombin time; PTT, partial thromboplastin time; RBC, red blood cell; SAH, subarachnoid hemorrhage; tPA, tissue plasminogen activator; TTP, thrombotic thrombocytoperic purpura; UL, microliter.

Data from: Hebert PC, Wells G, Blajchman MA, et al. A multicenter, randomized, controlled clinical trial of transfusion requirements in critical care. Transfusion Requirements in Critical Care Investigators, Canadian Critical Care Trials Group. N Engl J Med 1999;340(6):409–417.

Wu WC, Rathore SS, Wang Y, Radford MJ, Krumholz HM. Blood transfusion in elderly patients with acute myocardial infarction. N Engl J Med 2001;345(17): 1230–1236.

Corwin HL, Gettinger A, Fabian TC, et al; EPO Critical Care Trials Group. Efficacy and safety of epoetin alfa in critically ill patients. N Engl J Med 2007;357(10): 965–976.

Lauzier F, Cook D, Griffith L, Upton J, Crowther M. Fresh frozen plasma transfusion in critically ill patients. Crit Care Med 2007;35(7):1655–1659.

Gastric Ulcers

Prophylaxis is recommended in patients with the following conditions:[12]

- Coagulopathy
- Mechanical ventilation >48 hours
- Patients with at least two of the following: sepsis, intensive care unit (ICU) stay >1 week, occult bleeding >6 days or more, and use of high-dose corticosteroids (>250 mg/day of hydrocortisone or equivalent).
- Glasgow Coma Scale ≤10
- Thermal injuries to >35% body surface area
- Partial hepatectomy and/or hepatic failure
- Multiple trauma and spinal cord injuries
- Organ transplant patients

Enteral feeding is an effective, nonpharmacologic method for gastrointestinal (GI) prophylaxis. Histamin-2 receptor antagonist (H2A), sucralfate, proton-pump inhibitors (PPI), antacids, and prostaglandin analogues decrease the incidence of upper GI bleeding in ICU patients. H2A blockers should be used with caution in the neuro-ICU, as they may cause significant encephalopathy and interact with anticonvulsants. Concerns for higher incidence of nosocomial pneumonia associated with H2A use remain controversial. Both H_2 blockers and PPIs can aggravate *Clostridium difficile* colitis, and carafate or sulcrafate should be used preferentially in this context.

Pearls and Pitfalls

- Mobilize and prophylax *early*. VTE prophylaxis is important in all patients.
- Bundles can help limit nosocomial infection.
- *Use the gut.* Enteral nutrition is an effective prophylaxis for stress ulcers.

References

1. Geerts WH, Bergqvist D, Pineo GF, et al; American College of Chest Physicians. Prevention of venous thromboembolism: American College of Chest Physicians Evidence-Based Clinical Practice Guidelines (8th ed.). Chest 2008; 133(6, Suppl):381S–453S

2. Dettenkofer M, Ebner W, Hans FJ, Forster D, Babikir R, Zentner J, Pelz K, Daschner FD. Nosocomial infections in a neurosurgery intensive care unit. *Acta Neurochir (Wien)* 1999;141:1303–1308

3. Dettenkofer M, Ebner W, Els T, Babikir R, Lucking C, Pelz K, Ruden H, Daschner F. Surveillance of nosocomial infections in a neurology intensive care unit. *J Neurol.* 2001;248:959–964

4. Bota DP, Lefranc F, Vilallobos HR, Brimioulle S, Vincent JL. Ventriculostomy-related infections in critically ill patients: A 6-year experience. *J Neurosurg.* 2005;103:468–472

5. Zolldann D, Thiex R, Hafner H, Waitschies B, Lutticken R, Lemmen SW. Periodic surveillance of nosocomial infections in a neurosurgery intensive care unit. *Infection.* 2005;33:115–121

6. Cook D, Heyland D, Griffith L, Cook R, Marshall J, Pagliarello J. Risk factors for clinically important upper gastrointestinal bleeding in patients requiring mechanical ventilation. Canadian Critical Care *Trials* Group. Crit Care Med 1999;27(12):2812–2817

7. Spinal Cord Injury Thromboprophylaxis Investigators. Prevention of venous thromboembolism in the acute treatment phase after spinal cord injury: a randomized, multicenter trial comparing low-dose heparin plus intermittent pneumatic compression with enoxaparin. J Trauma 2003;54(6):1116–1124

8. Sherman DG, Albers GW, Bladin C, et al. PREVAIL Investigators. The efficacy and safety of enoxaparin versus unfractionated heparin for the prevention of venous thromboembolism after acute ischaemic stroke (PREVAIL Study): an open-label randomised comparison. Lancet 2007;369(9570):1347–1355

9. Agnelli G, Piovella F, Buoncristiani P, et al. Enoxaparin plus compression stockings compared with compression stockings alone in the prevention of venous thromboembolism after elective neurosurgery. N Engl J Med 1998;339(2):80–85

10. Broderick J, Connolly S, Feldmann E, et al; American Heart Association. American Stroke Association Stroke Council; High Blood Pressure Research Council; Quality of Care and Outcomes in Research Interdisciplinary Working Group. Guidelines for the management of spontaneous intracerebral hemorrhage in adults: 2007 update: a guideline from the American Heart Association/American Stroke Association Stroke Council, High Blood Pressure Research Council, and the Quality of Care and Outcomes in Research Interdisciplinary Working Group. Stroke 2007;38(6):2001–2023

11. Warkentin TE, Greinacher A, Koster A, Lincoff AM; American College of Chest Physicians. Treatment and prevention of heparin-induced thrombocytopenia: American College of Chest Physicians Evidence-Based Clinical Practice Guidelines (8th ed.). Chest 2008; 133(6, Suppl):340S–380S

12. Guidelines on Stress Ulcer Prophylaxis. ASHP Commission on Therapeutics and approved by the ASHP Board of Directors on November 14, 1998. Am J Health Syst Pharm 1999;56(4):347–379

19 Glucose Management and Nutrition

Jennifer A. Frontera

Hyperglycemia in critically ill patients, often referred to as stress hyperglycemia, is characterized by increased gluconeogenesis, elevated insulin levels, insulin resistance, and increased IGF-binding protein 1. Elevated catecholamines, cortisol, growth hormone, and glucagon also occur in the context of critical illness, contributing to hyperglycemia. Hyperglycemia has been shown to lead to worse outcomes among various critically ill populations and has the highest adjusted odds ratios for mortality among cardiac and neurologic patients.

Acute hyperglycemia is common after neurologic injury. It occurs in 30 to 70% of patients and may be mediated by an acute stress response, hypothalamic injury, or catecholamine surge at the time of neurologic injury. Animal models of brain ischemia suggest that hyperglycemia worsens acidosis, excitotoxicity, and breakdown of the blood–brain barrier with consequent edema or hemorrhagic transformation. Elevated admission glucose and prolonged hyperglycemia have been linked to worse outcomes in patients with ischemic stroke, intracerebral hemorrhage (ICH), subarachnoid hemorrhage (SAH), and traumatic brain injury (TBI).[3,4,6,7,8,9] Prolonged hypoglycemia, which can occur as a complication of glucose management, can also lead to neurologic deterioration. Finding the appropriate glucose range and the best way to maintain normoglycemia in the neurologically critically ill is an active area of research.

Case Example

You are called by the neuro-intensive care unit (NICU) nurse because a patient you recently admitted with subarachnoid hemorrhage has a point of care glucose level of 253 mg/dL.

Questions

- What was the patient's admission glucose?
- What was the last glucose value?
- Has the patient received any dextrose solutions or insulin?
- Is the patient receiving steroids or intravenous (IV) pressors?
- Is the patient being fed currently?

Urgent Orders

- Remove dextrose from any IV infusions, if possible.
- Initiate insulin infusion protocol or administer subcutaneous insulin.

■ History and Examination

History

Does the patient have a history of diabetes? Does the patient have a history of diabetic ketoacidosis (DKA) or hyperosmotic nonketotic hyperglycemia? Does the patient take oral hypoglycemics or insulin at home?

Physical Examination

- Vitals: Blood pressure, heart rate, respiratory rate, urine output
- General: Assess volume status (mucous membranes, skin tenting, ins and outs).
- Cardiovascular: Assess for tachycardia (evidence of possible volume depletion).
- Extremities: Assess for diabetic ulcers.

Neurologic Examination

- A full neurologic examination, including assessment of mental status, cranial nerves, motor skills, and reflexes, as well as a sensory and cerebellar exam, should be performed on all patients.
- Mental status: Assess for level of arousal, attention, orientation.

- Cranial nerve: Assess for funduscopic evidence of diabetes (macular degeneration).
- Motor skills: Standard assessment
- Sensory skills: Assess for evidence of diabetic neuropathy (stocking-glove sensory loss, including large fiber proprioception, vibration and light touch, and small fiber pain or temperature loss).
- Reflexes: May be decreased if evidence of diabetic neuropathy

■ Differential Diagnosis

1. *Stress hyperglycemia related to acute neurologic injury and critical illness*
2. *Underlying diabetes (check history and HgbA1c)*
3. *Hyperglycemia related to dextrose administration*

Life-Threatening Diagnoses Not to Miss

- *Prolonged untreated hyperglycemia* can worsen outcomes in neurologic patients.
- *Diabetic ketoacidosis* occurs more commonly in type I diabetics, but it also occurs in type II. If glucose is >400 mg/dL, this must be considered.
- *Hyperosmotic nonketotic hyperglycemia (HONK):* Similar laboratories for DKA, ketosis not seen.

■ Diagnostic Evaluation

- Serial point of care glucose, HgbA1c
- Microdialysis (if available):
  - Hyperglycemic: Elevated brain glucose
  - Hypoglycemic: Low brain glucose levels (<2 mmol/L)
  - When low brain glucose leads to metabolic distress: elevated glutamate (>5 μM) and elevated lactate/pyruvate (>25 to 40 mmol/L) are seen.

- If DKA or HONK suspected: Serial arterial blood gas (ABG; metabolic acidosis), serum osmolarity, chemistry panel (particularly K+, Na, HCO_3, creatinine), anion gap (>12 mEq/L is abnormal), urine and serum ketones (β-hydroxybutyrate if available).

Blood glucose should be monitored hourly until stable and other laboratories checked every 2 to 4 hours depending on the severity and clinical response.

■ Treatment

Insulin

- Changes in feeding, IV infusions, steroid and pressor use, sepsis, and liver or renal failure affect glucose control.
- Protocolized insulin infusions can allow for tight control.
- Blood glucose levels are checked every hour after admission. When two consecutive glucose levels an hour apart exceed a certain threshold (e.g., 110 mg/dL), an insulin infusion is initiated. A standard infusion contains 100 U of regular insulin in 100 mL of normal saline (NS).
- Some protocols will combine dextrose infusions with insulin to temper potential hypoglycemia. Glucose-insulin-potassium infusions are used in some centers, though potassium infusion can cause hypotension. Potassium levels should be checked regularly (at least daily) in patients on insulin infusion because insulin drives potassium intracellularly and can lead to hypokalemia.
- Subcutaneous insulin may have less reliable absorption in patients who are edematous.
- When patients are ready to leave the ICU and are receiving a regular feeding regimen, IV insulin can be converted to long-acting insulin.
  - To convert to neutral protamine Hagedorn (NPH insulin): Calculate the total regular insulin received over the last 24 hours. Two-thirds of the total dose received can be given as NPH (subcutaneously) divided every 6 hours. Sliding scale insulin should be instituted for additional coverage. NPH doses can be adjusted on a daily basis.

Feeding

- Glucose control can only be achieved when a feeding regimen is accounted for.
- Feeds should be initiated at 20 mL/h and increased by 15 mL every 8 hours until the goal rate is reached. Feeds should be held for elevated residuals ($2\times$ hourly rate of feeds).
- Replete electrolytes to normal levels prior to initiation and advancement of feeds. PO_4 should be maintained >2.5 mg/dL to avoid acute refeeding syndrome.
- Enteral nutrition (either orally [PO], via nasogastric tube [NGT], or via percutaneous endoscopic gastrostomy [PEG] tube) is generally preferred to parenteral nutrition because it limits gut translocation of bacteria, and the rates of infection (particularly fungemia) are higher with parenteral nutrition. However, in circumstances where enteral nutrition is not possible for prolonged periods of time (>7 days), parenteral nutrition may be necessary (**Table 19.1**).[1]

Treatment of DKA and HONK (Table 19.2)

- Complications of DKA/HONK treatment: Cerebral edema occurs in 0.5 to 1% of DKA episodes (less common in HONK) 12 to 24 hours after initiation of treatment and is more frequent in children. Mortality is 20 to 25%, and 15 to 35% of survivors have permanent neurologic sequelae. Treat with mannitol or hypertonic saline as with other intracranial pressure (ICP) crises. The 2006 American Diabetes Association (ADA) guidelines suggest a maximum reduction in plasma osmolality of 3 mOsm/kg/hour.[2]

■ Prognosis

- Admission and prolonged hyperglycemia affect outcome after neurologic injury:
  - Subarachnoid hemorrhage (SAH): Admission glucose and prolonged hyperglycemia are independently associated with death or severe disability, fewer independent activities of daily living, prolonged length of stay, and hospital complications including symptomatic vasospasm.[3,4]
  - Intracerebral hemorrhage (ICH): Hyperglycemia is associated with increased mortality and ICH expansion.[5,6]

Table 19.1 European Society for Clinical Nutrition and Metabolism Recommendations for Nutrition in Intensive Care Patients*

Recommendation	Grade
All patients who are not expected to be on a full oral diet within 3 days should receive enteral nutrition.	C
Hemodynamically stable critically ill patients who have a functioning GI tract should be fed early (<24 h) using an appropriate amount of feed.	C
During the acute and initial phase of critical illness, in excess of 20–25 kcal/kg BW/d may be associated with a less favorable outcome.	C
During the anabolic recovery phase, the aim is to provide 25–30 kcal/kg BW/d.	C
Patients with severe undernutrition should receive enteral nutrition up to 25–30 total kcal/kg BW/d. If these target values are not reached supplementary, parenteral nutrition should be given.	C
Supplementary intravenous metoclopramide or erythromycin can be administered to patients with intolerance to enteral feeding (i.e., high gastric residuals).	C
Use enteral nutrition in patients who can be fed via the enteral route.	C
There is no significant difference in the efficacy of jejunal vs gastric feeding in critically ill patients.	C
Avoid additional parenteral nutrition in patients who tolerate enteral nutrition and can be fed approximately to the target values.	A
Use supplemental parenteral nutrition in patients who cannot be fed sufficiently via the enteral route. Consider careful parenteral nutrition in patients intolerant to enteral nutrition at a level equal to but not exceeding the nutritional needs of the patient.	C
Whole protein formulas are appropriate in most patients because no clinical advantage of peptide-based formulas has been shown.	C
Immune-modulating formulas (enriched with arginine, nucleotides, and omega 3 fatty acids) are superior to standard enteral formulas in patients with elective upper GI surgery, mild sepsis (APACHE II<15), trauma, and ARDS. Patients with severe sepsis who do not tolerate more than 700 mL of enteral formula per day should not receive immune-modulating formulas.	A–B
Glutamine should be added to standard enteral formula in burn and trauma patients.	A

Abbreviations: ARDS, acute respiratory disease syndrome; BW, body weight; GI, gastrointestinal.
* See Chapter 22 for a summary of Grades of ESPEN evidence.

Data from: Kreymann KG, Berger MM, Deutz NE, et al. ESPEN Guidelines on Enteral Nutrition: intensive care. Clin Nutr 2006;25(2):210–223.

Table 19.2 Treatment of Diabetic Ketoacidosis (DKA) and Hyperosmotic Nonketotic Hyperglycemia (HONK)

Treatment	Comment
Fluid resuscitation	Volume deficit can be as high as 4–6 L because glucose acts as an osmotic diuretic. Replace with NS starting at 15–20 mL/kg BW/h.
Insulin	Begin intravenous infusion of regular insulin at 0.1 U/kg as IV bolus followed by 0.1 U/kg/h IV infusion. Check hourly blood glucose values and titrate as necessary. Replete potassium <3.3 mEq/dL prior to initiation of insulin infusion. If the serum glucose does not fall by 50–70 mg/dL from the initial value in the first hour, the bolus should be repeated, and the insulin infusion may be doubled every hour until glucose steadily declines. When glucose values are <200 mg/dL, IV fluids should be changed to D5NS and insulin continued until the anion gap is <12 mEq/L. Ketosis may persist for up to 24 hours. Do not discontinue the insulin infusion until the anion gap is closed. Correct the anion gap for the albumin level.
Potassium	May be normal or elevated at admission due to insulin deficiency. Potassium distribution is reversed (driven intracellularly) rapidly during insulin infusion. K+ 20 mEq/L is generally added to IV fluids and potassium levels carefully monitored and maintained between 4.0–5.0 mEq/L.
Bicarbonate	HCO_3 can lead to rise in pCO_2 resulting in paradoxic decline in cerebral pH as CO_2 rapidly crosses the blood–brain barrier. Patients with pH <7.0 or life-threatening hyperkalemia may benefit from HCO_3 administration.

Abbreviations: BW, body weight; D5NS, 5% dextrose in normal saline; IV, intravenous; NS, normal saline.

- Traumatic brain injury (TBI): Prolonged elevated glucose is associated with a worse neurologic examination, increased mortality, and prolonged length of stay.[7]
- Ischemic stroke: Hyperglycemia predicts hemorrhagic transformation after IV or intra-arterial thrombolysis, is associated with infarct expansion on magnetic resonance diffusion-weighted imaging, and is related to worse outcome, prolonged length of stay, and higher medical costs.[8,9]

A summary of the major trials and outcomes of glucose control is given in **Table 19.3**.[10-16]

Table 19.3 Major Trials and Outcomes of Glucose Control

Patient Population	Study	N	Findings
Surgical ICU	van den Berghe et al	1548	Randomized controlled single-center trial in mechanically ventilated patients of intensive insulin infusion targeted to 80–110 mg/dL compared with conventional insulin infusion initiated for a blood glucose >215 mg/dL and targeted to 180–200 mg/dL. ICU mortality was 8% in the conventional group compared with 4.6% in the intensive insulin group (p = .005). Hospital mortality decreased by 34% in the intensive insulin group (p = .01). Reduction in mortality was driven primarily by the long-staying group of patients in the ICU > 5 days. Bloodstream infection ↓ 45%, acute renal failure ↓ 41%, transfusion requirement ↓ 50%, and critical illness polyneuropathy ↓ 44%
Medical ICU	van den Berghe et al	1200	Randomized controlled single-center trial of patients requiring at least 3 days of ICU stay randomized to intensive and conventional insulin therapy as above Hypoglycemia <40 mg/dL occurred in 18.7% of intensive insulin-treated patients (25% of those staying >3 days) and 3.1% of conventionally treated patients. No difference in hospital mortality between the intensive insulin and conventional group Mortality among patients staying <3 days was actually higher in the intensive insulin group (56% vs 42% in the conventional group, p = .05), though this effect was lost when withdrawal of care patients were removed from analysis. In patients staying >3 days, mortality was 52.5% in the conventional group vs 43% in the intensive group (p = .009). Morbidity was reduced in the entire cohort, including decreased acute renal failure, accelerated weaning from mechanical ventilation, and accelerated discharge from the ICU and hospital.

(Continued on next page)

Table 19.3 Major Trials and Outcomes of Glucose Control *(continued)*

Patient Population	Study	N	Findings
Mixed ICU population	VISEP	537	Randomized controlled trial in critically ill patients with sepsis examining conventional vs intensive insulin infusion with 2×2 factorial design to also examine pentastarch vs modified lactated ringers for volume resuscitation
			No difference in mortality or organ failure rates at 28 days for conventional vs intensive insulin control (targeting glucose levels 80–110 mg/dL)
			Stopped early for excess hypoglycemia (17% in the intensive insulin group vs 4% in the conventional group)
			Interaction with insulin treatment and pentastarch study confounds the results of the insulin treatment study.
			Pentastarch led to higher rates of renal failure, which may confound the insulin study results.
			This study was underpowered to show a benefit of intensive vs conventional glucose control because it was stopped early.
	Glucontrol	1082	Randomized controlled multicenter trial of insulin infusion targeting glucose levels of 80–110 mg/dL vs 140–180 mg/dL
			No difference in mortality
			$7\times$ increased risk of hypoglycemia <60 mg/dL in the intensive insulin group
			Study stopped early, was powered to detect a mortality effect with 3500 patients; hence the truncated study is underpowered.
Neuro-ICU	van den Berghe et al	63	Substudy of van den Berghe SICU trial (above) including 4% of 1548 SICU patients with primary neurologic injury randomized to intensive insulin targeted to 80–110 mg/dL vs conventional therapy
			Intensive treatment group had significantly less critical illness polyneuropathy and a shorter duration of mechanical ventilation.
			The intensive group had lower mean and median ICP, though the difference of 2–3 mm Hg is not clinically meaningful.
			The intensive group had fewer seizures (insulin increases GABA receptor sensitivity and reduces GABA uptake).
			No difference in 6- or 12-month outcome in the intensive group compared with the

(Continued)

Table 19.3 Major Trials and Outcomes of Glucose Control *(continued)*

Patient Population	Study	N	Findings
			conventional group, though the intensive therapy group made greater neurologic improvement between 6 and 12 months.
	GIST-UK	899	Randomized controlled trial in 899 stroke patients (88% ischemic, 12% ICH) of GIK infusion with a goal glucose of 72–126 mg/dL vs saline infusion for 24 h. No difference in mortality or outcome at 90 d The mean glucose difference between the GIK and saline group was only 10 mg/dL, which may not be clinically significant. Study was stopped for slow enrollment; it enrolled less than 50% of the projected 2355 patients and was thus underpowered. 24 hours of treatment may have not been long enough to illicit an outcome effect. Sickest neurologic patients excluded from this study (i.e., SAH, posterior circulation strokes, comatose patients)
Medical ICU surgical ICU medical-surgical ICU	meta-ana-lysis	8432	29 randomized controlled trials analyzed. There was no difference in hospital mortality, or mortality stratified by glucose control in any population comparing tight and conventional glucose control. Tigh glucose control was not associated with decreased risk of dialysis, but was associated with less septicemia and increased risk of hypoglycemia.

Abbreviations: GABA, gamma-aminobutyric acid; GIK, glucose-insulin-potassium; ICH, intracerebral hemorrhage; ICP, intracranial pressure; ICU, intensive care unit; IV, intravenous; NS, normal saline; SAH, subarachnoid hemorrhage.

Data from: van den Berghe G, Wouters P, Weekers F, et al. Intensive insulin therapy in the critically ill patient. N Engl J Med 2001;345(19):1359–1367. van den Berghe G, Wilmer A, Hermans G, et al. Intensive insulin therapy in the medical ICU. N Engl J Med 2006;354(5):449–461. Brunkhorst FM, Engel C, Bloos F, et al. Intensive insulin therapy and pentastarch resuscitation in severe sepsis. N Engl J Med 2008;358(2):125–139. Preiser JC. Intensive glycemic control in med-surg patients (European Glucontrol trial). Paper presented at: the Society of Critical Care Medicine 36th Critical Care Congress; February 17–21, 2007; Orlando, FL. van den Berghe G, Schoonheydt K, Becx P, Bruyninckx F, Wouters PJ. Insulin therapy protects the central and peripheral nervous system of intensive care patients. Neurology 2005;64(8):1348–1353. Gray CS, Hildreth AJ, Sandercock PA, et al. Glucose-potassium-insulin infusions in the management of post-stroke hyperglycaemia: the UK Glucose Insulin in Stroke Trial (GIST-UK). Lancet Neurol 2007;6(5):397–406. Wiener RS, Wiener DC, Larson RJ. Benefits and risks of tight glucose control in critically ill adults: A meta-analysis. Jama. 2008;300:933–944.

Risk of Hypoglycemia

- Insulin protocols with lower glycemic targets pose higher risks of hypoglycemia.
- Risk factors for hypoglycemia include diabetes mellitus (DM), continuous venovenous hemodialysis (CVVHD), changes in feeds, sepsis, and inotropes.
- Neurologic patients may not tolerate hypoglycemia as well as patients without acute neurologic injury.
  - Brain glucose/blood glucose = 0.6 to 0.7, similar to cerebrospinal fluid (CSF) to serum glucose ratios. This ratio may be as low as 0.2 to 0.4 in acute brain injury. Smaller reductions in serum glucose may lead to inadequate brain glucose supply in the context of acute brain injury.
  - Microdialysis studies of traumatic brain injury patients have shown that intensive insulin therapy compared with conventional glucose control can lead to significant reductions in brain glucose with elevations in brain lactate/pyruvate and glutamate (markers of cellular distress).[17,18]

Symptoms of Hypoglycemia

- Short-term effects of hypoglycemia include seizures, confusion, coma, and focal deficits.

Long-term Effects of Hypoglycemia

- Hypoglycemia due to sepsis or renal or liver failure is associated with worse outcomes due to the underlying cause of the hypoglycemia. It is unclear if the negative effects of iatrogenic hypoglycemia (i.e., due to insulin infusion) are equivalent.
- In pediatric patients: Hypoglycemia is related to cognitive deficits, microcephaly, and epilepsy.
- In adults, a randomized controlled trial of 1144 outpatients with diabetes mellitus type 1 randomized to intensive insulin targeted to 70 to 120 mg/dL versus conventional insulin therapy with no target showed:[19]
  - Forty percent of patients had at least one episode of hypoglycemic coma or seizure.

- ◦ Neither the frequency of severe hypoglycemia nor treatment group assignment predicted cognitive decline in any domain.
- ◦ Worse long-term glucose control as measured by HgbA1c was associated with motor speed decline and psychomotor deficiency.
- The long-term effects of hypoglycemia incurred immediately after neurologic insults in neurocritical care patients are not known.

Pearls and Pitfalls

- Hyperglycemia contributes to worse outcomes in SAH, ICH, ischemic stroke, and TBI.
- Some trials suggest that long-staying ICU patients benefit from intensive glucose control.
- Tight glucose control comes at the expense of hypoglycemia, which may not be well tolerated in the context of acute brain injury.
- The ideal glucose target in neurologically critically ill patients is not known.
- Nutrition should be initiated 24 to 72 hours after admission.
- Enteral nutrition is preferred to parenteral, but patients who cannot meet caloric goals with enteral nutrition should receive parenteral feeds.

References

1. Kreymann KG, Berger MM, Deutz NE, et al. ESPEN Guidelines on Enteral Nutrition: intensive care. Clin Nutr 2006;25(2):210–223
2. Kitabchi AE, Umpierrez GE, Murphy MB, Kreisberg RA. Hyperglycemic crises in adult patients with diabetes: a consensus statement from the American Diabetes Association. Diabetes Care 2006;29(12):2739–2748
3. Frontera JA, Fernandez A, Claassen J, et al. Hyperglycemia after SAH: predictors, associated complications, and impact on outcome. Stroke 2006;37(1):199–203
4. Wartenberg KE, Schmidt JM, Claassen J, et al. Impact of medical complications on outcome after subarachnoid hemorrhage. Crit Care Med 2006;34(3):617–623 quiz 624

5. Broderick JP, Diringer MN, Hill MD, et al. Determinants of intracerebral hemorrhage growth: an exploratory analysis. Stroke 2007;38(3):1072–1075

6. Kimura K, Iguchi Y, Inoue T, et al. Hyperglycemia independently increases the risk of early death in acute spontaneous intracerebral hemorrhage. J Neurol Sci 2007;255(1–2):90–94

7. Jeremitsky E, Omert LA, Dunham CM, Wilberger J, Rodriguez A. The impact of hyperglycemia on patients with severe brain injury. J Trauma 2005;58(1):47–50

8. Bruno A, Levine SR, Frankel MR, et al. Admission glucose level and clinical outcomes in the NINDS rt-PA Stroke Trial. Neurology 2002;59(5):669–674

9. Capes SE, Hunt D, Malmberg K, Pathak P, Gerstein HC. Stress hyperglycemia and prognosis of stroke in nondiabetic and diabetic patients: a systematic overview. Stroke 2001;32(10):2426–2432

10. van den Berghe G, Wouters P, Weekers F, et al. Intensive insulin therapy in the critically ill patient. N Engl J Med 2001;345(19):1359–1367

11. van den Berghe G, Wilmer A, Hermans G, et al. Intensive insulin therapy in the medical ICU. N Engl J Med 2006;354(5):449–461

12. Brunkhorst FM, Engel C, Bloos F, et al. Intensive insulin therapy and pentastarch resuscitation in severe sepsis. N Engl J Med 2008;358(2):125–139

13. Preiser JC. Intensive glycemic control in med-surg patients (European Glucontrol trial). Paper presented at: the Society of Critical Care Medicine 36th Critical Care Congress; February 17–21, 2007; Orlando, FL

14. van den Berghe G, Schoonheydt K, Becx P, Bruyninckx F, Wouters PJ. Insulin therapy protects the central and peripheral nervous system of intensive care patients. Neurology 2005;64(8):1348–1353

15. Gray CS, Hildreth AJ, Sandercock PA, et al. Glucose-potassium-insulin infusions in the management of post-stroke hyperglycaemia: the UK Glucose Insulin in Stroke Trial (GIST-UK). Lancet Neurol 2007;6(5):397–406

16. Wiener RS, Wiener DC, Larson RJ. Benefits and risks of tight glucose control in critically ill adults: A meta-analysis. JAMA. 2008;300:933–944.

17. Vespa P, Boonyaputthikul R, McArthur DL, Miller C, Etchepare M, Bergsneider M, Glenn T, Martin N, Hovda D. Intensive insulin therapy reduces microdialysis glucose values without altering glucose utilization or improving the lactate/pyruvate ratio after traumatic brain injury. Crit Care Med. 2006;34:850–856

18. Vespa P, Bergsneider M, Hattori N, Wu HM, Huang SC, Martin NA, Glenn TC, McArthur DL, Hovda DA. Metabolic crisis without brain ischemia is common after traumatic brain injury: A combined microdialysis and positron emission tomography study. J Cereb Blood Flow Metab. 2005;25:763–774

19. Jacobson AM, Musen G, Ryan CM, et al. Long-term effect of diabetes and its treatment on cognitive function. N Engl J Med 2007;356(18):1842–1852

20 Induced Normothermia and Hypothermia

Katja E. Wartenberg and Stephan A. Mayer

Fever is very common among critically ill neurologic patients, occurring in 23 to 47% in patients admitted to the intensive care unit (ICU). Ischemic stroke is complicated by fever in 43% of patients during the first week, and 33 to 42% of patients with intracranial hemorrhage (ICH), 40 to 68% with traumatic brain injury (TBI), and 41 to 70% with subarachnoid hemorrhage (SAH) develop fever. Fever is associated with worse neurologic outcome in these patient populations. Therefore, maintaining normothermia (37°C) has become an essential part of ICU management of cerebrovascular disease and brain trauma. Temperature is tightly regulated within one-tenth of a degree by the anterior nucleus of the hypothalamus, particularly the preoptic nuclei. Prostaglandin E2 is the common mediator affecting the temperature set point.

Induced mild hypothermia (32 to 34°C) has neuroprotective effects and has been used in patients with elevated intracranial pressure (ICP) and anoxic brain injury postcardiac arrest, as well as in other select patient groups. The neuroprotective effects are listed in **Table 20.1**.

Table 20.1 Neuroprotective Effects of Induced Mild Hypothermia

Early: 0–30 minutes	Lowers metabolic demand Slows O_2 consumption, adenosine triphosphate (ATP) stores preserved Every 1°C reduction in body temperature reduces cerebral metabolic rate of O_2 ($CMRO_2$) by 6–7%
Intermediate: Hours	Inhibition of glutamate release, less excitotoxicity Suppression of oxygen-free radicals
Late: up to 24 hours	Decreased blood–brain barrier breakdown Less edema and hemorrhagic transformation of ischemic stroke

Case Example

A 54-year-old African American woman presented with a Hunt and Hess grade IV SAH and intraventricular hemorrhage (IVH). One day later she stopped following commands and was febrile to 39.5°C.

Questions

- Is there a source of infection?
- Does the patient have a rash to suggest drug fever or an allergic reaction?
- Has the patient recently received a transfusion?
- Is there evidence of deep vein thrombosis (DVT) causing fever?

Urgent Orders

- Fever work-up: Blood, sputum, and urine cultures; chest radiograph (CXR)
- Acetaminophen 500 to 1000 mg orally (PO) every 6 hours
- Temperature control to 37°C

■ History and Examination

History

- Inquire regarding sources of infection, including diarrhea, sputum production, sinus/nasal discharge, discharge from wound sites, indwelling catheter infections and/or decubitus ulcers.
- Inquire regarding recent transfusions or rashes.
- Look at the timing of the fever and the duration of fever.

Physical Examination

- Vitals signs, including core temperature (bladder, pulmonary artery, or other central catheter; airway; rectal; tympanic)
- Examination of the skin and mucous membranes for rashes, secretions, and fluid status

- Look for an infectious focus: Erythema, discharge around lines and tubes, appearance of urine or cerebrospinal fluid (CSF), auscultation of the lungs, auscultation and palpation of the abdomen.
- Examine upper and lower extremities for signs of swelling or DVT.

Neurologic Examination

- Assess for signs of meningismus or Kernig's and Brudzinski signs (see Chapter 10).

■ Differential Diagnosis

1. *Infection should always be assumed and thoroughly assessed.* The overall frequency of nosocomial infection in neuro-intensive care units ranges from 14 to 36 per 100 patients. The most commonly documented infections are pneumonia (3 to 12 per 100 patients), urinary tract infection (UTI; 3 to 9 per 100 patients), bloodstream infection (1 to 2 per 100 patients), and meningitis or ventriculitis (1 to 9 per 100 patients).[1,2,3,4]

2. *Drug-induced fever.* Phenytoin, carbamazepine, β-lactamase-antibiotics, sulfa drugs, etc.

3. *Transfusion reaction*

4. *Deep vein thrombosis*

5. *Central fever.* Clues include very high fever >40 to 42°C, early-onset fever and fever refractory to antibiotics. Central fever remains a diagnosis of exclusion, and 15 to 28% of fever episodes remain unexplained after an extensive fever work-up. Risk factors include intraventricular hemorrhage, SAH, placement of an external ventricular drain (EVD), and length of stay.[5]

6. *Malignant hyperthermia.* Syndrome presenting with muscular rigidity, hypermetabolic state with increased oxygen consumption, increased carbon dioxide production (hypercarbia), metabolic acidosis, tachycardia, hyperthermia (with temperatures increasing at a rate of up to 2°C per hour) and rhabdomyolysis (increase in myoglobin and creatinine kinase/creatinine phosphokinase [CK/CPK]). It can be triggered by exposure to halogenated volatile anesthetics and succinylcholine. Treatment includes IV dantrolene and correction of metabolic derangements. An episode of malignant hyperthermia can

be delayed up to 24 hours after exposure to offensive medications. It is related to a defect in ryanodine receptors of the sarcoplasmic reticulum which affects intracellular calcium levels. Malignant hyperthermia is genetically and phenotypically related to central core disease (central core myopathy).

7. *Serotonin syndrome.* Spontaneous drug reaction as a consequence of excess serotonergic activity at central nervous system (CNS) and peripheral serotonin receptors. Potential triggers include: monoamine oxidase [MAO] B inhibitors, selective serotonin reuptake inhibitors [SSRIs], tricyclic antidepressants, mirtazapine, venlafaxine, yohimbine, St. John's wort, clonazepam, methylphenidate, lysergic acid diethylamide [LSD], and cocaine, etc. Presents with a clinical triad of:

   • Cognitive effects: Confusion, hypomania, hallucinations, agitation, headache, coma

   • Autonomic effects: Shivering, sweating, fever, hypertension, tachycardia, nausea, diarrhea

   • Somatic effects: Myoclonus, clonus, hyperreflexia, tremor

   Treatment includes discontinuation of the offending medication and administration of serotonin antagonists (cyproheptadine or methysergide) and benzodiazepines.

8. *Neuroleptic malignant syndrome.* Presents with muscular rigidity, high fever, alteration of mental status, autonomic instability, confusion, coma, delirium, tremor along with elevated CPK, leukocytosis, elevated liver function tests, and metabolic acidosis. It is due to alteration of central dopamine neurotransmission and can be caused by dopamine agonists such as Haldol (Ortho-McNeil Pharmaceutical, Raritan, NJ) (all neuroleptics, though Clozaril [Novartis Pharmaceuticals, East Hanover, NJ] has the least potential), and antiemetics such as promethazine, metoclopramide, prochlorperazine, and droperidol. Therapy consists of discontinuation of the offensive agent, supportive care, and dantrolene, bromocriptine, and/or benzodiazepines.

9. *Heat stroke.* Body heat production or absorption is greater than the capacity for dissipation, usually due to excessive exposure to heat. Bringing the body temperature down and hydration are of utmost importance.

10. *Delirium tremens.* An acute episode of delirium caused by withdrawal or abstinence from alcohol, typically occurs within 48 to 72 hours from cessation of drinking or benzodiazepine use. Typical

presentation includes fever, tremor, confusion, disorientation, agitation, hallucinations, tachycardia, hypertension, and tachypnea. Treatment options include benzodiazepines (lorazepam, chlordiazepoxide, etc.).

■ Diagnostic Evaluation

- Laboratories: As above
- Consider evaluation of CSF (always measure opening and closing pressure).
- Consider evaluation for DVT with upper and lower extremity Doppler ultrasound, or pulmonary embolus with computed tomography (CT) angiography.
- Consider CXR or chest CT for interstitial pneumonia or bronchoscopy for bronchoalveolar lavage.
- Consider checking *Clostridium difficile* toxin for patients with diarrhea.
- Consider sinus CT to rule out sinusitis.

■ Treatment of Fever, Induced Normothermia (37°C) and Mild-Moderate Therapeutic Hypothermia (32–34°C) (Table 20.2)

Table 20.2 Methods of Inducing Normothermia (37°C) or Mild-Moderate Hypothermia (32–34°C)

Method	Efficacy	Pro	Con	Comments
Antipyretics: acetamino -phen, NSAIDs, steroids	0.3–0.4°C in 24 h	Inexpensive, readily available	Need oral access, minimal efficacy	Effects on CNS. Cox 1–2 inhibitors block PGE2 production, as do steroids. No difference in efficacy between acetaminophen and NSAIDs

(Continued on next page)

Table 20.2 Methods of Inducing Normothermia (37°C) or Mild-Moderate Hypothermia (32–34°C) *(continued)*

Method	Efficacy	Pro	Con	Comments
Ice packs	1.5°C/h	Inexpensive, readily available	Risk of skin lesions and frostbites, dangerous in patients who require defibrillation, labor intensive, overshoot possible/poor control	Applicable to the entire body or just neck, groin, axilla
Infusion of ice-cold normal saline (4°C)	0.6–4°C/h depending on speed and volume	Extremely rapid induction of cooling Very easy to apply in all situations and in combination with other methods Inexpensive	Ineffective for maintenance of temperature within a range Volume overload possible	30 mL/kg or 2 L over 30–60 min
Hydrogel-coated water-circulating pads	1.5–3°C/h	Effective, does not require central line, easy to initiate Temperature feedback system Displays water temperature (4–42°C), gradual rewarming	Slight risk of skin lesions and frostbites, should not be used with multiple pressors (risk of skin necrosis) Pads not reusable	Arctic Sun
Intravascular catheters	0.8–4.5°C/h	Highly reliable and rapid induction of cooling Temperature feedback system, efficacious in obese patients	Invasive procedure, associated with time loss and risk of procedure, deep vein thrombosis, and dissection risk Relatively expensive	Innercool Celsius Control, Alsius Intravascular Temperature Management, Reprieve Endovascular Temperature Therapy System, Femoral catheters recommended for 72–96 h

(Continued)

Table 20.2 Methods of Inducing Normothermia (37°C) or Mild-Moderate Hypothermia (32–34°C) *(continued)*

Method	Efficacy	Pro	Con	Comments
Helmets	1.5–1.6°C/h	Noninvasive, elegant method of cooling	Efficacious mainly in neonates, not in adults; scalp freezing and necrosis possible	Frigicap Hypotherm Gel Cap; caps filled with a solution of aqueous glycerol

Abbreviations: CNS, central nervous system; Cox, cyclooxygenase; NSAIDs, nonsteroidal antiinflammatory drugs; PGE2, prostaglandin E2.

Data from: Medivance Inc., Louisville, CO; Innercool Therapies, San Diego, CA; Alsius Corp., Irvine, CA; Radiant Medical, Inc., Redwood City, CA; Flexoversal, Hiden, Germany.

■ Applications and Complications of Hypothermia

- The major application of hypothermia in critical care includes neuroprotection after cardiac arrest (specifically after arrest from ventricular fibrillation/pulseless ventricular tachycardia), for neonates with hypoxic ischemic injury and in controlling elevated ICP refractory to medical management (see Chapter 15).[6–8] Two randomized, controlled trials provided level I evidence and led to the recommendation of hypothermia as an effective therapy after cardiac arrest in the ILCOR (International Liaison Committee on Resuscitation) Advisory Statement in 2003.[9] The American Heart Association (AHA) guidelines state that "unconscious adult patients with spontaneous circulation after out-of-hospital cardiac arrest should be cooled to 32°C to 34°C for 12 to 24 hours when the initial rhythm was ventricular fibrillation (VF) (class IIa). Such cooling may also be beneficial to other rhythms or in-hospital cardiac arrest (class IIb)."[10] Studies pertinent to induced hypothermia in various clinical contexts are listed in **Table 20.3**.[11–16]

- An example of a hypothermia protocol can be seen in **Fig. 20.1**.

Table 20.3 Studies on Induced Hypothermia in Various Clinical Contexts

Cardiac Arrest

Study	Location	Study Design	Inclusion	Number of Patients	Intervention	Outcome Measure	Results
Bernard et al, 2002	Ambulance, ED, ICU	Prospective, randomized	Out-of-hospital cardiac arrest with ventricular fibrillation	77	33°C with ice packs to head, neck, torso, and limbs for 12 h, active rewarming over 18 h	Good outcome at discharge (home or rehabilitation facility)	Better neurologic outcome (49 vs 26%) with intervention, no significant difference in mortality, time to target temperature 150 min
HACA Study Group, 2002	ED, ICU	Prospective, randomized	Out-of-hospital cardiac arrest with ventricular fibrillation/ ventricular tachycardia	275	32–34°C with cold air circulating mattress ± ice packs for 24 h, passive rewarming over 8 h	CPC and mortality at 6 mo	Better neurologic outcome (CPC 1,2) 55 vs 39%, $p = .009$), less mortality (41 vs 55%, $p = .02$) with intervention, time to target temperature 480 min

Traumatic Brain Injury

Study	Study Design	Number of Patients	Duration of Cooling	Effect on ICP	Good Outcome (GOS 4 or 5)		
					Hypothermia	**Normothermia**	**Significant Differences**
Marion et al, 1997	Randomized, controlled	82	24 h	→	62%	38%	$p = .05$
NABISH Clifton et al, 2001	Randomized, controlled	392	48 h	→	43% Mortality: 28%	43% Mortality: 27%	NS
Zhi et al, 2003	Randomized, controlled	396	1–7 d	→	62% 74% survival	38% 64% survival	$p < .05$ $p < .05$
McIntyre et al, 2003	Meta-analysis of 12 randomized controlled trials	1069	24 to >48 h	NA	19% (CI = 0.69–0.96) reduction in death 22% (CI = 0.63–0.98) reduction in poor outcome Hypothermia for 48 h had mortality and neurologic benefit Hypothermia for 24 h had only neurologic benefit		
					PCPO**		
					Hypothermia	**Normothermia**	**Significant Differences**
Hutchison et al, 2008	Randomized, controlled in pediatric patients aged 1–17 years with severe TBI	225	24h	No significant difference	PCPO** 31% mortality 21%	PCPO** 22% mortality 12%	$p = 0.14$ $p = 0.06$

(Continued on next page)

Table 20.3 Studies on Induced Hypothermia in Various Clinical Contexts (*continued*)

Ischemic Stroke

Study	Location	Study Design	Inclusion	Number of Patients	Intervention	Outcome Measure	Results
COOLAID De Georgia et al, 2004	Neuro-ICU	Prospective, randomized, controlled	Patients with MCA or ACA infarctions within 12 h after symptom onset	740	Hypothermia with endovascular cooling device to 33°C for 24 h vs normothermia	Infarct size by DWI 3–5 days after symptom onset MRS and NIHSS at 90 d	No difference in any outcome measures

Neuroprotection during Aneurysm Surgery

Study	Location	Study Design	Inclusion	Number of Patients	Intervention	Outcome Measure	Results
IHAST Todd et al, 2005	Operating room	Prospective, randomized	Good grade SAH patients (WFNS grades 1–3) within 14 days of aneurysm rupture	1001	Intraoperative hypothermia (target temperature 33°C by surface cooling) vs normothermia (36.5°C)	GOS at 90 days	No difference in good outcome between the two groups Bacteremia was more common after hypothermia (5% vs. 3%, $p = .05$)

Abbreviations: ACA, anterior cerebral artery; CI, confidence interval; CPC, Glasgow-Pittsburgh Cerebral Performance Category; DWI, diffusion weighted magnetic resonance image; ED, emergency department; GOS, Glasgow Outcome Score; ICP, intracranial pressure; ICU, intensive care unit; MCA, middle cerebral artery; mRS, modified Rankin Score; NA, nonapplicable; NIHSS, National Institute of Health Stroke Scale; NS, nonsignificant; OR, odds ratio; SAH, subarachnoid hemorrhage; WFNS, World Federation of Neurological Surgeons.
** PCPO, Pediatric Cerebral Performance Outcome at 6 months (severe disability, pesistent vegetative state or death)

Neonatal Encephalopathy

Study	Location	Study Design	Inclusion	Number of Patients	Intervention	Outcome Measure	Results
Shankaran et al, 2005	Neonatal ICU	Prospective, randomized, controlled	Gestational age of 36 weeks, within 6 h of birth with either severe acidosis or perinatal complications and resuscitation who had moderate or severe encephalopathy	208	Whole-body hypothermia to 33.5°C for 72 h (surface cooling, Blanketrol II) vs normothermia	Severe, moderate disability and death at 18 and 22 mo	44% death, severe or moderate disability in the hypothermia group and 62% in the control group (OR = 0.72; 95% CI = 0.54–0.95, p = .01)

Data from: Hypo-Hyperthermia System, Cincinnati Subzero, Cincinnati, OH. Bernard SA, Gray TW, Buist MD, et al. Treatment of comatose survivors of out-of-hospital cardiac arrest with induced hypothermia. N Engl J Med 2002;346(8): 557–563. Group THS. Mild therapeutic hypothermia to improve the neurologic outcome after cardiac arrest. N Engl J Med 2002;346(8):549–556. Marion DW, Penrod LE, Kelsey SF, et al. Treatment of traumatic brain injury with moderate hypothermia. N Engl J Med 1997;336(8):540–546. Clifton GL, Miller ER, Choi SC, et al. Lack of effect of induction of hypothermia after acute brain injury. N Engl J Med 2001;344(8):556–563. Zhi D, Zhang S, Lin X. Study on therapeutic mechanism and clinical effect of mild hypothermia in patients with severe head injury. Surg Neurol 2003;59(5):381–385. McIntyre LA, Fergusson DA, Hebert PC, Moher D, Hutchison JS. Prolonged therapeutic hypothermia after traumatic brain injury in adults: a systematic review. JAMA 2003;289(22):2992–2999. Hutchison JS, Ward RE, Lacroix J, Hebert PC, Barnes MA, Bohn DJ, Dirks PB, Doucette S, Fergusson D, Gottesman R, Joffe AR, Kirpalani HM, Meyer PG, Morris KP, Moher D, Singh RN, Skippen PW: Hipothermia theraphy after traumatic brain injury in children. N Engl J Med 2008;358:2447–2456. De Georgia M, Krieger DW, Abou-Chebl A, et al. Cooling for acute ischemic brain damage (COOL AID). Neurology 2004;63:312–317. Todd MM, Hindman BJ, Clarke WR, Torner JC. Mild intraoperative hypothermia during surgery for intracranial aneurysm. N Engl J Med 2005;352(2):135–145. Shankaran S, Laptook AR, Ehrenkranz RA, et al. Whole-body hypothermia for neonates with hypoxic-ischemic encephalopathy. N Engl J Med 2005;353(15): 1574–1584

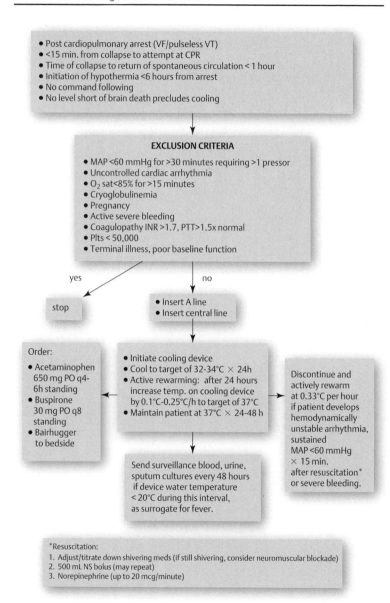

- Post cardiopulmonary arrest (VF/pulseless VT)
- <15 min. from collapse to attempt at CPR
- Time of collapse to return of spontaneous circulation < 1 hour
- Initiation of hypothermia <6 hours from arrest
- No command following
- No level short of brain death precludes cooling

EXCLUSION CRITERIA

- MAP <60 mmHg for >30 minutes requiring >1 pressor
- Uncontrolled cardiac arrhythmia
- O_2 sat<85% for >15 minutes
- Cryoglobulinemia
- Pregnancy
- Active severe bleeding
- Coagulopathy INR >1.7, PTT>1.5x normal
- Plts < 50,000
- Terminal illness, poor baseline function

yes

no

stop

- Insert A line
- Insert central line

Order:

- Acetaminophen 650 mg PO q4-6h standing
- Buspirone 30 mg PO q8 standing
- Bairhugger to bedside

- Initiate cooling device
- Cool to target of 32-34°C × 24h
- Active rewarming: after 24 hours increase temp. on cooling device by 0.1°C-0.25°C/h to target of 37°C
- Maintain patient at 37°C × 24-48 h

Discontinue and actively rewarm at 0.33°C per hour if patient develops hemodynamically unstable arrhythmia, sustained MAP <60 mmHg × 15 min. after resuscitation* or severe bleeding.

Send surveillance blood, urine, sputum cultures every 48 hours if device water temperature < 20°C during this interval, as surrogate for fever.

*Resuscitation:
1. Adjust/titrate down shivering meds (if still shivering, consider neuromuscular blockade)
2. 500 mL NS bolus (may repeat)
3. Norepinephrine (up to 20 mcg/minute)

Fig. 20.1 An example of a hypothermia protocol. CPR, cardiopulmonary resuscitation; INR, international normalized ratio; MAP, mean arterial pressure; NS, normal saline; Plts, platelets; PO, orally; PTT, partial thromboplastin time; q, every; sat, saturation; VF, ventricular fibrillation; VT, ventricular tachycardia.

- Complications of hypothermia: Shivering is the most important and most common complication of hypothermia and must be managed aggressively. Because shivering can increase O_2 consumption by 30% and can increase ICP, prolonged shivering is not only detrimental, but can undermine any positive effects of hypothermia. Shivering begins on the neck and thorax and may only initially be identified by a wavering electrocardiogram (ECG) baseline. As shivering worsens, it progresses to include the thorax and extremities. Shivering is maximal at 34°C and becomes less pronounced/absent at 32°C (**Table 20.4** and **Table 20.5**).

Table 20.4 Antishivering Protocol

Method	Dosage	Mechanism
Basic Management		
Acetaminophen	650–1000 mg PO q 6 h	Central fever control
Buspirone	30 mg PO q 8 h	5HT1A and D2 agonist
Skin counterwarming	BAIR Hugger Polar Air Cooling System	Vasodilatation, hypothalamic feedback
Advanced Management for Persistent Shivering		
Propofol	0.1–0.2 mg/kg/min IV Patient must be intubated.	Impairs vasoconstriction and shivering threshold
Dexmedetomidine	0.2–1.0 µg/kg/h IV Do not use with heart block, care with bradycardia, hypotension	Alpha-2 receptor agonist
Fentanyl	50–200 µg/h IV	Opioid receptor agonist
Midazolam	0.02–0.10 mg/kg/h IV	GABA agonist
Magnesium sulfate	0.5–1.0 g per h for target serum magnesium of 1–2 mmol/L (3–4 g/dL) (20 g in 1000 mL) Check Mg every 4–6 h, daily K+ and Ca+2 Monitor for toxicity: hypotension, muscle weakness, respiratory paralysis	Vasodilatation Calcium and magnesium absorption at the renal level (loop of Henle) are linked to one another and should be repleted together
Meperidine	25–100 mg IV q 4 h (or 0.5–1.0 mg/kg/h) Do not use if MAOI (including MAO-B selegiline) use in <14 d, recent seizures, or elevated Cr >1.2 mg/dL	Kappa receptor agonist NMDA receptor antagonism Inhibition of biogenic amine reuptake

(Continued on next page)

Table 20.4 Antishivering Protocol *(continued)*

Method	Dosage	Mechanism
Advanced Management for Refractory Shivering		
Cisatracurium	Usually not needed and should be avoided because of increased incidence of critical illness polyneuropathy Should always be used in combination with a hypnotic/sedating medication	Paralysis, cisatracurium undergoes Hoffman elimination: not renally or hepatically cleared.

Abbreviations: GABA, gamma-aminobutyric acid; IV, intravenous; MAOI, monoamine oxidase inhibitor; NMDA, N-methy-D-aspartate; PO, orally; q, every.

Data from: Arizant Healthcare, Eden Prairie, MN.

Table 20.5 Other Complications of Hypothermia

Metabolic	Decreased basal metabolic rate Plasma concentration increased for morphine, fentanyl, propofol Duration of action increased for vecuronium, atracurium
Electrolytes	During cooling: hypokalemia, hypomagnesemia, hypophosphatemia, hyperglycemia (insulin resistance) During rewarming: rebound hyperkalemia
Neurologic	Slurred speech, confusion, stupor, coma with progressing hypothermia, elevated ICP and cerebral edema upon rewarming
Cardiac	Atrial fibrillation ≤32°C; ventricular arrhythmias at ≤30°C Note: Arrhythmias often refractory to conventional therapy—must rewarm to treat; ECG repolarization abnormalities, Osborne waves
Hemodynamic	Cold diuresis; ↑SVR, ↓BP, ↓HR, ↓CO
Hematologic	Coagulopathy: platelet dysfunction, prolonged bleeding time, DIC, enhanced fibrinolysis, leukopenia, thrombocytopenia. Must rewarm to treat refractory or life-threatening bleeding.
Renal	Renal tubular acidosis (ATN)
Pulmonary	Increased pulmonary edema
Infection	Increased sepsis/bacteremia, pneumonia, wound infection
GI	Ileus, stress ulcer, elevated lipase/amylase

Abbreviations: ATN, acute tubercular necrosis; BP, blood pressure; CO, cardiac output; DIC, disseminated intravascular coagulopathy; ECG, electrocardiogram; GI, gastrointestinal; HR, heart rate; ICP, intracranial pressure; SVR, systemic vascular resistance.

In cases of accidental hypothermia (exposure), patients can suffer all of the above complications of hypothermia. In fact, to adequately assess the neurologic exam, patients with accidental hypothermia should be passively rewarmed (as in TBI) or rewarmed with a BAIR Hugger (Arizant Healthcare, Eden Prairie, MN) (as for postoperative patients).

- Complications of rewarming: Rebound cerebral edema and elevated ICP, systemic inflammatory response syndrome (SIRS), hypotension due to peripheral vasodilation, arrhythmias, pulmonary edema, disseminated intravascular coagulation (DIC), rebound hyperkalemia, hypermagnesemia, hyperphosphatemia, rhabdomyolysis, and acute tubercular necrosis (ATN). Rewarm slowly (0.1–0.25°C per hour) to a goal of 37°C and lock the patient at normothermia for 24 hours before discontinuing a cooling device.

■ Prognosis

Hyperthermia has a detrimental impact on outcome after neurologic injury. In ischemic stroke, higher admission temperature is associated with increased mortality and infarct size. The relative risk of poor functional outcome doubles with each degree increase in temperature. Fever also impairs functional and cognitive outcome after SAH, has been associated with symptomatic vasospasm, increased mortality, and functional disability after ICH and TBI. Induced hypothermia after cardiac arrest improves clinical outcomes.

Pearls and Pitfalls

- The application of hypothermia (32 to 34°C) 12 to 24 hours after cardiac arrest is crucial to improving neurologic outcome.
- Hypothermia is effective in ICP control.
- Fever is associated with worse functional outcome after acute neurological injury, therefore, fever control is essential.

References
1. Bota DP, Lefranc F, Villalobos HR, Brimioulle S, Vincent JL. Ventriculostomy-related infections in critically ill patients: A 6-year experience. *J Neurosurg.* 2005;103:468–472

2. Dettenkofer M, Ebner W, Els T, Babikir R, Lucking C, Pelz K, Ruden H, Daschner F. Surveillance of nosocomial infections in a neurology intensive care unit. *J Neurol.* 2001;248:959–964

3. Dettenkofer M, Ebner W, Hans FJ, Forster D, Babikir R, Zentner J, Pelz K, Daschner FD. Nosocomial infections in a neurosurgery intensive care unit. *Acta Neurochir (Wien).* 1999;141:1303–1308

4. Zolldann D, Thiex R, Hafner H, Waitschies B, Lutticken R, Lemmen SW. Periodic surveillance of nosocomial infections in a neurosurgery intensive care unit. *Infection.* 2005;33:115–121

5. Commichau C, Scarmeas N, Mayer SA. Risk factors for fever in the neurologic intensive care unit. Neurology 2003;60(5):837–841

6. Group THS. Mild therapeutic hypothermia to improve the neurologic outcome after cardiac arrest. N Engl J Med 2002;346(8):549–556

7. Bernard SA, Gray TW, Buist MD, et al. Treatment of comatose survivors of out-of-hospital cardiac arrest with induced hypothermia. N Engl J Med 2002;346(8): 557–563

8. Shankaran S, Laptook AR, Ehrenkranz RA, et al. Whole-body hypothermia for neonates with hypoxic-ischemic encephalopathy. N Engl J Med 2005;353(15): 1574–1584

9. Nolan JP, Morley PT, Vanden Hoek TL, et al. Therapeutic hypothermia after cardiac arrest: an advisory statement by the Advanced Life Support Task Force of the International Liaison Committee on Resuscitation. Circulation 2003;108(1):118–121

10. Committee ECC, Subcommittees and Task Forces of the American Heart Association. 2005 American Heart Association Guidelines for Cardiopulmonary Resuscitation and Emergency Cardiovascular Care. Circulation 2005; 112(24, Suppl):IV1–IV203

11. Marion DW, Penrod LE, Kelsey SF, et al. Treatment of traumatic brain injury with moderate hypothermia. N Engl J Med 1997;336(8):540–546

12. Clifton GL, Miller ER, Choi SC, et al. Lack of effect of induction of hypothermia after acute brain injury. N Engl J Med 2001;344(8):556–563

13. Zhi D, Zhang S, Lin X. Study on therapeutic mechanism and clinical effect of mild hypothermia in patients with severe head injury. Surg Neurol 2003;59(5):381–385

14. McIntyre LA, Fergusson DA, Hebert PC, Moher D, Hutchison JS. Prolonged therapeutic hypothermia after traumatic brain injury in adults: a systematic review. JAMA 2003;289(22):2992–2999

15. De Georgia M, Krieger DW, Abou-Chebl A, et al. Cooling for acute ischemic brain damage (COOL AID). Neurology 2004;63:312–317

16. Todd MM, Hindman BJ, Clarke WR, Torner JC. Mild intraoperative hypothermia during surgery for intracranial aneurysm. N Engl J Med 2005;352(2):135–145

21 Basics of Neuroimaging

Chitra Venkatasubramanian
and Christine A. Wijman

Imaging of the central nervous system (CNS) has undergone exciting advances in the last decade, and one can now choose from a variety of imaging techniques to detect, monitor, and treat neurologic diseases. However, this has also led to increasing challenges with regard to which imaging modality to choose for a particular disease, when to order a study, what to look for in a scan, and how to recognize critical information that needs immediate attention. The imaging studies that are most commonly ordered in the neuro-intensive care unit (NICU) are CT (computed tomography), CTA (CT angiography), MRI (magnetic resonance imaging), MRA (MR angiography), and digital subtraction angiography (DSA).

■ Imaging Modalities

Computed Tomography

CT uses x-rays and radiation detectors to measure the degree of attenuation of x-rays during passage through tissues and a computer to transform the information into a cross-sectional image. Helical CT involves continuous rotation of the x-ray tube during simultaneous movement of the CT table. Three-dimensional (3D) data are acquired and then divided into individual slices of variable thickness. The absorption coefficients (or degree of attenuation) are measured in Hounsfield units (HU) with the resultant image in varying shades of black, gray, and white, depending on the HU of the tissues (**Fig. 21.1**). Tissues with higher HU appear bright on CT (e.g., bone, acute blood), and those with lower HU appear dark (e.g., cerebrospinal fluid [CSF], air, fat) as compared with the brain parenchyma. Bone is $+1000$ HU, water is 0, and air is -1000 HU.

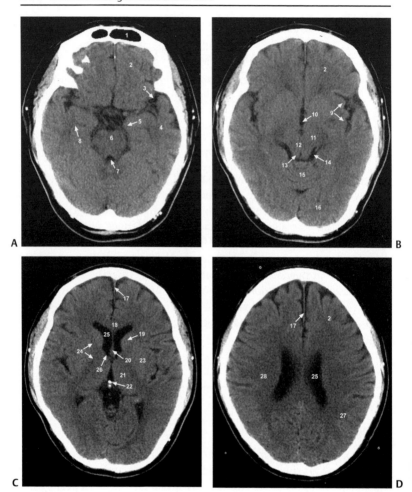

Fig. 21.1 Noncontrast-enhanced head computed tomography (CT) scan showing normal anatomy. **(A)** Level of the rostral pons, **(B)** level of the third ventricle, **(C)** level of the pineal gland, and **(D)** level of the corona radiate. (1) Frontal sinus, (2) frontal lobe, (3) sylvian fissure, (4) temporal lobe, (5) uncus, (6) pons, (7) fourth ventricle, (8) temporal horn of lateral ventricle, (9) insula, (10) third ventricle, (11) cerebral peduncle, (12) midbrain, (13) superior colliculus, (14) quadrigeminal cistern, (15) vermis of the cerebellum, (16) occipital lobe, (17) falx cerebri, (18) genu of corpus callosum, (19) caudate, (20) septum pellucidum, (21) thalamus, (22) pineal gland (calcified), (23) putamen, (24) internal capsule, (25) lateral ventricle, (26) foramen of Monro, (27) parietal lobe, (28) corona radiata.

Noncontrast-Enhanced Head Computed Tomography

Noncontrast-enhanced CT is readily available, noninvasive, and cheap and is the first choice for scanning in emergency situations. With a short acquisition time and low susceptibility to motion, it is particularly advantageous for postoperative, critically ill, and restless patients. It can be used in patients with MRI contraindications (e.g., pacemakers, large body habitus, metallic fragments near the eye). It can also accommodate ancillary equipment (e.g., ventilators). Furthermore, the recent introduction of portable CT scanners offers the option to image the brain in patients who are too unstable to be transported.

Clinical Indications and Uses

- *Acute stroke:* To differentiate between acute ischemic stroke (**Fig. 21.2A**) and intracerebral hemorrhage (ICH) (**Fig. 21.3A, Fig. 21.4A, Fig. 21.5A**) and to monitor complications of stroke/therapy (e.g., edema, tissue shifts, herniation, hemorrhagic transformation, and hydrocephalus, **Fig. 21.3B**).
- *Trauma:* CT is the modality of choice to detect brain contusions, epidural (**Fig. 21.4A**) and subdural hematoma, skull fractures (**Fig. 21.4B**), and air and metallic foreign bodies, and also to verify placement of external ventricular drains and intracranial pressure monitors.
- *Subarachnoid hemorrhage (SAH):* To screen for blood in the subarachnoid space (**Fig. 21.6A**)

Limitations

- Poor resolution of posterior fossa structures due to bone artifacts and beam hardening
- Poor contrast between normal and injured tissue (e.g., detection of early ischemia)
- False-negatives in SAH when there is very little blood confined only to the basal cisterns
- Less sensitive for the detection of diffuse axonal injury (DAI) and spinal cord injury
- Ionizing radiation (use with caution in first trimester of pregnancy)

Contrast-Enhanced Head Computed Tomography

Contrast-enhanced CT involves intravenous injection of iodinated contrast, which appears bright on CT. Contrast-enhanced CT is useful for

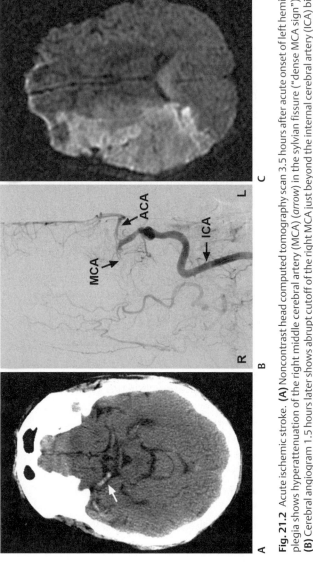

Fig. 21.2 Acute ischemic stroke. **(A)** Noncontrast head computed tomography scan 3.5 hours after acute onset of left hemiplegia shows hyperattenuation of the right middle cerebral artery (MCA) (*arrow*) in the sylvian fissure ("dense MCA sign"). **(B)** Cerebral angiogram 1.5 hours later shows abrupt cutoff of the right MCA just beyond the internal cerebral artery (ICA) bifurcation into the MCA and anterior cerebral artery (ACA). **(C)** Axial diffusion weighted magnetic resonance imaging scan 24 hours after stroke onset demonstrates restricted diffusion (bright area) involving the entire right MCA territory.

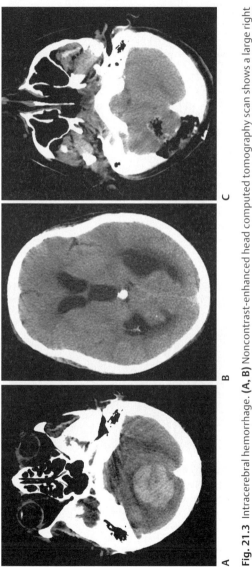

Fig. 21.3 Intracerebral hemorrhage. **(A, B)** Noncontrast-enhanced head computed tomography scan shows a large right cerebellar hemorrhage, extending into the cerebellar vermis with brainstem compression, obliteration of the fourth ventricle, and obstructive hydrocephalus. **(C)** The patient subsequently underwent emergent right suboccipital craniotomy and hematoma evacuation.

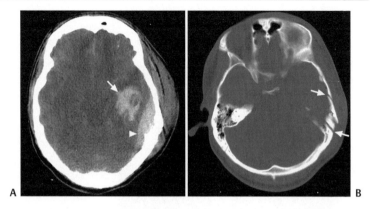

Fig. 21.4 Head trauma. **(A)** Noncontrast-enhanced head computed tomography (CT) scan in a patient with traumatic brain injury shows a left temporal contusion (*arrow*) and epidural hematoma (*arrowhead*), diffuse subarachnoid hemorrhage, and cerebral edema with obliteration of the basal cisterns. **(B)** CT (bone window) shows multiple fractures of the temporal bone and mastoid (*arrows*), underlying the epidural hematoma.

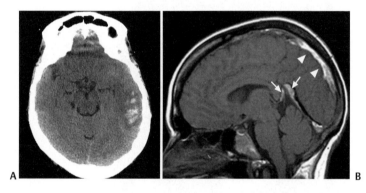

Fig. 21.5 Cerebral venous thrombosis. **(A)** Noncontrast-enhanced head computed tomography (CT) scan shows a left temporal hemorrhagic venous infarct secondary to transverse sinus thrombosis, which was diagnosed by CT and magnetic resonance (MR) venogram. **(B)** Sagittal T1-weighted MR image from a different patient shows bright signal along the posterior two-thirds of the superior sagittal sinus (*arrowheads*), the straight sinus, and the vein of Galen (*arrows*), consistent with (subacute to early chronic phase of) cerebral venous thrombosis.

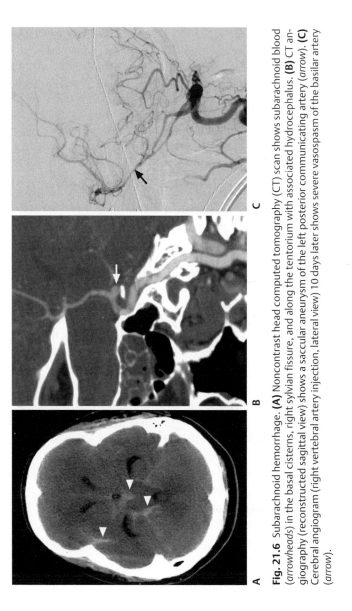

Fig. 21.6 Subarachnoid hemorrhage. **(A)** Noncontrast head computed tomography (CT) scan shows subarachnoid blood (*arrowheads*) in the basal cisterns, right sylvian fissure, and along the tentorium with associated hydrocephalus. **(B)** CT angiography (reconstructed sagittal view) shows a saccular aneurysm of the left posterior communicating artery (*arrow*). **(C)** Cerebral angiogram (right vertebral artery injection, lateral view) 10 days later shows severe vasospasm of the basilar artery (*arrow*).

visualizing blood vessels and studying diseases that result in blood–brain barrier (BBB) leakage (e.g., meningitis, brain tumors, brain abscesses). Iodinated contrast is contraindicated in patients with a serum creatinine >2 mg/dL (unless the patient is already receiving renal replacement therapy) and in those with a history of allergic reactions to contrast, iodine, or shellfish. Pretreatment can be given in those with a contrast allergy (methylprednisolone 50 mg intravenously [IV] x 1 prior to contrast administration and 50 mg IV 6 hours later, along with diphenhydramine 50 mg 1 hour prior to contrast). The most important measures to prevent nephrotoxicity are adequate hydration and discontinuation of nephrotoxic medications.

Computed Tomography Angiography

CTA involves the administration of a time-optimized bolus of contrast through a peripheral vein (typically an 18- or 20-gauge IV). Blood vessels (up to 1 mm) are enhanced, and the resultant information is processed by a computer and displayed as 2D or 3D black-and-white or color images. CTA can be acquired in minutes and is ideal for vascular imaging of neuro-ICU patients. The venous phase of CTA gives excellent anatomical detail of the cerebral veins and sinuses for diagnosis of cerebral venous thrombosis (CVT). However, CTA is a structural study, not a dynamic study, and does not provide information about blood flow. A blood vessel may opacify fully with contrast but still have impaired flow.

Clinical Indications and Uses

- *Subarachnoid hemorrhage:* Quick screening for intracranial aneurysms (**Fig. 21.6B**) and vascular malformations can be performed with CTA. Computer 3D modeling of aneurysm anatomy allows a detailed view of the aneurysm neck and base and is useful for selecting patients for aneurysm clipping versus coiling.

- *Ischemic stroke:* Detection of stroke etiology (e.g., carotid dissection, carotid stenosis, vessel cut-off due to embolic material); selection of patients for advanced reperfusion techniques beyond the 3-hour time window (e.g., mechanical or intraarterial thrombolysis).[1]

- *Intracranial hemorrhage:* Screening for etiology of ICH (e.g., vascular malformations, CVT).

Computed Tomography Perfusion

CT perfusion (CTP)[2] is a newer technique for qualitative and quantitative assessment of brain perfusion. CTP uses a bolus injection of IV contrast with dynamic acquisition of sequential CT slices to track the "first pass" of the contrast through the head and neck vasculature. Cerebral blood flow, blood volume, and mean transit time maps are obtained. Brain areas with decreased perfusion appear as a change in intensity/color on these maps. Quantification of cerebral blood flow, blood volume and transit time is possible with specialized software. Though some scanners only provide information at 2 levels, newer scanners can provide information over multiple levels. The total body dose of radiation delivered from CTP is slightly more than that of non-contrast HCT (2.8 mSV vs 1.5–2.5 mSV respectively).

Clinical Indications and Uses

- In acute ischemic stroke or vasospasm, CTP can detect the presence of hypoperfused but viable tissue, presumed to be the "penumbra" around the core of the infarct. These patients may benefit from reperfusion therapies.

Magnetic Resonance Imaging

Water and fat in body tissues have weakly magnetic hydrogen protons. These align briefly with a strong external magnetic field from the MRI scanner and are subsequently disturbed with a radiofrequency (RF) pulse. Once this pulse is turned off, the proton "relaxes" back to its original alignment and emits a weak radio signal. A computer combines all such signals to create an magnetic resonance (MR) image.[3] The following are the routinely obtained MR sequences.

T1- and T2-Weighted MRI Scans

These sequences are based on measures of independent proton relaxation mechanisms obtained by varying the RF pulse. The different T1 and T2 times of body tissues result in contrast between tissues. T1 gives excellent anatomical detail (**Fig. 21.5B, Fig. 21.7A**), whereas T2 is especially sensitive to tissue water (**Fig. 21.7B, Fig. 21.8**). Most pathologic processes of the brain are associated with increased water (edema) and appear "dark" on T1 and "bright" on T2 (**Table 21.1**).

MRI is especially useful in multiplanar imaging of the posterior fossa, orbit, optic nerves, and temporal bone due to the absence of bony artifacts. Rapidly flowing protons in arterial blood reduce MR signal, creating a flow "void," which is used to identify blood vessels. T1 is also used in conjunction with gadolinium, which is a strongly paramagnetic, noniodinated contrast agent. Areas of BBB disruption (e.g., certain tumors, inflammation) "leak" gadolinium and appear bright (i.e., "enhance"). Complications of gadolinium include nephrogenic

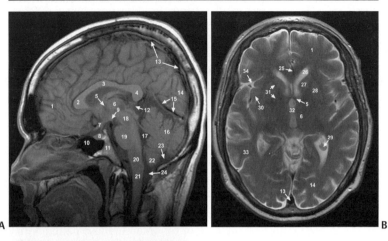

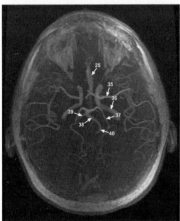

Fig. 21.7 Magnetic resonance imaging (MRI) of the brain showing normal anatomy. **(A)** Sagittal T1 weighted image through corpus callosum, **(B)** Axial T2 weighted image at the level of the third ventricle, **(C)** Time of flight magnetic resonance angiography (MRA) depicting the circle of Willis. (1) Frontal lobe, (2) genu of corpus callosum, (3) body of corpus callosum, (4) splenium of corpus callosum, (5) foramen of Monro, (6) thalamus, (7) optic chiasm, (8) pituitary gland, (9) mammillary body, (10) sphenoid sinus, (11) clivus, (12) pineal gland, (13) superior sagittal sinus, (14) occipital lobe, (15) straight sinus, (16) cerebellum, (17) 4th ventricle, (18) midbrain, (19) pons, (20) medulla, (21) cervical spinal cord, (22) cerebellar tonsil, (23) cisterna magna, (24) foramen magnum, (25) anterior cerebral artery, (26) frontal horn of the lateral ventricle, (27) caudate, (28) putamen, (29) choroid plexus, (30) insula, (31) internal capsule, (32) 3rd ventricle, (33) parietal lobe, (34) Sylvian fissure, (35) middle cerebral artery, (36) internal carotid artery, (37) posterior cerebral artery, (38) basilar artery, (39) superior cerebellar artery, (40) vertebral artery.

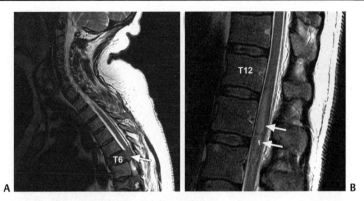

Fig. 21.8 Spinal cord. **(A)** Sagittal T2-weighted magnetic resonance image (MRI) scan of the cervical and thoracic spine from a patient with multiple myeloma shows a destructive mass lesion of the T6 vertebral body extending extradurally to cause severe cord compression (*arrow*). **(B)** Sagittal T2-weighted MRI of the thoracic spine in a patient with sudden onset of paraplegia with preserved sensation shows hyperintense signal within the spinal cord (*arrows*) extending from T12 to the conus medullaris (not shown), consistent with acute spinal cord infarction.

Table 21.1 Appearance of Pathologies on T1- and T2-Weighted Magnetic Resonance Imaging

Disease/Structure	T1	T2
Cerebrospinal fluid	Dark	Bright
Calcium/mineralization	Dark	Dark
Air	Dark	Dark
Edema & most pathologic lesions	Dark	Bright
Fat	Bright	Dark
Gadolinium	Bright	Bright

systemic fibrosis, which occurs in patients with renal insufficiency who receive gadolinium. It is characterized by fibrosis of the skin and internal organs and resembles scleroderma clinically.

Fluid-Attenuated Inversion Recovery (FLAIR)

This is a modified T2 sequence in which the CSF signal is attenuated (**Fig. 21.9B**) and is ideal for the detection of lesions adjacent to the CSF spaces (ventricles and sulci).

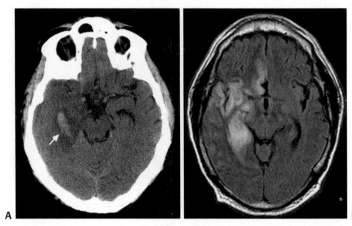

Fig. 21.9 Herpes encephalitis. **(A)** Noncontrast-enhanced head computed tomography scan shows a hemorrhagic lesion in the right temporal lobe (*arrow*) with surrounding edema, sulcal effacement, and mass effect on the right temporal horn. **(B)** Corresponding brain magnetic resonance imaging scan (axial fluid-attenuated inversion recovery [FLAIR]) shows bright signal involving the right insula and the medial temporal and orbitofrontal gray matter across multiple vascular territories. This radiologic appearance is classic for herpes encephalitis.

Gradient Echo (GRE)

This is a fast scanning sequence generated by varying the RF pulse and angle on T2-weighted images. Blood (of any age) and calcium appear dark on GRE. However, GRE tends to "overestimate" the extent of such lesions due to "blooming" artifact.

Diffusion Weighted Imaging (DWI)

DWI detects brain areas with "restricted" diffusion of hydrogen molecules caused by a shift of water from the interstitial compartment to the intracellular space. Certain diseases, like acute stroke, result in failure of high-energy metabolism and ion exchange pumps, resulting in "restricted" diffusion of water. Areas with restricted diffusion have less signal decay and appear "bright" on DWI (**Fig. 21.2C, Fig. 21.10A**). False-positive artifact or "T2 shine through" occurs when a bright lesion on T2 also appears bright on DWI. Confusion can be avoided by obtaining ADC (apparent diffusion coefficient) maps, which are based on quantitative differences of tissue diffusion and are independent of T2 effects (**Fig. 21.10B**). DWI and ADC are particularly useful in acute stroke imaging (**Fig. 21.2C**), as ischemic areas may generate signal changes in less than 1 hour after stroke onset ("bright" on DWI and

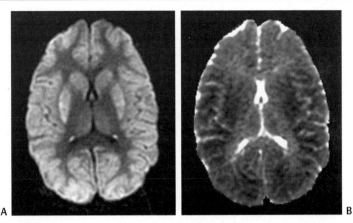

Fig. 21.10 Cardiac arrest. **(A)** Axial diffusion weighted magnetic resonance image scan and **(B)** corresponding apparent diffusion coefficient (ADC) map 4 days after cardiac arrest demonstrate widespread cortical areas of restricted diffusion (bright on diffusion-weighted image, dark on ADC), consistent with severe postanoxic injury.

"dark" on ADC). These changes last up to a week on ADC and a month on DWI. Restricted diffusion can also occur in other disease processes, including seizure, brain abscesses (both bacterial and fungal), brain tumors (e.g., lymphoma), and hypoxic-ischemic brain injury (**Fig. 21.10**).

Perfusion Weighted Imaging

Perfusion weighted imaging (PWI)[4] is the MRI counterpart of CTP and is used to assess the state of brain perfusion after injection of gadolinium. PWI data can be postprocessed to provide color maps of time to peak, cerebral blood volume, and cerebral blow flow, which facilitate qualitative interpretation.

Magnetic Resonance Angiography

The objectives of MRA is to maximize the signal from rapidly flowing blood and to minimize the signal from the background stationary tissues. The two commonly used techniques are time of flight (TOF) (**Fig. 21.7C**) and contrast-enhanced MRA (Time-Resolved Imaging of Contrast Kinetics, or TRICKS). TOF is a dynamic study that provides information about flow rather than structure (the converse of CTA) and does not require contrast. In contrast-enhanced MRA, 3D images are obtained during the arterial phase of intravenous gadolinium bolus injection. These data are subtracted from the precontrast background data after eliminating background fat signal, giving information about anatomical structure rather than flow. The venous phase (MR venogram) is used to detect abnormal flow in the cerebral veins and sinuses. MRA is inferior to conventional angiography for the evaluation of lesions in small and medium-sized blood vessels (e.g., vasospasm, vasculitis).

Clinical Indications and Uses

- *Acute ischemic stroke:* The combination of DWI and PWI is particularly useful in determining the presence of salvageable "penumbral" tissue and can guide reperfusion therapies. In large middle cerebral artery (MCA) infarcts, the DWI lesion volume may help identify patients who might benefit from early decompressive hemicraniectomy.

- *SAH:* Although MRA is good for aneurysm screening, CTA gives better anatomical and 3D detail. Aneurysm clips and coils will result in artifacts in both techniques.

- *ICH:* Although CT is still preferred for emergent diagnosis,[5] MRI is equally sensitive in the detection of acute blood and superior in the detection of subacute blood. MRI may be particularly useful in determining ICH etiology (e.g., cerebral microbleeds in amyloid angiopathy, hemorrhagic conversion of an ischemic or venous infarct). Because blood products age over time and change susceptibility, it is important to analyze both T1 and T2 sequences to date blood products (**Table 21.2**).

- *Infections:* FLAIR, DWI, and T1-weighted MRI with gadolinium are particularly useful in detecting abscesses, meningeal enhancement, cerebritis, and encephalitis (**Fig. 21.9B**), especially when the CT appears normal.

- *Leukoencephalopathy:* FLAIR is a useful sequence for detecting white matter changes (microvascular ischemia, posterior re-

Table 21.2 Appearance of Blood Products on T1- and T2-Weighted Magnetic Resonance Imaging

Phase	Time	T1	T2	Hemoglobin
Hyperacute	<24 h	Gray/black	White	Oxyhemoglobin (intracellular)
Acute	1–3 d	Gray/black	Black	Deoxyhemoglobin (intracellular)
Early subacute	3–7 d	White	Black	Methemoglobin (intracellular)
Late subacute	7–14 d	White	White	Methemoglobin (extracellular)
Chronic	>14 d	Black/gray	Black	Hemosiderin (extracellular)

versible leukoencephalopathy as seen in hypertensive crisis or with cyclosporin or tacrolimus, drug-induced white matter changes such as that seen after smoking heroin, etc.)

- *Trauma:* FLAIR, T2, and DWI sequences are more sensitive than CT in detecting diffuse axonal injury (DAI).[6]
- *Coma:* Because of its superb sensitivity, MRI is very useful in determining the etiology of coma, especially when the CT appears normal (DAI, postanoxic [**Fig. 21.10**], encephalitis, etc.).
- *Spinal cord:* MRI is superior to CT in providing details of cord pathology (e.g., spinal cord contusion, compression [**Fig. 21.8A**], ischemia [**Fig. 21.8B**], or demyelination).

Limitations

- Long scan times (unsuitable for restless or hemodynamically unstable patients); motion artifacts (especially on the FLAIR sequence)
- Contraindicated in patients with pacemakers, defibrillators, and metallic fragments
- Needs ferromagnetic-compatible life support devices (e.g., infusion pumps, ventilators, ICP monitors, Foley catheters, aneurysm clips)
- Not ideal for bone imaging
- Unsuitable for patients weighing >300 lbs (need "open" MRI, which has lower resolution)
- Rare cases of skin and organ fibrosis have occurred after administration of gadolinium in patients with advanced renal failure and/or on hemodialysis.

Digital Subtraction Angiography

Conventional cerebral DSA utilizes the combination of x-rays and selective injection of a radio-opaque iodinated contrast into the blood vessels of interest. Images are viewed in real time. DSA is a dynamic study and gives relative information about blood flow based on the distribution and dispersion of contrast. It is performed by femoral artery catheterization, with selective cannulation and contrast injection into either the carotid or vertebral arteries (**Fig. 21.11**). Computerized digital subtraction is then used to produce images with high resolution by minimizing bony artifacts. 3D images can also be constructed.

Clinical Indications and Uses

- Gold standard for the diagnosis of cerebral vascular diseases (**Fig. 21.2B, Fig. 21.6C**)

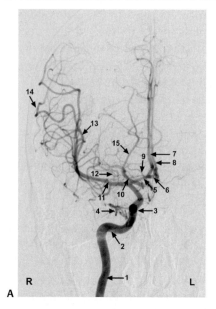

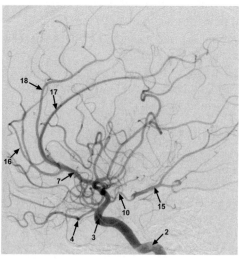

Fig. 21.11 Digital subtraction cerebral angiogram showing normal anatomy. **(A)** Right internal carotid artery (ICA) injection, anteroposterior (AP) view; **(B)** right internal carotid artery injection, lateral view; **(C)** right vertebral artery injection, AP view; **(D)** right vertebral artery injection, lateral view. (1) ICA (cervical segment), (2) ICA (petrous segment), (3) ICA (cavernous segment), (4) opthalmic artery, (5) anterior cerebral artery (ACA; A1 segment), (6) anterior communicating artery, (7) right ACA (A2 segment), (8) left ACA (A2 segment), (9) recurrent artery of Heubner, (10) posterior communicating artery, (11) middle cerebral artery (MCA; M1 segment), (12)

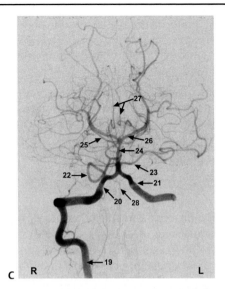

C R L

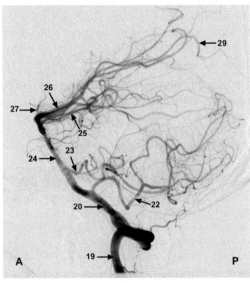

D A P

lenticulostriate branches from MCA, (13) MCA (insular branch), (14) MCA (opercular branches), (15) posterior cerebral artery, (16) ACA (frontopolar branch), (17) ACA (pericallosal branch), (18) ACA (callosomarginal branch), (19) vertebral artery (extracranial segment), (20) right vertebral artery (intracranial segment), (21) left vertebral artery (intracranial segment), (22) posterior inferior cerebellar artery (PICA), (23) anterior inferior cerebellar artery (AICA), (24) basilar artery, (25) superior cerebellar artery, (26) posterior cerebral artery (PCA), (27) thalamoperforating arteries, (28) anterior spinal artery, (29) PCA (calcarine branch).

- Allows for the performance of therapeutic endovascular procedures, such as mechanical clot retrieval, intra-arterial thrombolysis, angioplasty with/without stenting, aneurysm coiling, and intra-arterial vasodilator injection.

- Provides a road map of collateral circulation prior to neurosurgical procedures, such as external carotid to internal carotid (EC-IC) bypass surgery

- Ancillary test for detecting brain death (i.e., no intracranial blood flow indicates brain death)

Limitations

- Invasive technique: Local complications include bleeding, arterial dissection, pseudoaneurysm, and arteriovenous fistula formation. Neurologic complications include rupture of intracranial vessels leading to SAH/ ICH, ischemic stroke, and air embolism.

- Needs special angiographic suite, equipment, and highly trained personnel. Some procedures need anesthesia and critical care nursing.

- Iodinated contrast can trigger either a systemic allergic reaction with anaphylaxis or a neurologic reaction, such as seizure, encephalopathy, or reversible neurologic deficits.

- Contrast induced nephrotoxicity occurs in 2–4% of patients and can be mitigated with hydration.

References

1. Köhrmann M, Jüttler E, Huttner HB, Nowe T, Schellinger PD. Acute stroke imaging for thrombolytic therapy—an update. Cerebrovasc Dis 2007;24:161–169
2. Latchaw RE, Kucharczyk J, Moseley ME, eds. Imaging of the Nervous System. Philadelphia, PA: Elsevier Mosby; 2005:273–295
3. Symms M, Jäger HR, Schmierer K, Yousry TA. A review of structural magnetic resonance neuroimaging. J Neurol Neurosurg Psychiatry 2004;75:1235–1244
4. Perez-Arjona EA, DelProposto Z, Sehgal V, Fessler RD. New techniques in cerebral imaging. Neurol Res 2002;24:S17–S26
5. Gilman S. Imaging the brain. First of two parts. N Engl J Med 1998;338:812–820
6. Gilman S. Imaging the brain. Second of two parts. N Engl J Med 1998;338:889–896

22 Grades of Recommendations Based on Level of Evidence

Jennifer A. Frontera

Table 22.1 The American Academy of Neurology's Classification Scheme for Rating a Prognostic Article

Class I	Evidence provided by a prospective study of a broad spectrum of persons who may be at risk for developing the outcome (e.g., target disease, work status). The study measures the predictive ability using an independent gold standard for case definition. The predictor is measured in an evaluation that is masked to clinical presentation, and the outcome is measured in an evaluation that is masked to the presence of the predictor. All patients have the predictor and outcome variables measured.
Class II	Evidence provided by a prospective study of a narrow spectrum of persons at risk for having the condition, or by a retrospective study of a broad spectrum of persons with the condition compared with a broad spectrum of controls. The study measures the prognostic accuracy of the risk factor using an acceptable independent gold standard for case definition. The risk factor is measured in an evaluation that is masked to the outcome.
Class III	Evidence provided by a retrospective study where either the persons with the condition or the controls are of narrow spectrum. The study measures the predictive ability using an acceptable independent gold standard for case definition. The outcome, if not objective, is determined by someone other than the person who measured the predictor.
Class IV	Any design where the predictor is not applied in an independent evaluation OR evidence provided by expert opinion or case series without controls.

Data from: Wijdicks EF, Hijdra A, Young GB, Bassetti CL, Wiebe S. Practice parameter: prediction of outcome in comatose survivors after cardiopulmonary resuscitation (an evidence-based review): report of the Quality Standards Subcommittee of the American Academy of Neurology. Neurology 2006;67(2):203–210.

Table 22.2 The American Academy of Neurology's Classification of Recommendation

A	Established as effective, ineffective, or harmful for the given condition in the specified population. (Level A rating requires at least two consistent class I studies.)
B	Probably effective, ineffective, or harmful for the given condition in the specified population. (Level B rating requires at least one class I study or at least two consistent class II studies.)
C	Possibly effective, ineffective, or harmful for the given condition in the specified population. (Level C rating requires at least one class II study or two consistent class III studies.)
U	Data inadequate or conflicting; given current knowledge, predictor is unproven

Data from: Wijdicks EF, Hijdra A, Young GB, Bassetti CL, Wiebe S. Practice parameter: prediction of outcome in comatose survivors after cardiopulmonary resuscitation (an evidence-based review): report of the Quality Standards Subcommittee of the American Academy of Neurology. Neurology 2006;67(2):203–210.

Table 22.3 The American College of Chest Physicians' Classification of Recommendation

Grade of Recommendation	Clarity of Risk/ Benefit	Methodological Strength of Supporting Evidence	Implications
1A	Clear; high quality evidence	Randomized controlled trials (RCTs) without important limitations	Strong recommendation; can apply to most patients in most circumstances without reservation
1B	Clear; moderate quality evidence	RCTs with important limitations (inconsistent results, methodological flaws, indirect or imprecise) or very strong evidence from observational studies	Strong recommendation; likely to apply to most patients. Higher quality research may change the confidence in the estimate of effect or may change the estimate

(Continued)

Table 22.3 The American College of Chest Physicians' Classification of Recommendation *(continued)*

Grade of Recommen- dation	Clarity of Risk/ Benefit	Methodological Strength of Supporting Evidence	Implications
1C	Clear; low or very low quality evidence	Evidence for at least one critical outcome from observational studies, case series, or from RCTs with serious flaws or indirect evidence	Strong recommendation; can apply to most patients in many circumstances. Higher quality research is likely to change the confidence in the estimate of effect or may change the estimate.
2A	Unclear; high quality evidence	RCTs without important limitations or exceptionally strong evidence from observational studies	Weak recommendation; best action may differ depending on circumstances or patients' or societal values
2B	Unclear; moderate quality evidence	RCTs with important limitations (inconsistent results, methodological flaws, indirect or imprecise) or very strong evidence from observational studies	Weak recommendation; best action may differ depending on circumstances or patient or society values. Higher quality research may change the confidence in the estimate of effect or may change the estimate
2C	Unclear; low or very low quality evidence	Evidence for at least one critical outcome from observational studies, case series, or from RCTs with serious flaws or indirect evidence	Weak recommendations; other alternatives may be equally reasonable. Higher quality research is likely to change the confidence in the estimate of effect or may change the estimate

Abbreviation: RCT, randomized controlled trial.

Data from: Guyatt GH, et al. *Grades of recommendation for antithrombotic agents: American College of Chest Physicians Evidence-Based Clinical Practice Guidelines (8th Edition)*. Chest 2008; 133(6 Suppl): p.123S–131S.

Table 22.4 The American Heart Association and the American Stroke Association's Classification of Recommendation

Class I	Conditions for which there is evidence for and/or general agreement that the procedure or treatment is useful and effective
Class II	Conditions for which there is conflicting evidence and/or a divergence of opinion about the usefulness/efficacy of a procedure or treatment
Class IIa	The weight of evidence or opinion is in favor of the procedure or treatment
Class IIb	Usefulness/efficacy is less well established by evidence or opinion
Class III	Conditions for which there is evidence and/or general agreement that the procedure or treatment is not useful/effective and in some cases may be harmful
Therapeutic recommendation	
Level of evidence A	Data derived from multiple randomized clinical trials
Level of evidence B	Data derived from a single randomized trial or nonrandomized studies
Level of evidence C	Consensus opinion of experts
Diagnostic recommendation	
Level of evidence A	Data derived from multiple prospective cohort studies employing a reference standard applied by a masked evaluator
Level of evidence B	Data derived from a single grade A study or 1 or more case-control studies or studies employing a reference standard applied by an unmasked evaluator
Level of evidence C	Consensus opinion of experts

Data from: Broderick J, Connolly S, Feldmann E, et al. Guidelines for the management of spontaneous intracerebral hemorrhage in adults: 2007 update: a guideline from the American Heart Association/American Stroke Association Stroke Council, High Blood Pressure Research Council, and the Quality of Care and Outcomes in Research Interdisciplinary Working Group. Stroke 2007;38(6):2001–2023.

Table 22.5 The Brain Trauma Foundation's Classification of Recommendation

Class of Evidence	Study Design	Quality Criteria
I	Good-quality RCT	Adequate random assignment method Allocation concealment Groups similar at baseline Outcome assessors blinded Adequate sample size Intention-to-treat analysis Follow-up rate 85% No differential loss to follow-up Maintenance of comparable groups
II	Moderate-quality RCT	Violation of one or more of the criteria for a good-quality RCT
II	Good-quality cohort	Blind or independent assessment in a prospective study, or use of reliable data in a retrospective study Nonbiased selection Follow-up rate 85% Adequate sample size Statistical analysis of potential confounders
II	Good-quality case-control	Nonbiased selection of cases/controls with exclusion criteria applied equally to both Adequate response rate Appropriate attention to potential confounding variables
III	Poor-quality RCT	Major violations of the criteria for a good- or moderate-quality RCT
III	Moderate- or poor-quality cohort	Violation of one or more criteria for a good-quality cohort
III	Moderate- or poor-quality case-control	Violation of one or more criteria for a good-quality case-control
III	Case series, databases, or registries	—

Abbreviation: RCT, randomized controlled trial.

Data from: Brain Trauma Foundation; American Association of Neurological Surgeons; Congress of Neurological Surgeons. Guidelines for the management of severe traumatic brain injury. J Neurotrauma 2007;24(Suppl 1):S1–S106.

Table 22.6 The European Society for Clinical Nutrition and Metabolism (ESPEN) Classification of Recommendation

Grade of Recommendation	Level of Evidence	Requirement
A	Ia	Meta-analysis of RCTs
	Ib	At least one RCT
B	IIa	At least one well-designed controlled trial without randomization
	IIb	At least one other type of well-designed, quasi-experimental study
	III	Well-designed nonexperimental descriptive studies such as comparative studies, correlation studies, case-control studies
C	IV	Expert opinions and/or clinical experience of respected authorities

Abbreviation: RCT, randomized controlled trial.

Data from: Schutz T, Herbst B, Koller M. Methodology for the development of the ESPEN Guidelines on Enteral Nutrition. Clin Nutr 2006;25(2):203–209.

Index

Note: Page numbers followed by *f* and *t* indicate figures and tables, respectively.

A